SUPPLEMENT I
TO
THE JAPANESE
PHARMACOPOEIA
EIGHTEENTH EDITION

Official from December 12, 2022

English Version

PMRJ   PHARMACEUTICAL AND MEDICAL DEVICE
REGULATORY SCIENCE SOCIETY OF JAPAN

Published 2023 by

PHARMACEUTICAL AND MEDICAL DEVICE REGULATORY SCIENCE SOCIETY OF JAPAN

2–12–15, Shibuya, Shibuya-ku, Tokyo, 150–0002 JAPAN

Distributed by

YAKUJI NIPPO, LTD.

1, Kanda Izumicho, Chiyoda-ku, Tokyo, 101–8648 JAPAN

Notice: This *English Version* of the Japanese Pharmacopoeia is published for the convenience of users unfamiliar with the Japanese language. When and if any discrepancy arises between the Japanese original and its English translation, the former is authentic.

ISBN978-4-8408-1625-0 C3047

Printed in Japan

The Ministry of Health, Labour and Welfare Ministerial Notification No. 355

Pursuant to Paragraph 1, Article 41 of Act on Securing Quality, Efficacy and Safety of Products Including Pharmaceuticals and Medical Devices (Law No. 145, 1960), we hereby revise a part of the Japanese Pharmacopoeia (Ministerial Notification No. 220, 2021) as follows*.

KATO Katsunobu
The Minister of Health, Labour and Welfare

December 12, 2022

Japanese Pharmacopoeia
(The text referred to by the term ''as follows'' are omitted here. All of the revised Japanese Pharmacopoeia in accordance with this notification are made available for public exhibition at the Pharmaceutical Evaluation Division, Pharmaceutical Safety and Environmental Health Bureau, Ministry of Health, Labour and Welfare, at each Regional Bureau of Health and Welfare, and at each Prefectural Office in Japan, and made public by publishing it on the website of the Ministry of Health, Labour and Welfare.)

Supplementary Provisions
(Effective Date)

Article 1　This Notification is applied from the date of the notification. (referred to as the ''notification date'' in the next and third articles)

(Transitional measures)

Article 2　In the case of drugs which are listed in the Japanese Pharmacopoeia (hereinafter referred to as ''previous Pharmacopoeia'') [limited to those listed in the Japanese Pharmacopoeia whose standards are changed in accordance with this notification (hereinafter referred to as ''new Pharmacopoeia'')] and drugs which have been approved as of the notification date as prescribed under Paragraph 1, Article 14 of the same law [including drugs the Minister of Health, Labour and Welfare specifies (the Ministry of Health and Welfare Ministerial Notification No. 104, 1994) as of the day before the notification date as those exempted from marketing approval pursuant to Paragraph 1, Article 14 of the same law (hereinafter referred to as ''drugs exempted from approval'')], the Name and Standards established in the previous Pharmacopoeia (limited to part of the Name and Standards for the drugs concerned) may be accepted to conform to the Name and Standards established in the new Pharmacopoeia before and on June 30, 2024.

Article 3　In the case of drugs which are listed in the new Pharmacopoeia (excluding those listed in the previous Pharmacopoeia) and drugs which have been approved as of the notification date as prescribed under the Paragraph 1, Article 14 of the same law (including those exempted from approval), they may be accepted as those being not listed in the new Pharmacopoeia before and on June 30, 2024.

*The term ''as follows'' here indicates the content of Supplement I to the Japanese Pharmacopoeia Eighteenth Edition from General Tests, Processes and Apparatus to Ultraviolet-visible Reference Spectra (pp. 2807 – 2930).

CONTENTS

Preface i
Supplement I to The Japanese Pharmacopoeia,
Eighteenth Edition **2807–2930**
General Tests, Processes and Apparatus ... 2807
2.00 Chromatography........................... 2807
2.01 Liquid Chromatography 2816
2.02 Gas Chromatography.................... 2819
2.22 Fluorometry................................ 2820
2.27 Near Infrared Spectrometry............ 2821
2.28 Circular Dichroism Spectroscopy...... 2824
2.58 X-Ray Powder Diffraction Method... 2825
3.04 Particle Size Determination 2830
9.01 Reference Standards 2833
9.41 Reagents, Test Solutions................. 2833
9.42 Solid Supports/Column Packings for
Chromatography........................... 2844

Official Monographs 2845
Crude Drugs and Related Drugs.............. 2907

Infrared Reference Spectra **2925–2927**

Ultraviolet-visible Reference Spectra **2929–2930**

General Information
G0 Basic Concepts on Pharmaceutical Quality
Concept on Impurities in Chemically
Synthesized Drug Substances and
Drug Products ⟨G0-3-181⟩ 2931
G1 Physics and Chemistry
System Suitability ⟨G1-2-181⟩ 2934
Near Infrared Spectrometry ⟨G1-3-161⟩
.... 2935
Instrumental Measurement of Colora-
tion of Liquids ⟨G1-4-181⟩................ 2935
Control Strategies and Change Control
Concepts at Each Stage of Chro-
matography Lifecycle (Change Con-
trol in Chromatography Lifecycle)
⟨G1-5-181⟩ 2937
G2 Solid-state Properties
Measurement of Powder Flow Proper-
ties by Shear Cell Methods ⟨G2-5-181⟩
.... 2939
G4 Microorganisms
Biorisk Management of the Handling of
Microorganisms in Microbial Tests
⟨G4-11-181⟩ 2942
G5 Crude Drugs
On the Scientific Names of Crude Drugs
listed in the JP ⟨G5-1-181⟩................ 2948
G6 Drug Formulation
Tablet Friability Test ⟨G6-5-181⟩........... 2949
G9 Pharmaceutical Excipients
Functionality-Related Characteristics of
Excipients Relevant to Preparations
⟨G9-1-181⟩ 2949
GZ Others
Quality Control of Water for Phar-
maceutical Use ⟨GZ-2-181⟩ 2950

Index... 2955
Index in Latin Name............................. 2975
Index in Japanese................................. 2977

PREFACE

The 18th Edition of the Japanese Pharmacopoeia (JP) was promulgated by Ministerial Notification No. 220 of the Ministry of Health, Labour and Welfare (MHLW) on June 7, 2021.

In July 2021, the Committee on JP established the basic principles for the preparation of the JP 19th Edition, setting out the roles and characteristics of the JP, the definite measures for the revision, and the date of the revision.

It was agreed that the JP should be an official document that defines the specifications, criteria and standard test methods necessary to properly assure the quality of medicines in Japan in response to the progress of science and technology and medical demands, in order to contribute to ensuring public health. It should define the standards for specifications, as well as the methods of testing to assure overall quality of all drugs in principle, and it should have a role in clarifying the criteria for quality assurance of drugs that are recognized to be essential for medical treatment. The JP has been prepared with the aid of the knowledge and experience of many professionals in the pharmaceutical field. Therefore, the JP should have the characteristics of an official standard, which might be widely used by all parties concerned, and it should play an appropriate role of providing information and understanding about the quality of drugs to the public. Moreover, as a pharmaceutical quality standard in the international community, it should play an appropriate role and contribute to the utilization of advanced technology and the promotion of international consistency in order to ensure the quality of drugs beyond the national level.

As the policy of the JP, the five basic principles, which we refer to as the "five pillars", were established as follows: 1) Enhancing listed articles by prioritizing drugs which are important from the viewpoint of health care and medical treatment; 2) Making qualitative improvement by introducing the latest science and technology; 3) Further promoting internationalization in response to globalization of drug market; 4) Making prompt partial revision as necessary and facilitating smooth administrative operation; and 5) Ensuring transparency regarding the revision, and disseminating the JP to the public domestically and internationally. It was agreed that the Committee on JP should make efforts, on the basis of these principles, to ensure that the JP is used more effectively in the fields of health care and medical treatment by taking appropriate measurements, including getting the understanding and cooperation of other parties concerned.

It was also agreed that JP articles should cover drugs, which are important from the viewpoint of health care and medical treatment, clinical performance or merits and frequency of use, as soon as possible after they reach the market.

The target date for the publication of JP 19th Edition (the Japanese edition) was set as April 2026.

JP drafts are discussed in the following committees that were established in the Pharmaceuticals and Medical Devices Agency: Expert Committee; Sub-committee on Manufacturing Process-related Matters; Committee on Chemicals; Committee on Antibiotics; Committee on Biologicals; Committee on Crude Drugs; Committee on Pharmaceutical Excipients; Committee on Physico-Chemical Methods; Committee on Drug Formulation; Committee on Physical Methods; Committee on Biological Methods; Committee on Nomenclature for Pharmaceuticals; Committee on International Harmonization; and Committee on Reference Standards. Furthermore, working groups are established under the Expert Committee, Committee on Biologicals, Committee on Pharmaceutical Excipients and Committee on Drug Formulation.

The committees initiated deliberations on the several revision. Draft revisions covering subjects in General Tests and Monographs, Ultraviolet-visible Reference Spectra, Infrared Reference Spectra, for which discussions were finished between September 2020 and June 2022, were prepared for a supplement to the JP 18.

Numbers of discussions in the committees to prepare the supplement drafts were as follows: Expert Committee (17, including working group); Sub-committee on Manufacturing Process-related Matters (1); Committee on Chemicals (23); Committee on Antibiotics (4); Committee on Biologicals (7); Committee on Crude Drugs (16); Committee on Pharmaceutical Excipients (13, including working group); Committee on Physico-Chemical Methods (8); Committee on Drug Formulation (17, including working group); Committee on Physical Methods (6); Committee on Biological Methods (6); Committee on Nomenclature for Pharmaceuticals (4); Committee on International Harmonization (7); and Committee on Reference

ii   *Preface*

Standards (3, including working group).

It should be noted that in the preparation of the drafts for the supplement, generous cooperation was given by the Pharmaceutical Technology Committee of the Kansai Pharmaceutical Manufacturers Association, the Pharmacopeia and CMC Committee of the Pharmaceutical Manufacturers' Association of Tokyo, the Tokyo Crude Drugs Association, the International Pharmaceutical Excipients Council Japan, the Home Medicine Association of Japan, the Japan Kampo Medicines Manufacturers Association, the Japan Flavor and Fragrance Materials Association, the Japan Natural Medicines Association, the Japan Pharmaceutical Manufacturers Association, the Federation of Pharmaceutical Manufacturers' Association of Japan, the Parenteral Drug Association Japan Chapter, the Japan Reagent Association, the Japan Oilseed Processors Association, the Japan Analytical Instruments Manufacturers' Association, and the Asian Society of Innovative Packaging Technology.

The draft revisions were examined by the Committee on JP in July 2022, followed by the Pharmaceutical Affairs and Food Sanitation Council (PAFSC) in September 2022, and then submitted to the Minister of Health, Labour and Welfare. In the committee on JP, Mitsuru Hashida took the role of the chairman from January 2011 to December 2020, and Shigeru Ohta from January 2021 to December 2022.

In consequence of this revision, the Supplement I to the JP 18th Edition carries 2042 articles, owing to the addition of 11 articles and the deletion of 2 articles.

The principles of description and the salient points of the revision in this volume are as follows:

1. The Supplement I to the JP 18th Edition comprises the following items, in order: Notification of MHLW; Contents; Preface; General Tests, Processes and Apparatus; Official Monographs; then followed by Infrared Reference Spectra and Ultraviolet-visible Reference Spectra; General Information; and; as an appendix a Cumulative Index containing references to the main volume and Supplement I.

2. The articles in Official Monographs, Infrared Reference Spectra and Ultraviolet-visible Reference Spectra are respectively placed in alphabetical order in principle.

3. The following items in each monograph are put in the order shown below, except that unnecessary items are omitted depending on the nature of the drug:
 (1) English title
 (2) Commonly used name(s)
 (3) Latin title (only for crude drugs)
 (4) Title in Japanese
 (5) Structural formula or empirical formula
 (6) Molecular formula and molecular mass
 (7) Chemical name
 (8) Chemical Abstracts Service (CAS) Registry Number
 (9) Origin
 (10) Limits of the content of the ingredient(s) and/or the unit of potency
 (11) Labeling requirements
 (12) Method of preparation
 (13) Manufacture
 (14) Description
 (15) Identification tests
 (16) Specific physical and/or chemical values
 (17) Purity tests
 (18) Potential adulteration
 (19) Loss on drying or Ignition, or Water
 (20) Residue on ignition, Total ash or Acid-insoluble ash
 (21) Tests being required for pharmaceutical preparations
 (22) Other special tests
 (23) Assay
 (24) Containers and storage
 (25) Shelf life
 (26) Others

4. In each monograph, the following physical and chemical values representing the properties and quality of the drug are given in the order indicated below, except that unnecessary items are omitted depending on the nature of drug:
 (1) Alcohol number
 (2) Absorbance
 (3) Congealing point
 (4) Refractive index
 (5) Osmolar ratio
 (6) Optical rotation
 (7) Constituent amino acids
 (8) Viscosity
 (9) pH
 (10) Content ratio of the active ingredients
 (11) Specific gravity
 (12) Boiling point
 (13) Melting point
 (14) Acid value
 (15) Saponification value
 (16) Ester value
 (17) Hydroxyl value
 (18) Iodine value

Supplement I, JP XVIII   *Preface*   iii

5. Identification tests comprise the following items, which are generally put in the order given below:
(1) Coloration reactions
(2) Precipitation reactions
(3) Decomposition reactions
(4) Derivatives
(5) Infrared and/or ultraviolet-visible absorption spectrometry
(6) Nuclear magnetic resonance spectrometry
(7) Chromatography
(8) Special reactions
(9) Cations
(10) Anions

6. Purity tests comprise the following items, which are generally put in the order given below, except that unnecessary items are omitted depending on the nature of drug:
(1) Color
(2) Odor
(3) Clarity and/or color of solution
(4) Acidity or alkalinity
(5) Acidity
(6) Acidity Alkalinity
(7) Chloride
(8) Sulfate
(9) Sulfite
(10) Nitrate
(11) Nitrite
(12) Carbonate
(13) Bromide
(14) Iodide
(15) Soluble halide
(16) Thiocyanate
(17) Selenium
(18) Cationic salts
(19) Ammonium
(20) Heavy metals
(21) Iron
(22) Manganese
(23) Chromium
(24) Bismuth
(25) Tin
(26) Aluminum
(27) Zinc
(28) Cadmium
(29) Mercury
(30) Copper
(31) Lead
(32) Silver
(33) Alkaline earth metals
(34) Arsenic
(35) Free phosphoric acid

(36) Foreign matters
(37) Related substances
(38) Isomer
(39) Enantiomer
(40) Diastereomer
(41) Polymer
(42) Residual solvent
(43) Other impurities
(44) Residue on evaporation
(45) Readily carbonizable substances

7. The following item was newly added to General Tests, Processes and Apparatus:
(1) 2.00 Chromatography
(2) 2.27 Near Infrared Spectrometry
(3) 2.28 Circular Dichroism Spectroscopy

8. The following items in General Tests, Processes and Apparatus were revised:
(1) 2.01 Liquid Chromatography
(2) 2.02 Gas Chromatography
(3) 2.22 Fluorometry
(4) 2.58 X-Ray Powder Diffraction Method
(5) 3.04 Particle Size Determination
(6) 9.01 Reference Standards
(7) 9.41 Reagents, Test Solutions
(8) 9.42 Solid Supports/Column Packings for Chromatography

9. The following Reference Standards were newly added:
(1) Anastrozole RS
(2) Budesonide RS
(3) Temozolomide RS

10. The following Reference Standards was deleted.
(1) Nartograstim RS

11. The following Reference Standards were deleted from the list of "9.01 (2) The reference standards which are prepared by National Institute of Infectious Diseases" and added to the list of "9.01 (1) The reference standards which are prepared by those who have been registered to prepare them by the Minister of Health, Labour and Welfare, according to the Ministerial ordinance established by the Minister separately":
(1) Amikacin Sulfate RS
(2) Cefaclor RS
(3) Cefalexin RS
(4) Clindamycin Phosphate RS
(5) Doxorubicin Hydrochloride RS

iv   *Preface*   *Supplement I, JP XVIII*

12. The following substances were newly added to the Official Monographs:
(1) Anastrozole
(2) Anastrozole Tablets
(3) Bicalutamide Tablets
(4) Budesonide
(5) Oxybutynin Hydrochloride
(6) Temozolomide
(7) Temozolomide Capsules
(8) Temozolomide for Injection
(9) Voglibose Orally Disintegrating Tablets
(10) Saikokeishikankyoto Extract
(11) Yokukansankachimpihange Extract

13. The following monographs were revised:
(1) Amphotericin B for Injection
(2) Amphotericin B Tablets
(3) Ampicillin Sodium and Sulbactam Sodium for Injection
(4) Benzyl Alcohol
(5) Bromhexine Hydrochloride
(6) Butropium Bromide
(7) Butyl Parahydroxybenzoate
(8) Croscarmellose Sodium
(9) Cefoperazone Sodium and Sulbactam Sodium for Injection
(10) Powdered Cellulose
(11) Enviomycin Sulfate
(12) Epoetin Beta (Genetical Recombination)
(13) Ethanol
(14) Anhydrous Ethanol
(15) Ethyl Parahydroxybenzoate
(16) Formoterol Fumarate Hydrate
(17) Glyceryl Monostearate
(18) Hypromellose Phthalate
(19) Imipenem and Cilastatin Sodium for Injection
(20) Insulin Human (Genetical Recombination)
(21) Insulin Human (Genetical Recombination) Injection
(22) Isophane Insulin Human (Genetical Recombination) Injectable Aqueous Suspension
(23) Biphasic Isophane Insulin Human (Genetical Recombination) Injectable Aqueous Suspension
(24) Magnesium Stearate
(25) D-Mannitol
(26) *dl*-Menthol
(27) *l*-Menthol
(28) Methyl Parahydroxybenzoate
(29) White Petrolatum
(30) Yellow Petrolatum
(31) Polysorbate 80
(32) Propyl Parahydroxybenzoate
(33) Sarpogrelate Hydrochloride Fine Granules
(34) Sodium Chloride
(35) Spectionomycin Hydrochloride for Injection
(36) Wheat Starch
(37) Stearic Acid
(38) Voglibose Tablets
(39) Achyranthes Root
(40) Akebia Stem
(41) Apricot Kernel
(42) Artemisia Capillaris Flower
(43) Artemisia Leaf
(44) Bearberry Leaf
(45) Bitter Cardamon
(46) Burdock Fruit
(47) Cardamon
(48) Cimicifuga Rhizome
(49) Clove
(50) Clove Oil
(51) Cnidium Monnieri Fruit
(52) Cornus Fruit
(53) Corydalis Tuber
(54) Powdered Corydalis Tuber
(55) Gardenia Fruit
(56) Ginger
(57) Powdered Ginger
(58) Glehnia Root and Rhizome
(59) Goshajinkigan Extract
(60) Goshuyuto Extract
(61) Hachimijiogan Extract
(62) Hangekobokuto Extract
(63) Keishibukuryogan Extract
(64) Leonurus Herb
(65) Magnolia Bark
(66) Maoto Extract
(67) Mukoi-Daikenchuto Extract
(68) Nutmeg
(69) Peach Kernel
(70) Powdered Peach Kernel
(71) Picrasma Wood
(72) Powdered Picrasma Wood
(73) Plantago Herb
(74) Prepared Glycyrrhiza
(75) Processed Ginger
(76) Senna Leaf
(77) Powdered Senna Leaf
(78) Shimbuto Extract
(79) Sinomenium Stem and Rhizome
(80) Tokakujokito Extract
(81) Turmeric
(82) Uncaria Hook

14. Several items of Purity were deleted from the following monographs:
(1) Acebutolol Hydrochloride

Supplement I, JP XVIII   *Preface*   v

(2) Acemetacin
(3) Acetaminophen
(4) Acetazolamide
(5) Acetic Acid
(6) Glacial Acetic Acid
(7) Acetohexamide
(8) Acetylcholine Chloride for Injection
(9) Acetylcysteine
(10) Aciclovir
(11) Aclarubicin Hydrochloride
(12) Acrinol Hydrate
(13) Adrenaline
(14) Afloqualone
(15) Alacepril
(16) L-Alanine
(17) Aldioxa
(18) Alendronate Sodium Hydrate
(19) Alimemazine Tartrate
(20) Allopurinol
(21) Alprazolam
(22) Alprenolol Hydrochloride
(23) Alprostadil Injection
(24) Dried Aluminum Hydroxide Gel
(25) Aluminum Monostearate
(26) Aluminum Potassium Sulfate Hydrate
(27) Natural Aluminum Silicate
(28) Synthetic Aluminum Silicate
(29) Amantadine Hydrochloride
(30) Ambenonium Chloride
(31) Amidotrizoic Acid
(32) Amikacin Sulfate
(33) Aminophylline Hydrate
(34) Amiodarone Hydrochloride
(35) Amitriptyline Hydrochloride
(36) Amlexanox
(37) Amlodipine Besilate
(38) Ammonia Water
(39) Amobarbital
(40) Amosulalol Hydrochloride
(41) Amoxapine
(42) Amoxicillin Hydrate
(43) Anhydrous Ampicillin
(44) Ampicillin Hydrate
(45) Ampicillin Sodium
(46) Ampiroxicam
(47) Antipyrine
(48) Aprindine Hydrochloride
(49) Arbekacin Sulfate
(50) Argatroban Hydrate
(51) L-Arginine
(52) L-Arginine Hydrochloride
(53) Arotinolol Hydrochloride
(54) Ascorbic Acid

(55) L-Aspartic Acid
(56) Aspirin
(57) Aspoxicillin Hydrate
(58) Atenolol
(59) Atorvastatin Calcium Hydrate
(60) Auranofin
(61) Azathioprine
(62) Azelastine Hydrochloride
(63) Azelnidipine
(64) Azithromycin Hydrate
(65) Azosemide
(66) Aztreonam
(67) Bacampicillin Hydrochloride
(68) Bacitracin
(69) Baclofen
(70) Bamethan Sulfate
(71) Barbital
(72) Barium Sulfate
(73) Beclometasone Dipropionate
(74) Bekanamycin Sulfate
(75) Benidipine Hydrochloride
(76) Benserazide Hydrochloride
(77) Benzbromarone
(78) Benzoic Acid
(79) Benzylpenicillin Benzathine Hydrate
(80) Benzylpenicillin Potassium
(81) Bepotastine Besilate
(82) Berberine Chloride Hydrate
(83) Betahistine Mesilate
(84) Betamethasone
(85) Betamethasone Dipropionate
(86) Betamipron
(87) Betaxolol Hydrochloride
(88) Bethanechol Chloride
(89) Bezafibrate
(90) Bicalutamide
(91) Bifonazole
(92) Biotin
(93) Biperiden Hydrochloride
(94) Bisacodyl
(95) Bismuth Subgallate
(96) Bisoprolol Fumarate
(97) Bleomycin Hydrochloride
(98) Bleomycin Sulfate
(99) Boric Acid
(100) Bromazepam
(101) Bromfenac Sodium Hydrate
(102) Bromhexine Hydrochloride
(103) Bromocriptine Mesilate
(104) Bromovalerylurea
(105) Brotizolam
(106) Bucillamine
(107) Bucumolol Hydrochloride

(108) Bufetolol Hydrochloride	(161) Cefbuperazone Sodium
(109) Buformin Hydrochloride	(162) Cefcapene Pivoxil Hydrochloride Hydrate
(110) Bumetanide	(163) Cefdinir
(111) Bunazosin Hydrochloride	(164) Cefditoren Pivoxil
(112) Bupivacaine Hydrochloride Hydrate	(165) Cefepime Dihydrochloride Hydrate
(113) Bupranolol Hydrochloride	(166) Cefmenoxime Hydrochloride
(114) Buprenorphine Hydrochloride	(167) Cefmetazole Sodium
(115) Busulfan	(168) Cefminox Sodium Hydrate
(116) Butenafine Hydrochloride	(169) Cefodizime Sodium
(117) Butropium Bromide	(170) Cefoperazone Sodium
(118) Butyl Parahydroxybenzoate	(171) Cefotaxime Sodium
(119) Cabergoline	(172) Cefotetan
(120) Cadralazine	(173) Cefotiam Hexetil Hydrochloride
(121) Anhydrous Caffeine	(174) Cefotiam Hydrochloride
(122) Caffeine Hydrate	(175) Cefozopran Hydrochloride
(123) Caffeine and Sodium Benzoate	(176) Cefpiramide Sodium
(124) Precipitated Calcium Carbonate	(177) Cefpirome Sulfate
(125) Calcium Chloride Hydrate	(178) Cefpodoxime Proxetil
(126) Calcium Folinate Hydrate	(179) Cefroxadine Hydrate
(127) Calcium Gluconate Hydrate	(180) Cefsulodin Sodium
(128) Calcium Hydroxide	(181) Ceftazidime Hydrate
(129) Calcium Lactate Hydrate	(182) Cefteram Pivoxil
(130) Calcium Levofolinate Hydrate	(183) Ceftibuten Hydrate
(131) Calcium Pantothenate	(184) Ceftizoxime Sodium
(132) Calcium Paraaminosalicylate Hydrate	(185) Ceftriaxone Sodium Hydrate
(133) Anhydrous Dibasic Calcium Phosphate	(186) Cefuroxime Axetil
(134) Dibasic Calcium Phosphate Hydrate	(187) Celecoxib
(135) Monobasic Calcium Phosphate Hydrate	(188) Cellacefate
(136) Calcium Polystyrene Sulfonate	(189) Microcrystalline Cellulose
(137) Calcium Sodium Edetate Hydrate	(190) Powdered Cellulose
(138) Calcium Stearate	(191) Cetirizine Hydrochloride
(139) Camostat Mesilate	(192) Cetotiamine Hydrochloride Hydrate
(140) Candesartan Cilexetil	(193) Cetraxate Hydrochloride
(141) Captopril	(194) Chenodeoxycholic Acid
(142) Carbamazepine	(195) Chloramphenicol
(143) Carbazochrome Sodium Sulfonate Hydrate	(196) Chloramphenicol Palmitate
(144) Carbidopa Hydrate	(197) Chloramphenicol Sodium Succinate
(145) L-Carbocisteine	(198) Chlordiazepoxide
(146) Carmellose	(199) Chlorhexidine Hydrochloride
(147) Carmellose Calcium	(200) Chlormadinone Acetate
(148) Carmellose Sodium	(201) Chlorphenesin Carbamate
(149) Croscarmellose Sodium	(202) Chlorpheniramine Maleate
(150) Carmofur	(203) d-Chlorpheniramine Maleate
(151) Carteolol Hydrochloride	(204) Chlorpromazine Hydrochloride
(152) Carumonam Sodium	(205) Chlorpropamide
(153) Carvedilol	(206) Cibenzoline Succinate
(154) Cefaclor	(207) Ciclacillin
(155) Cefadroxil	(208) Ciclosporin
(156) Cefalexin	(209) Cilastatin Sodium
(157) Cefalotin Sodium	(210) Cilazapril Hydrate
(158) Cefatrizine Propylene Glycolate	(211) Cilnidipine
(159) Cefazolin Sodium	(212) Cilostazol
(160) Cefazolin Sodium Hydrate	(213) Cimetidine

Supplement I, JP XVIII   *Preface*   vii

(214) Cinoxacin
(215) Ciprofloxacin
(216) Ciprofloxacin Hydrochloride Hydrate
(217) Citicoline
(218) Anhydrous Citric Acid
(219) Citric Acid Hydrate
(220) Clarithromycin
(221) Clebopride Malate
(222) Clemastine Fumarate
(223) Clindamycin Hydrochloride
(224) Clindamycin Phosphate
(225) Clinofibrate
(226) Clobetasol Propionate
(227) Clocapramine Hydrochloride Hydrate
(228) Clofedanol Hydrochloride
(229) Clofibrate
(230) Clomifene Citrate
(231) Clomipramine Hydrochloride
(232) Clonazepam
(233) Clonidine Hydrochloride
(234) Cloperastine Fendizoate
(235) Cloperastine Hydrochloride
(236) Clopidogrel Sulfate
(237) Clorazepate Dipotassium
(238) Clotiazepam
(239) Clotrimazole
(240) Cloxacillin Sodium Hydrate
(241) Cloxazolam
(242) Colestimide
(243) Colistin Sodium Methanesulfonate
(244) Copovidone
(245) Croconazole Hydrochloride
(246) Crospovidone
(247) Cyanamide
(248) Cyclopentolate Hydrochloride
(249) Cyclophosphamide Hydrate
(250) Cycloserine
(251) Cyproheptadine Hydrochloride Hydrate
(252) L-Cysteine
(253) L-Cysteine Hydrochloride Hydrate
(254) L-Cystine
(255) Cytarabine
(256) Danazol
(257) Dantrolene Sodium Hydrate
(258) Daunorubicin Hydrochloride
(259) Deferoxamine Mesilate
(260) Dehydrocholic Acid
(261) Purified Dehydrocholic Acid
(262) Dehydrocholic Acid Injection
(263) Demethylchlortetracycline Hydrochloride
(264) Dexamethasone
(265) Dextran 40
(266) Dextran 70

(267) Dextran Sulfate Sodium Sulfur 5
(268) Dextran Sulfate Sodium Sulfur 18
(269) Dextrin
(270) Dextromethorphan Hydrobromide Hydrate
(271) Diazepam
(272) Dibekacin Sulfate
(273) Dibucaine Hydrochloride
(274) Diclofenac Sodium
(275) Diethylcarbamazine Citrate
(276) Difenidol Hydrochloride
(277) Diflorasone Diacetate
(278) Diflucortolone Valerate
(279) Dihydroergotoxine Mesilate
(280) Dilazep Hydrochloride Hydrate
(281) Diltiazem Hydrochloride
(282) Dimemorfan Phosphate
(283) Dimercaprol
(284) Dimorpholamine
(285) Diphenhydramine
(286) Diphenhydramine Hydrochloride
(287) Diphenhydramine Tannate
(288) Dipyridamole
(289) Disopyramide
(290) Distigmine Bromide
(291) Disulfiram
(292) Dobutamine Hydrochloride
(293) Docetaxel Hydrate
(294) Domperidone
(295) Donepezil Hydrochloride
(296) Dopamine Hydrochloride
(297) Doripenem Hydrate
(298) Dorzolamide Hydrochloride
(299) Doxapram Hydrochloride Hydrate
(300) Doxazosin Mesilate
(301) Doxifluridine
(302) Doxycycline Hydrochloride Hydrate
(303) Droperidol
(304) Droxidopa
(305) Dydrogesterone
(306) Ebastine
(307) Ecabet Sodium Hydrate
(308) Ecothiopate Iodide
(309) Edaravone
(310) Edrophonium Chloride
(311) Emedastine Fumarate
(312) Emorfazone
(313) Enalapril Maleate
(314) Enoxacin Hydrate
(315) Entacapone
(316) Enviomycin Sulfate
(317) Epalrestat
(318) Eperisone Hydrochloride
(319) Ephedrine Hydrochloride

viii   *Preface*

(320) Epirizole
(321) Epirubicin Hydrochloride
(322) Eplerenone
(323) Eribulin Mesilate
(324) Erythromycin
(325) Estazolam
(326) Estriol
(327) Etacrynic Acid
(328) Ethambutol Hydrochloride
(329) Ethenzamide
(330) Ethionamide
(331) Ethosuximide
(332) Ethyl Aminobenzoate
(333) Ethylcellulose
(334) Ethyl L-Cysteine Hydrochloride
(335) Ethylenediamine
(336) Ethyl Icosapentate
(337) Ethyl Loflazepate
(338) Ethyl Parahydroxybenzoate
(339) Etidronate Disodium
(340) Etilefrine Hydrochloride
(341) Etizolam
(342) Etodolac
(343) Etoposide
(344) Famotidine
(345) Faropenem Sodium Hydrate
(346) Felbinac
(347) Felodipine
(348) Fenbufen
(349) Fenofibrate
(350) Fentanyl Citrate
(351) Ferrous Sulfate Hydrate
(352) Fexofenadine Hydrochloride
(353) Flavin Adenine Dinucleotide Sodium
(354) Flavoxate Hydrochloride
(355) Flecainide Acetate
(356) Flomoxef Sodium
(357) Flopropione
(358) Fluconazole
(359) Flucytosine
(360) Fludiazepam
(361) Fludrocortisone Acetate
(362) Flunitrazepam
(363) Fluorometholone
(364) Fluorouracil
(365) Fluphenazine Enanthate
(366) Flurazepam Hydrochloride
(367) Flurbiprofen
(368) Flutamide
(369) Flutoprazepam
(370) Fluvoxamine Maleate
(371) Formoterol Fumarate Hydrate
(372) Fosfomycin Calcium Hydrate

(373) Fosfomycin Sodium
(374) Fradiomycin Sulfate
(375) Fructose
(376) Fructose Injection
(377) Fudosteine
(378) Furosemide
(379) Fursultiamine Hydrochloride
(380) Gabexate Mesilate
(381) β-Galactosidase (Aspergillus)
(382) β-Galactosidase (Penicillium)
(383) Gatifloxacin Hydrate
(384) Gefarnate
(385) Gefitinib
(386) Gelatin
(387) Purified Gelatin
(388) Gentamicin Sulfate
(389) Glibenclamide
(390) Gliclazide
(391) Glimepiride
(392) Glucose
(393) Glucose Hydrate
(394) Purified Glucose
(395) L-Glutamic Acid
(396) L-Glutamine
(397) Glutathione
(398) Glycerin
(399) Concentrated Glycerin
(400) Glycine
(401) Guaifenesin
(402) Guanabenz Acetate
(403) Guanethidine Sulfate
(404) Haloperidol
(405) Haloxazolam
(406) Heparin Calcium
(407) Heparin Sodium
(408) Heparin Sodium Injection
(409) L-Histidine
(410) L-Histidine Hydrochloride Hydrate
(411) Homochlorcyclizine Hydrochloride
(412) Hydralazine Hydrochloride
(413) Hydrochloric Acid
(414) Dilute Hydrochloric Acid
(415) Hydrochlorothiazide
(416) Hydrocortisone Butyrate
(417) Hydrocortisone Sodium Phosphate
(418) Hydrocotarnine Hydrochloride Hydrate
(419) Hydrogenated Oil
(420) Hydroxyethylcellulose
(421) Hydroxypropylcellulose
(422) Low Substituted Hydroxypropylcellulose
(423) Hydroxyzine Hydrochloride
(424) Hydroxyzine Pamoate
(425) Hymecromone

Supplement I, JP XVIII   *Preface*   ix

(426) Hypromellose
(427) Hypromellose Acetate Succinate
(428) Hypromellose Phthalate
(429) Ibudilast
(430) Ibuprofen
(431) Ibuprofen Piconol
(432) Idarubicin Hydrochloride
(433) Idoxuridine
(434) Ifenprodil Tartrate
(435) Imidapril Hydrochloride
(436) Imipenem Hydrate
(437) Indapamide
(438) Indenolol Hydrochloride
(439) Indigocarmine
(440) Indometacin
(441) Iohexol
(442) Iopamidol
(443) Iotalamic Acid
(444) Iotroxic Acid
(445) Ipratropium Bromide Hydrate
(446) Ipriflavone
(447) Irbesartan
(448) Irinotecan Hydrochloride Hydrate
(449) Irsogladine Maleate
(450) Isepamicin Sulfate
(451) L-Isoleucine
(452) Isomalt Hydrate
(453) Isoniazid
(454) *l*-Isoprenaline Hydrochloride
(455) Isopropylantipyrine
(456) Isosorbide
(457) Isosorbide Dinitrate
(458) Isosorbide Mononitrate 70%/Lactose 30%
(459) Isoxsuprine Hydrochloride
(460) Itraconazole
(461) Josamycin
(462) Josamycin Propionate
(463) Kainic Acid Hydrate
(464) Kanamycin Monosulfate
(465) Kanamycin Sulfate
(466) Ketamine Hydrochloride
(467) Ketoconazole
(468) Ketoprofen
(469) Ketotifen Fumarate
(470) Kitasamycin Tartrate
(471) Labetalol Hydrochloride
(472) Lactic Acid
(473) L-Lactic Acid
(474) Anhydrous Lactose
(475) Lactose Hydrate
(476) Lactulose
(477) Lafutidine
(478) Lanoconazole

(479) Lansoprazole
(480) Latamoxef Sodium
(481) Lenampicillin Hydrochloride
(482) L-Leucine
(483) Levallorphan Tartrate
(484) Levodopa
(485) Levofloxacin Hydrate
(486) Levomepromazine Maleate
(487) Lidocaine
(488) Lincomycin Hydrochloride Hydrate
(489) Lisinopril Hydrate
(490) Lithium Carbonate
(491) Lobenzarit Sodium
(492) Lorazepam
(493) Losartan Potassium
(494) Loxoprofen Sodium Hydrate
(495) L-Lysine Acetate
(496) L-Lysine Hydrochloride
(497) Lysozyme Hydrochloride
(498) Magnesium Aluminosilicate
(499) Magnesium Aluminometasilicate
(500) Magnesium Carbonate
(501) Magnesium Oxide
(502) Magnesium Stearate
(503) Magnesium Sulfate Hydrate
(504) Maltose Hydrate
(505) Manidipine Hydrochloride
(506) D-Mannitol
(507) Maprotiline Hydrochloride
(508) Meclofenoxate Hydrochloride
(509) Medazepam
(510) Medicinal Carbon
(511) Medicinal Soap
(512) Medroxyprogesterone Acetate
(513) Mefenamic Acid
(514) Mefloquine Hydrochloride
(515) Mefruside
(516) Meglumine
(517) Melphalan
(518) Menatetrenone
(519) Mepenzolate Bromide
(520) Mepitiostane
(521) Mepivacaine Hydrochloride
(522) Mequitazine
(523) Mercaptopurine Hydrate
(524) Meropenem Hydrate
(525) Mesalazine
(526) Mestranol
(527) Metenolone Acetate
(528) Metenolone Enanthate
(529) Metformin Hydrochloride
(530) L-Methionine
(531) Methoxsalen

(532) Methylcellulose
(533) Methyldopa Hydrate
(534) *dl*-Methylephedrine Hydrochloride
(535) Methyl Parahydroxybenzoate
(536) Methylprednisolone Succinate
(537) Methyl Salicylate
(538) Meticrane
(539) Metildigoxin
(540) Metoclopramide
(541) Metoprolol Tartrate
(542) Metronidazole
(543) Metyrapone
(544) Mexiletine Hydrochloride
(545) Miconazole
(546) Miconazole Nitrate
(547) Micronomicin Sulfate
(548) Midecamycin
(549) Midecamycin Acetate
(550) Miglitol
(551) Migrenin
(552) Minocycline Hydrochloride
(553) Mitiglinide Calcium Hydrate
(554) Mizoribine
(555) Montelukast Sodium
(556) Mosapride Citrate Hydrate
(557) Mupirocin Calcium Hydrate
(558) Nabumetone
(559) Nadolol
(560) Nafamostat Mesilate
(561) Naftopidil
(562) Nalidixic Acid
(563) Naphazoline Nitrate
(564) Naproxen
(565) Nateglinide
(566) Nicardipine Hydrochloride
(567) Nicergoline
(568) Niceritrol
(569) Nicomol
(570) Nicorandil
(571) Nicotinamide
(572) Nicotinic Acid
(573) Nifedipine
(574) Nilvadipine
(575) Nitrazepam
(576) Nitrendipine
(577) Nizatidine
(578) Norfloxacin
(579) Norgestrel
(580) Nortriptyline Hydrochloride
(581) Noscapine
(582) Nystatin
(583) Ofloxacin
(584) Olmesartan Medoxomil

(585) Olopatadine Hydrochloride
(586) Omeprazole
(587) Orciprenaline Sulfate
(588) Oxapium Iodide
(589) Oxaprozin
(590) Oxazolam
(591) Oxethazaine
(592) Oxprenolol Hydrochloride
(593) Oxybuprocaine Hydrochloride
(594) Oxydol
(595) Oxytetracycline Hydrochloride
(596) Ozagrel Sodium
(597) Panipenem
(598) Pantethine
(599) Paraffin
(600) Liquid Paraffin
(601) Light Liquid Paraffin
(602) Parnaparin Sodium
(603) Paroxetine Hydrochloride Hydrate
(604) Pazufloxacin Mesilate
(605) Pemirolast Potassium
(606) Penbutolol Sulfate
(607) Pentazocine
(608) Pentobarbital Calcium
(609) Pentoxyverine Citrate
(610) Peplomycin Sulfate
(611) Perphenazine
(612) Perphenazine Maleate
(613) White Petrolatum
(614) Yellow Petrolatum
(615) Phenethicillin Potassium
(616) Phenobarbital
(617) L-Phenylalanine
(618) Phenylbutazone
(619) Phenytoin
(620) Phenytoin Sodium for Injection
(621) Phytonadione
(622) Pilsicainide Hydrochloride Hydrate
(623) Pimaricin
(624) Pimozide
(625) Pindolol
(626) Pioglitazone Hydrochloride
(627) Pipemidic Acid Hydrate
(628) Piperacillin Hydrate
(629) Piperacillin Sodium
(630) Piperazine Adipate
(631) Piperazine Phosphate Hydrate
(632) Pirarubicin
(633) Pirenoxine
(634) Pirenzepine Hydrochloride Hydrate
(635) Piroxicam
(636) Pitavastatin Calcium Hydrate
(637) Pivmecillinam Hydrochloride

Supplement I, JP XVIII   *Preface*   xi

(638) Polaprezinc
(639) Polymixin B Sulfate
(640) Polyoxyl 40 Stearate
(641) Polysorbate 80
(642) Potassium Bromide
(643) Potassium Canrenoate
(644) Potassium Carbonate
(645) Potassium Chloride
(646) Potassium Clavulanate
(647) Potassium Hydroxide
(648) Potassium Iodide
(649) Potassium Permanganate
(650) Potassium Sulfate
(651) Povidone
(652) Povidone-Iodine
(653) Pranlukast Hydrate
(654) Pranoprofen
(655) Prasterone Sodium Sulfate Hydrate
(656) Pravastatin Sodium
(657) Prazepam
(658) Prazosin Hydrochloride
(659) Prednisolone
(660) Prednisolone Sodium Phosphate
(661) Primidone
(662) Probenecid
(663) Probucol
(664) Procainamide Hydrochloride
(665) Procaine Hydrochloride
(666) Procarbazine Hydrochloride
(667) Procaterol Hydrochloride Hydrate
(668) Prochlorperazine Maleate
(669) Proglumide
(670) L-Proline
(671) Promethazine Hydrochloride
(672) Propafenone Hydrochloride
(673) Propiverine Hydrochloride
(674) Propranolol Hydrochloride
(675) Propylene Glycol
(676) Propyl Parahydroxybenzoate
(677) Prothionamide
(678) Protirelin
(679) Protirelin Tartrate Hydrate
(680) Pullulan
(681) Pyrantel Pamoate
(682) Pyrazinamide
(683) Pyridostigmine Bromide
(684) Pyridoxal Phosphate Hydrate
(685) Pyridoxine Hydrochloride
(686) Quetiapine Fumarate
(687) Quinapril Hydrochloride
(688) Quinine Ethyl Carbonate
(689) Quinine Sulfate Hydrate
(690) Rabeprazole Sodium

(691) Ranitidine Hydrochloride
(692) Rebamipide
(693) Ribavirin
(694) Riboflavin Butyrate
(695) Ribostamycin Sulfate
(696) Rifampicin
(697) Rilmazafone Hydrochloride Hydrate
(698) Ringer's Solution
(699) Risperidone
(700) Ritodrine Hydrochloride
(701) Rosuvastatin Calcium
(702) Roxatidine Acetate Hydrochloride
(703) Roxithromycin
(704) Saccharin
(705) Saccharin Sodium Hydrate
(706) Salazosulfapyridine
(707) Salbutamol Sulfate
(708) Salicylic Acid
(709) Sarpogrelate Hydrochloride
(710) Scopolamine Butylbromide
(711) L-Serine
(712) Purified Shellac
(713) White Shellac
(714) Light Anhydrous Silicic Acid
(715) Silodosin
(716) Silver Nitrate
(717) Simvastatin
(718) Sitagliptin Phosphate Hydrate
(719) Sivelestat Sodium Hydrate
(720) Sodium Acetate Hydrate
(721) Sodium Aurothiomalate
(722) Sodium Benzoate
(723) Sodium Bicarbonate
(724) Sodium Bisulfite
(725) Sodium Borate
(726) Sodium Bromide
(727) Dried Sodium Carbonate
(728) Sodium Carbonate Hydrate
(729) Sodium Chloride
(730) Isotonic Sodium Chloride Solution
(731) Sodium Citrate Hydrate
(732) Sodium Cromoglicate
(733) Disodium Edetate Hydrate
(734) Sodium Fusidate
(735) Purified Sodium Hyaluronate
(736) Sodium Hydroxide
(737) Sodium Iodide
(738) Sodium L-Lactate Solution
(739) Sodium L-Lactate Ringer's Solution
(740) Dibasic Sodium Phosphate Hydrate
(741) Sodium Picosulfate Hydrate
(742) Sodium Polystyrene Sulfonate
(743) Sodium Pyrosulfite

xii   *Preface*

(744) Sodium Risedronate Hydrate
(745) Sodium Salicylate
(746) Sodium Starch Glycolate
(747) Dried Sodium Sulfite
(748) Sodium Thiosulfate Hydrate
(749) Sodium Valproate
(750) Sorbitan Sesquioleate
(751) D-Sorbitol
(752) D-Sorbitol Solution
(753) Spiramycin Acetate
(754) Stearic Acid
(755) Streptomycin Sulfate
(756) Sucralfate Hydrate
(757) White Soft Sugar
(758) Sulbactam Sodium
(759) Sulbenicillin Sodium
(760) Sulfamethizole
(761) Sulfamethoxazole
(762) Sulfamonomethoxine Hydrate
(763) Sulfisoxazole
(764) Sulfobromophthalein Sodium
(765) Sulfur
(766) Sulindac
(767) Sulpiride
(768) Sulpyrine Hydrate
(769) Sultamicillin Tosilate Hydrate
(770) Sultiame
(771) Tacrolimus Hydrate
(772) Talampicillin Hydrochloride
(773) Taltirelin Hydrate
(774) Tamoxifen Citrate
(775) Tamsulosin Hydrochloride
(776) Tartaric Acid
(777) Taurine
(778) Tazobactam
(779) Tegafur
(780) Teicoplanin
(781) Telmisartan
(782) Temocapril Hydrochloride
(783) Teprenone
(784) Terbinafine Hydrochloride
(785) Terbutaline Sulfate
(786) Tetracaine Hydrochloride
(787) Tetracycline Hydrochloride
(788) Theophylline
(789) Thiamazole
(790) Thiamine Chloride Hydrochloride
(791) Thiamine Nitrate
(792) Thiamylal Sodium
(793) Thiopental Sodium
(794) Thiopental Sodium for Injection
(795) Thioridazine Hydrochloride
(796) L-Threonine

(797) Tiapride Hydrochloride
(798) Tiaramide Hydrochloride
(799) Ticlopidine Hydrochloride
(800) Timepidium Bromide Hydrate
(801) Timolol Maleate
(802) Tinidazole
(803) Tipepidine Hibenzate
(804) Tizanidine Hydrochloride
(805) Tobramycin
(806) Tocopherol
(807) Tocopherol Acetate
(808) Tocopherol Nicotinate
(809) Todralazine Hydrochloride Hydrate
(810) Tofisopam
(811) Tolbutamide
(812) Tolnaftate
(813) Tolperisone Hydrochloride
(814) Tosufloxacin Tosilate Hydrate
(815) Tramadol Hydrochloride
(816) Tranexamic Acid
(817) Tranilast
(818) Trapidil
(819) Trehalose Hydrate
(820) Trepibutone
(821) Triamcinolone
(822) Triamcinolone Acetonide
(823) Triamterene
(824) Triazolam
(825) Trichlormethiazide
(826) Triclofos Sodium
(827) Trientine Hydrochloride
(828) Trihexyphenidyl Hydrochloride
(829) Trimebutine Maleate
(830) Trimetazidine Hydrochloride
(831) Trimethadione
(832) Trimetoquinol Hydrochloride Hydrate
(833) Tropicamide
(834) Troxipide
(835) L-Tryptophan
(836) Tulobuterol
(837) Tulobuterol Hydrochloride
(838) L-Tyrosine
(839) Ubenimex
(840) Ubidecarenone
(841) Ulinastatin
(842) Urapidil
(843) Urea
(844) Urokinase
(845) Ursodeoxycholic Acid
(846) Valaciclovir Hydrochloride
(847) L-Valine
(848) Valsartan
(849) Vancomycin Hydrochloride

Supplement I, JP XVIII *Preface* xiii

(850) Verapamil Hydrochloride
(851) Voglibose
(852) Voriconazole
(853) Warfarin Potassium
(854) Wine
(855) Xylitol
(856) Zaltoprofen
(857) Zidovudine
(858) Zinc Chloride
(859) Zinc Oxide
(860) Zinc Sulfate Hydrate
(861) Zolpidem Tartrate
(862) Zonisamide
(863) Zopiclone

15. The following monographs were deleted:
(1) Nartograstim (Genetical Recombination)
(2) Nartograstim for Injection (Genetical Recombination)

16. The following articles were newly added to Ultraviolet-visible Reference Spectra:
(1) Anastrozole
(2) Budesonide
(3) Oxybutynine Hydrochloride
(4) Temozolomide

17. The following articles were newly added to Infrared Reference Spectra:
(1) Anastrozole
(2) Budesonide
(3) Croscarmellose Sodium
(4) Oxybutynine Hydrochloride
(5) White Petrolatum
(6) Yellow Petrolatum
(7) Temozolomide

Those who were engaged in the preparation of the Supplement I to the JP 18th Edition are as follows:

ABE Misato
ABE Yasuhiro
AMAKURA Yoshiaki
ARATO Teruyo
ARUGA Naoki
ASAI Yumi
ASHIKAGA Takao
ASHIZAWA Kazuhide
DEMIZU Yosuke
EMURA Makoto
FUCHINO Hiroyuki
FUJII Hirosato
FUJII Makiko
FUJII Norikazu
FUJII Shinya
FUKAMI Toshiro
FUKASAWA Masayoshi
FUKAZAWA Hidesuke
FUKUHARA Kiyoshi
FURUKAWA Hiromitsu
GODA Yukihiro
GOTO Takashi
GOTO Tamami
HA Hyeonseong
HAISHIMA Yuji
HAKAMATA Hideki
HAKAMATSUKA Takashi
HANAJIRI Ruri
HARAYA Yuki
HARAZONO Akira
HASEGAWA Atsuhiro
HASHII Noritaka
HAYAKAWA Masako
HAYASHI Ai
HAYASHI Akira
HAYASHI Katsuhiko
HAYASHI Yoshinori
HIGANO Taro
HIGUCHI Kenji
HIGUCHI Yasuhiko
HIRATA Mao
HONMA Masamitsu**
HYUGA Masashi
ICHIKAWA Hiroyuki
ICHINOSE Koji
IKARASHI Yoshiaki
IKEDA Koji
IKEDO Shingo
IKEMATSU Yasuhito
INOUE Takayuki
ISHIDA Masato
ISHIDA Seiichi
ISHII Akiko
ITO Michiho
ITO Ryoichi
IZUTANI Yusuke
IZUTSU Kenichi
KAIDA Naoki
KAKINUMA Sayaka
KAMMOTO Toshihiro
KATAYAMA Hirohito
KATO Hiroshi
KATO Kumiko
KATORI Noriko
KAWAGUCHI Masami
KAWAHARA Nobuo
KAWAI Tamotsu
KAWANO Noriaki
KAWARASAKI Yoshihiko
KIKUCHI Yutaka
KIMURA Noritaka
KINOSHITA Eiji
KINOSHITA Mitsuhiro
KITAJIMA Akihito
KITTAKA Atsushi
KIUCHI Fumiyuki
KOCHI Rika
KOHAMA Ai
KOHITA Hideki
KOIDE Tatsuo
KOMATSU Katsuko
KONDO Ryo
KONDO Seizo
KUBOTA Kiyoshi
KUDO Yukiko
KUMASAKA Kenichi
KURIHARA Masaaki
KUROIWA Yuki
KUROKAWA Junko
KUSUNOKI Hideki
KUSUNOSE Naoto
MAEKAWA Keiko
MAEKAWA Naoya
MAKIURA Toshinobu
MARUYAMA Takuro
MASADA Sayaka
MASUMOTO Naoko
MATSUMOTO Kazuhiro
MATSUMOTO Makoto
MATSUURA Tadashi
MISAWA Takashi
MITSUHASHI Takao
MIYAZAKI Takashi
MIYAZAKI Tamaki
MIZUNO Ryoichi
MIZUNO Takeshi
MOCHIDA Kimiko
MORI Mitsuo
MORIBE Kunikazu
MORIMOTO Takashi
MORISAKI Takahito
MORIYASU Takako
MURABAYASHI Mika
MURATA Takahisa
MUROI Masashi
NAGUMO Seishin
NAKAGAWA Hidehiko
NAKAGAWA Shinsaku
NAKAGAWA Tsutomu
NAKAGAWA Yukari
NAKAKO Mayumi
NAKANO Tatsuya
NAKAOKA Kyohei
NAMIKAWA Nobuhiro
NARIAI Ryosuke
NOGUCHI Shuji
OBARA Sakae
OCHIAI Masaki
OGAWA Kiyoshi
OGAWA Toru
OGURA Yasumitsu
OGURI Kazuki
OHGAMI Yasutaka
OHTA Shigeru*

OHYA Kenji
OKUBO Tsuneo
OKUDA Akihiro
OKUDA Haruhiro
OMURA Koichi
ONODA Hiroshi
SAITO Hideyuki
SAITO Yoshiro
SAKAI Eiji
SAKAMOTO Tomoaki
SANTA Tomofumi
SASAKI Yuko
SATO Koji
SATO Kyoko
SHIBATA Hiroko
SHIBAZAKI Keiko
SHIDA Shizuka
SHIMAZAWA Rumiko
SHIMOKAWA Sayuri
SHINOZAKI Yoko
SHIRATORI Makoto
SHIROTA Osamu
SHODA Takuji
SHOKEN Saori
SUDO Hirotaka
SUGIMOTO Chishio
SUGIMOTO Naoki
SUGIMOTO Satoshi
SUZUKI Mikio
SUZUKI Noriyuki
SUZUKI Ryoji
SUZUKI Shigeo
TADA Minoru
TADAKI Shinichi
TAGAMI Takaomi
TAKAI Yoshiaki
TAKANO Akihito
TAKAO Masaki

TAKATANI Kazuhiro
TAKAYANAGI Yoichiro
TAKEBAYASHI Kenji
TAKEDA Tomoko
TAKEUCHI Hirohumi
TAKEUCHI Hisashi
TANAKA Masakazu
TANAKA Rie
TANAKA Satoshi
TANIMOTO Tsuyoshi
TAOKA Yukako
TOKUMOTO Hiroko
TOKUOKA Shogo
TOYODA Taichi
TSUCHIYA Aya
TSUDA Shigeki
TSUDA Tsubasa
TSUJI Genichiro
TSUNEHIRO Masaya
UCHIDA Eriko
UCHIYAMA Nahoko
USHIRODA Osamu
WATANABE Eiji
WATANABE Takumi
YAMADA Yuko
YAMAGUCHI Shigeharu
YAMAGUCHI Tetsuji
YAMAMOTO Eiichi
YAMAMOTO Hiromitsu
YAMAMOTO Yutaka
YAMANE Emiko
YAMASHITA Chikamasa
YASUHARA Masato
YONEDA Sachiyo
YONEMOCHI Etsuo
YOSHIDA Hiroyuki
YOSHIMATSU Kayo
ZHANG Hongyan

*: Chairman, the Committee on JP
**: Acting Chairman, the Committee on JP

Supplement I to
The Japanese
Pharmacopoeia
Eighteenth Edition

GENERAL TESTS, PROCESSES AND APPARATUS

Add the following:

2.00 Chromatography

This test is harmonized with the European Pharmacopoeia and the U.S. Pharmacopeia.

The corresponding part of the attributes/provisions which are agreed as non-harmonized within the scope of the harmonization is marked with symbols (♦ ♠) and the corresponding parts which are agreed as the JP local requirement other than the scope of the harmonization are marked with symbols (◇ ◊).

Information on the harmonization with the European Pharmacopoeia and the U.S. Pharmacopeia is available on the website of the Pharmaceuticals and Medical Devices Agency.

1. Introduction

Chromatographic separation techniques are multi-stage separation procedures in which the components of a sample are distributed between 2 phases, one of which is stationary, while the other is mobile. The stationary phase may be a solid or a liquid supported on a solid or a gel. The stationary phase may be packed in a column, spread as a layer, or distributed as a film, etc. The mobile phase may be gaseous or liquid or supercritical fluid. The separation may be based on adsorption, mass distribution (partition), ion exchange, etc., or may be based on differences in the physico-chemical properties of the molecules such as size, mass, volume, etc. This chapter contains definitions and calculations of common parameters and generally applicable requirements for system suitability. ◇The prescription described in Liquid Chromatography <2.01> other than the prescription of this test can be applied to the system suitability of liquid chromatography.◊ Principles of separation, apparatus and methods are given in the corresponding general tests.

2. Definitions

The system suitability and acceptance criteria in monographs have been set using parameters as defined below. With some equipment, certain parameters, such as the signal-to-noise ratio and resolution, can be calculated using software provided by the manufacturer. It is the responsibility of the user to ensure that the calculation methods used in the software are equivalent to the requirements of the Japanese Pharmacopoeia and to make any necessary corrections if this is not the case.

Chromatogram

A graphical or other representation of detector response, effluent concentration or other quantity used as a measure of effluent concentration, versus time or volume. Idealized chromatograms are represented as a sequence of Gaussian peaks on a baseline (Fig. 2.00-1).

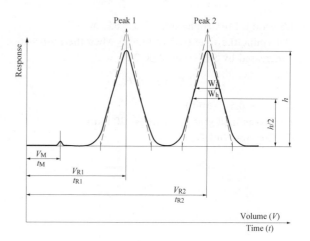

Fig. 2.00-1

V_M: Hold-up volume
t_M: Hold-up time
V_{R1}: Retention volume of peak 1
t_{R1}: Retention time of peak 1
V_{R2}: Retention volume of peak 2
t_{R2}: Retention time of peak 2
W_h: Peak width at half-height
W_i: Peak width at the inflexion point
h: Height of the peak
$h/2$: Half-height of peak

Distribution constant (K_0)

In size-exclusion chromatography, the elution characteristics of a component in a particular column may be given by the distribution constant (also referred to as distribution coefficient), which is calculated using the following equation:

$$K_0 = \frac{t_R - t_0}{t_t - t_0}$$

t_R: Retention time
t_0: Retention time of an unretained compound
t_t: Total mobile phase time

Dwell volume (D) (also referred to as V_D):

The dwell volume (also known as gradient delay volume) is the volume between the point at which the eluents meet and the inlet of the column. It can be determined using the following procedure.

Column: replace the chromatographic column by an appropriate capillary tubing (e.g. 1 m × 0.12 mm).

Mobile phase.

Mobile phase A: water.
Mobile phase B: 0.1 vol% solution of acetone in water.

Time (min)	Mobile phase A (vol%)	Mobile phase B (vol%)
0 – 20	100 → 0	0 → 100
20 – 30	0	100

Flow rate: Set to obtain sufficient back-pressure (e.g. 2 mL/min).
Detection: Spectrophotometer at 265 nm.
Determine the time ($t_{0.5}$) (minutes) when the absorbance has increased by 50% (Fig. 2.00-2).

$$D = t_D \times F$$

t_D: $t_{0.5} - 0.5\ t_G$ (min)
t_G: Pre-defined gradient time (= 20 min)
F: Flow rate (mL/min)

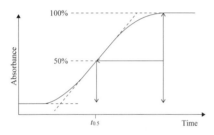

Fig. 2.00-2

Note: Where applicable, this measurement is performed with the autosampler in the inject position so as to include the injection loop volume in the dwell volume.

Hold-up time (t_M)
Time required for elution of an unretained component (Fig. 2.00-1, baseline scale being in minutes or seconds).
In size-exclusion chromatography, the term retention time of an unretained compound (t_0) is used.

Hold-up volume (V_M)
Volume of the mobile phase required for elution of an unretained component. It may be calculated from the hold-up time and the flow rate (F) in mL/minute using the following equation:

$$V_M = t_M \times F$$

In size-exclusion chromatography, the term retention volume of an unretained compound (V_0) is used.

Peak
Portion of a chromatogram recording the detector response when a single component (or 2 or more unresolved components) is eluted from the column.
The peak response may be represented by the peak area or the peak height (h).

Peak-to-valley ratio (p/v)
The peak-to-valley ratio may be employed as a system suitability criterion when baseline separation between two peaks is not achieved (Fig. 2.00-3).

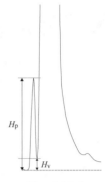

Fig. 2.00-3

$$p/v = \frac{H_p}{H_v}$$

H_p: Height above the extrapolated baseline of the minor peak
H_v: Height above the extrapolated baseline at the lowest point of the curve separating the minor and major peaks

Plate height (H) (synonym: Height equivalent to one theoretical plate (HETP))
Ratio of the column length (L) (μm) to the plate number (N):

$$H = \frac{L}{N}$$

Plate number (N)
A number indicative of column performance (column efficiency). It can only be calculated from data obtained under either isothermal, isocratic or isodense conditions, depending on the technique, as the plate number, using the following equation, the values of t_R and w_h being expressed in the same units.

$$N = 5.54 \left(\frac{t_R}{w_h}\right)^2$$

t_R: Retention time of the peak corresponding to the component;
w_h: Peak width at half-height ($h/2$).

The plate number varies with the component as well as with the column, the column temperature, the mobile phase and the retention time.

Reduced plate height (h)
Ratio of the plate height (H) (μm) to the particle diameter (d_p) (μm):

$$h = \frac{H}{d_p}$$

Relative retardation (R_{rel})
The relative retardation, used in thin-layer chromatography, is calculated as the ratio of the distances travelled by the spot of the compound of interest and a reference com-

pound (Fig. 2.00-4).

$$R_{rel} = b/c$$

a: Migration distance of the mobile phase
b: Migration distance of the compound of interest
c: Migration distance of the reference compound

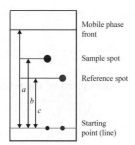

Fig. 2.00-4

Relative retention (r)

Relative retention is calculated as an estimate using the following equation:

$$r = \frac{t_{Ri} - t_M}{t_{Rst} - t_M}$$

t_{Ri}: Retention time of the peak of the component of interest
t_{Rst}: Retention time of the reference peak (usually the peak corresponding to the substance to be examined)
t_M: Hold-up time

Relative retention, unadjusted (r_G) or (RRT)

Unadjusted relative retention is calculated using the following equation:

$$r_G = \frac{t_{Ri}}{t_{Rst}}$$

Unless otherwise indicated, values for relative retention stated in monographs correspond to unadjusted relative retention.

Relative retention time (RRT):
see Relative retention, unadjusted.

Resolution (R_S)

The resolution between peaks of 2 components (Fig. 2.00-1) may be calculated using the following equation:

$$R_S = \frac{1.18 (t_{R2} - t_{R1})}{w_{h1} + w_{h2}}$$

t_{R1}, t_{R2}: Retention times of the peaks, $t_{R2} > t_{R1}$
w_{h1}, w_{h2}: Peak widths at half-height

◇Complete separation means the resolution of not less than 1.5, and is also referred to as baseline separation.◇

In quantitative thin-layer chromatography, using densitometry, the migration distances are used instead of retention times and the resolution between peaks of 2 components may be calculated using the following equation:

$$R_S = \frac{1.18a (R_{F2} - R_{F1})}{w_{h1} + w_{h2}}$$

$R_{F2} > R_{F1}$
R_{F1}, R_{F2}: Retardation factors of the peaks
w_{h1}, w_{h2}: Peak widths at half-height
a: Migration distance of the solvent front

Retardation factor (R_F)

The retardation factor, used in thin-layer chromatography, is the ratio of the distance from the point of application to the center of the spot and the distance simultaneously travelled by the solvent front from the point of application (Fig. 2.00-4).

$$R_F = \frac{b}{a}$$

b: Migration distance of the compound of interest
a: Migration distance of the solvent front

Retention factor (k)

The retention factor (also known as mass distribution ratio (D_m) or capacity factor (k')) is defined as:

$$k = \frac{\text{amount of component in stationary phase}}{\text{amount of component in mobile phase}} = K_C \frac{V_S}{V_M}$$

K_C: Distribution constant (also known as equilibrium distribution coefficient);
V_S: Volume of the stationary phase
V_M: Volume of the mobile phase

The retention factor of a component may be determined from the chromatogram using the following equation:

$$k = \frac{t_R - t_M}{t_M}$$

t_R: Retention time
t_M: Hold-up time

Retention time (t_R)

Time elapsed between the injection of the sample and the appearance of the maximum peak response of the eluted sample zone (Fig. 2.00-1, baseline scale being in minutes or seconds).

Retention volume (V_R)

Volume of the mobile phase required for elution of a component. It may be calculated from the retention time and the flow rate (F: mL/minute) using the following equation:

$$V_R = t_R \times F$$

Retention time of an unretained compound (t_0)

In size-exclusion chromatography, retention time of a component whose molecules are larger than the largest gel pores (Fig. 2.00-5).

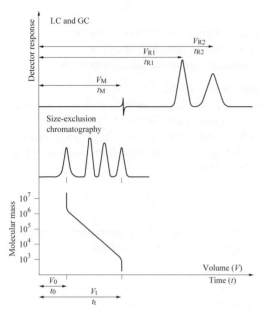

Fig. 2.00-5

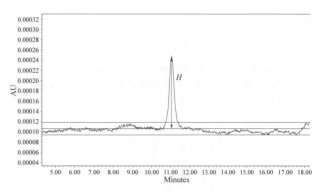

Fig. 2.00-6. Chromatogram of the reference solution

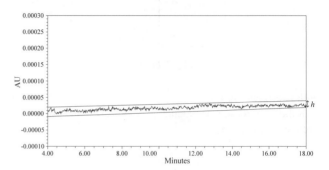

Fig. 2.00-7. Chromatogram of a blank

Retention volume of an unretained compound (V_0)

In size-exclusion chromatography, retention volume of a component whose molecules are larger than the largest gel pores. It may be calculated from the retention time of an unretained compound and the flow rate (F: mL/minute) using the following equation:

$$V_0 = t_0 \times F$$

Separation factor (α)

Relative retention calculated for two adjacent peaks (by convention, the value of the separation factor is always > 1):

$$\alpha = k_2/k_1$$

k_1: Retention factor of the first peak
k_2: Retention factor of the second peak

Signal-to-noise ratio (S/N)

The short-term noise influences the precision and accuracy of quantitation. The signal-to-noise ratio is calculated using the following equation:

$$S/N = \frac{2H}{h}$$

H: Height of the peak (Fig. 2.00-6) corresponding to the component concerned, in the chromatogram obtained with the prescribed reference solution, measured from the maximum of the peak to the extrapolated baseline of the signal observed over a distance equal to 20 times the width at half-height

h: Range of the noise in a chromatogram obtained after injection of a blank (Fig. 2.00-7), observed over a distance equal to 20 times the width at half-height of the peak in the chromatogram obtained with the prescribed reference solution and, if possible, situated equally around the place where this peak would be found.

If a baseline of 20 times the width at half-height is not obtainable because of peaks due to the solvents or reagents, or arising from the mobile phase or the sample matrix, or due to the gas chromatographic temperature program, a baseline of at least 5 times the width at half-height is permitted.

Symmetry factor (A_S)

The symmetry factor of a peak (also known as the asymmetry factor or tailing factor) (Fig. 2.00-8) is calculated using the following equation:

$$A_S = \frac{w_{0.05}}{2d}$$

$w_{0.05}$: Width of the peak at one-twentieth of the peak height
d: Distance between the perpendicular dropped from the peak maximum and the leading edge of the peak at one-twentieth of the peak height

An A_S value of 1.0 signifies symmetry. When $A_S > 1.0$, the peak is tailing. When $A_S < 1.0$, the peak is fronting.

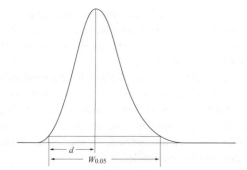

Fig. 2.00-8

System repeatability

The repeatability of response is expressed as an estimated percentage relative standard deviation (%RSD) of a consecutive series of measurements for not fewer than 3 injections or applications of a reference solution, and is calculated using the following equation.

$$\%\text{RSD} = \frac{100}{\bar{y}} \sqrt{\frac{\Sigma (y_i - \bar{y})^2}{n-1}}$$

y_i: Individual values expressed as peak area, peak height, or ratio of areas by the internal standardization method;
$\bar{y}$: Mean of individual values
n: Number of individual values

Total mobile phase time (t_t)

In size-exclusion chromatography, retention time of a component whose molecules are smaller than the smallest gel pores (Fig. 2.00-5).

Total mobile phase volume (V_t)

In size-exclusion chromatography, retention volume of a component whose molecules are smaller than the smallest gel pores. It may be calculated from the total mobile phase time and the flow rate (F) (mL/minute) using the following equation.

$$V_t = t_t \times F$$

3. System suitability

This section only covers liquid chromatography and gas chromatography.

The various components of the equipment employed must be qualified and be capable of achieving the performance required to conduct the test or assay.

The system suitability tests represent an integral part of the analytical procedure and are used to ensure adequate performance of the chromatographic system. Column plate number, retention factor (mass distribution ratio), system repeatability, signal-to-noise, symmetry factor and resolution/peak-to-valley ratio are the parameters that may be employed in assessing the performance of the chromatographic system. When stated in the individual monograph, in cases of complex chromatographic profiles (e.g., for biotechnological/biological products), visual comparison of the profiles can be used as a system suitability test.

Factors that may affect the chromatographic behavior include:
- Composition and temperature of the mobile phase;
- Ionic strength and pH of the aqueous component of the mobile phase;
- Flow rate, column dimensions, column temperature and pressure;
- Stationary phase characteristics including type of chromatographic support (particle-based or monolithic), particle or pore size, porosity, specific surface area;
- Reversed phase and other surface-modification of the stationary phases, the extent of chemical modification (as expressed by end-capping, carbon loading etc.).

Retention times and relative retentions may be provided in monographs for information purposes only. There are no acceptance criteria applied to relative retentions.

Compliance with the system suitability criteria is required throughout the chromatographic procedure. No sample analysis is acceptable unless the suitability of the system has been demonstrated.

◇When the following criteria are specified in the system suitability tests, each requirement is to be fulfilled unless otherwise prescribed.◇

System repeatability — assay of an active substance or an excipient

In an assay of an active substance or an excipient, where the target value is 100% for a pure substance, and a system repeatability requirement is not specified, the maximum permitted relative standard deviation (%RSD$_{max}$) for the defined limits is calculated for a series ($n = 3$ to 6) of injections of the reference solution.

The maximum permitted relative standard deviation of the peak response does not exceed the appropriate value given in Table 2.00-1.

$$\%\text{RSD}_{max} = \frac{KB\sqrt{n}}{t_{90\%,\, n-1}}$$

K: Constant (0.349), obtained from the expression,
$K = \dfrac{0.6}{\sqrt{2}} \times \dfrac{t_{90\%,\,5}}{\sqrt{6}}$ in which $\dfrac{0.6}{\sqrt{2}}$ represents the required relative standard deviation (percentage) determined on 6 injections for $B = 1.0$
B: (Upper limit given in the definition of the individual monograph − 100) %
N: Number of replicate injections of the reference solution ($3 \leq n \leq 6$);
$t_{90\%,\,n-1}$: Student's t at the 90% probability level (double sided) with $n - 1$ degrees of freedom.

2812   *General Tests, Processes and Apparatus*

Table 2.00-1 Maximum permitted relative standarddeviation (assay)

B (%)	Number of individual injections n			
	3	4	5	6
	Maximum permitted relative standard deviation (%)			
2.0	0.41	0.59	0.73	0.85
2.5	0.52	0.74	0.92	1.06
3.0	0.62	0.89	1.10	1.27

B: (Upper limit of content given in the individual monograph – 100) %.

System sensitivity

The signal-to-noise ratio is used to define the system sensitivity. The limit of quantitation (corresponding to a signal-to-noise ratio of 10) is equal to or less than the reporting threshold.

Peak symmetry

Unless otherwise stated, in a test or assay, the symmetry factor (tailing factor) of the peak used for quantitation is 0.8 to 1.8.

4. Adjustment of chromatographic conditions

The chromatographic conditions described have been validated during the elaboration of the monograph.

The extent to which the various parameters of a chromatographic test may be adjusted without fundamentally modifying the pharmacopoeial analytical procedures are listed below. Changes other than those indicated require revalidation of the procedure.

Multiple adjustments can have a cumulative effect on the performance of the system and are to be properly evaluated by the users. This is particularly important in cases where the separation pattern is described as a profile. In those cases, a risk assessment has to be carried out.

Any adjustments must be made on the basis of the pharmacopoeial procedure.

If adjustments are made to the procedure, additional verification tests may be required. To verify the suitability of the adjusted pharmacopoeial procedure, assess the relevant analytical performance characteristics potentially affected by the change.

When a pharmacopoeial analytical procedure has been adjusted according to the requirements stated below, no further adjustments are allowed without appropriate revalidation.

Compliance with the system suitability criteria is required to verify that conditions for satisfactory performance of the test or assay are achieved.

Adjustment of conditions with gradient elution (HPLC) or temperature programming (GC) is more critical than with isocratic (HPLC) or isothermal (GC) elution, since it may shift some peaks to a different step of the gradient or to different elution temperatures, potentially causing partial or complete coelution of adjacent peaks or peak inversion, and thus leading to the incorrect assignment of peaks, and to the masking of peaks or a shift such that elution occurs beyond the prescribed elution time.

◇In the tests of biotechnological/biological products such as peptide mapping, glycosylation analysis and tests related to molecular heterogeneity, the separation pattern obtained by liquid chromatography may be set for acceptance criteria as a profile. In such a test method, the method shown in this section may not be applicable.◇

◇Crude drugs and related drugs are outside the scope of this section.◇

4.1.   Liquid chromatography: isocratic elution
Column parameters and flow rate

• Stationary phase: No change of the identity of the substituent (e.g. no replacement of C18 by C8); the other physico-chemical characteristics of the stationary phase, i.e. chromatographic support, surface modification and extent of chemical modification must be similar; a change from Totally Porous Particle (TPP) columns to Superficially Porous Particle (SPP) columns is allowed provided the above-mentioned requirements are met.

• Column dimensions (particle size, length): The particle size and/or length of the column may be modified provided that the ratio of the column length (L) to the particle size (d_p) remains constant or in the range between -25% to $+50\%$ of the prescribed L/d_p ratio.

• Adjustment from totally porous to superficially porous particles: For the application of particle-size adjustment from totally porous to superficially porous particles, other combinations of L and d_p can be used provided that the plate number (N) is within -25% to $+50\%$, relative to the prescribed column. These changes are acceptable provided system suitability criteria are fulfilled, and selectivity and elution order of the specified impurities to be controlled are demonstrated to be equivalent.

• Internal diameter: In absence of a change in particle size and/or length, the internal diameter of the column may be adjusted.

Caution is necessary when the adjustment results in smaller peak volumes, due to a smaller particle size or a smaller internal diameter, a situation which may require adjustments to minimize extra-column band broadening by factors such as instrument connections, detector cell volume and sampling rate, and injection volume.

When the particle size is changed, the flow rate ◇may require◇ adjustment, because smaller-particle columns will require higher linear velocities for the same performance (as measured by reduced plate height). The flow rate ◇can be adjusted◇ for both the change in column diameter and particle size using the following equation:

$$F_2 = F_1 \times [(d_{c2}{}^2 \times d_{p1})/(d_{c1}{}^2 \times d_{p2})]$$

F_1: Flow rate (mL/minute) indicated in the monograph
F_2: Adjusted flow rate (mL/minute)
d_{c1}: Internal diameter (mm) of the column indicated in the monograph

---

The JP Drugs are to be tested according to the provisions given in the pertinent monographs, General Notices, General Rules for Crude Drugs, General Rules for Preparations, and General Tests for their conformity to the Japanese Pharmacopoeia. (See the General Notices 5.)

Supplement I, JP XVIII

d_{c2}: Internal diameter (mm) of the column used
d_{p1}: Particle size (μm) indicated in the monograph
d_{p2}: Particle size (μm) of the column used

When a change is made from $\geq 3\ \mu$m to $< 3\ \mu$m particles in isocratic separations, an additional increase in linear velocity (by adjusting the flow rate) may be justified, provided that the column performance does not drop by more than 20%. Similarly, when a change is made from $< 3\ \mu$m to $\geq 3\ \mu$m particles, an additional reduction of linear velocity (flow rate) may be justified to avoid reduction in column performance by more than 20%.

After an adjustment due to a change in column dimensions, an additional change in flow rate of $\pm 50\%$ is permitted.

Column temperature: $\pm 10°C$, where the operating temperature is specified, unless otherwise prescribed.

Further adjustments in analytical procedure conditions (mobile phase, temperature, pH, etc.) may be required, within the permitted ranges described under System Suitability and Adjustment of chromatographic conditions in this test method.

Mobile phase:
- Composition: The amount of the minor solvent components may be adjusted by $\pm 30\%$ relative. For a minor component at 10% of the mobile phase, a 30% relative adjustment allows a range of 7 – 13%. For a minor component at 5% of the mobile phase, a 30% relative adjustment allows a range of 3.5 – 6.5%. No component is altered by more than 10% absolute. A minor component comprises less than or equal to (100/n) %, n being the total number of components of the mobile phase.
- pH of the aqueous component of the mobile phase: ± 0.2 pH units, unless otherwise prescribed
- Concentration of salts in the buffer component of a mobile phase: $\pm 10\%$
- Flow rate: In absence of a change in column dimensions, an adjustment of the flow rate by $\pm 50\%$ is permitted.

Detector wavelength: No adjustment permitted.

Injection volume: When the column dimensions are changed, the following equation may be used for adjusting the injection volume.

$$V_{inj2} = V_{inj1}\ (L_2 d_{c2}^2)/(L_1 d_{c1}^2)$$

V_{inj1}: Injection volume (μL) indicated in the monograph
V_{inj2}: Adjusted injection volume (μL)
L_1: Column length (cm) indicated in the monograph
L_2: New column length (cm)
d_{c1}: Column internal diameter (mm) indicated in the monograph
d_{c2}: New column internal diameter (mm)

This equation may not be applicable to changes from TPP columns to SPP columns.

Even in the absence of any column dimension change, the injection volume may be varied provided System Suitability criteria remain within their established acceptability limits.

When the injection volume is decreased, special attention is given to (limit of) detection and repeatability of the peak response(s) to be determined. An increase is permitted provided, in particular, linearity and resolution of the peak(s) to be determined remain satisfactory.

4.2. Liquid chromatography: gradient elution

Adjustment of chromatographic conditions for gradient systems requires greater caution than for isocratic systems.

Column parameters and flow rate
- Stationary phase: No change of the identity of the substituent (e.g. no replacement of C18 by C8). The other physico-chemical characteristics of the stationary phase, i.e. chromatographic support; surface modification and extent of chemical modification must be similar. A change from Totally Porous Particle (TPP) columns to Superficially Porous Particle (SPP) columns is allowed provided the above-mentioned requirements are met.
- Column dimensions (particle size, length): The particle size and/or length of the column may be modified provided that the ratio of the column length (L) to the particle size (d_p) remains constant or in the range between -25% to $+50\%$ of the prescribed L/d_p ratio.

Adjustments from totally porous to superficially porous particles: For the application of particle-size adjustment from totally porous to superficially porous particles, other combinations of L and d_p can be used provided that the ratio $(t_R/w_h)^2$ is within -25% to $+50\%$, relative to the prescribed column, for each peak used to check the system suitability, as stated in this chapter and the individual monograph.

These changes are acceptable provided system suitability criteria are fulfilled, and selectivity and elution order of the specified impurities to be controlled are demonstrated to be equivalent.
- Internal diameter: In absence of a change in particle size and/or length, the internal diameter of the column may be adjusted.

Caution is necessary when the adjustment results in smaller peak volumes, due to a smaller particle size or a smaller internal diameter, a situation which may require adjustments to minimize extra-column band broadening by factors such as instrument connections, detector cell volume and sampling rate, and injection volume.

When the particle size is changed, the flow rate $^\diamond$may require$_\diamond$ adjustment, because smaller-particle columns will require higher linear velocities for the same performance (as measured by reduced plate height). The flow rate $^\diamond$can be adjusted$_\diamond$ for both the change in column diameter and particle size using the following equation:

$$F_2 = F_1 \times [(d_{c2}^2 \times d_{p1})/(d_{c1}^2 \times d_{p2})]$$

F_1: Flow rate (mL/minute) indicated in the monograph
F_2: Adjusted flow rate (mL/minute)
d_{c1}: Internal diameter (mm) of the column indicated in the monograph
d_{c2}: Internal diameter (mm) of the column used
d_{p1}: Particle size (μm) indicated in the monograph

The JP Drugs are to be tested according to the provisions given in the pertinent monographs, General Notices, General Rules for Crude Drugs, General Rules for Preparations, and General Tests for their conformity to the Japanese Pharmacopoeia. (See the General Notices 5.)

2814 General Tests, Processes and Apparatus

d_{p2}: Particle size (μm) of the column used

A change in column dimensions, and thus in column volume, impacts the gradient volume which controls selectivity. Gradients are adjusted to the column volume by changing the gradient volume in proportion to the column volume. This applies to every gradient segment volume. Since the gradient volume is the gradient time, t_G, multiplied by the flow rate, F, the gradient time for each gradient segment needs to be adjusted to maintain a constant ratio of the gradient volume to the column volume (expressed as $L \times d_c^2$). Thus, the new gradient time, t_{G2} can be calculated from the original gradient time, t_{G1}, the flow rate(s), and the column dimensions as follows.

$$t_{G2} = t_{G1} \times (F_1/F_2) [(L_2 \times d_{c2}^2)/(L_1 \times d_{c1}^2)]$$

Thus, the change in conditions for gradient elution requires three steps:
(1) adjust the column length and particle size according to L/d_p,
(2) adjust the flow rate for changes in particle size and column diameter, and
(3) adjust the gradient time of each segment for changes in column length, diameter and flow rate. The example below illustrates this process.

Variable	Original Conditions	Adjusted Conditions	Comment
Column length (L) (mm)	150	100	User's choice
Column diameter (d_c) (mm)	4.6	2.1	User's choice
Particle size (d_p) (μm)	5	3	User's choice
L/d_p	30.0	33.3	(1)
Flow rate (mL/min)	2.0	0.7	(2)
Gradient adjustment factor (t_{G2}/t_{G1})		0.4	(3)
Gradient conditions			
B (%)	Time (min)	Time (min)	
30	0	0	
30	3	$(3 \times 0.4) = 1.2$	
70	13	$[1.2 + (10 \times 0.4)] = 5.2$	
30	16	$[5.2 + (3 \times 0.4)] = 6.4$	

(1) 11% increase within allowed L/d_p change of -25% to $+50\%$

(2) calculated using $F_2 = F_1 [(d_{c2}^2 \times d_{p1})/(d_{c1}^2 \times d_{p2})]$
(3) calculated using $t_{G2} = t_{G1} \times (F_1/F_2) [(L_2 \times d_{c2}^2)/(L_1 \times d_{c1}^2)]$

- Column temperature: $\pm 5°C$, where the operating temperature is specified, unless otherwise prescribed.

Further adjustments in analytical procedure conditions (mobile phase, temperature, pH, etc.) may be required, within the permitted ranges described under System Suitability and Adjustment of Chromatographic Conditions in this chapter.

Mobile phase
- Composition/gradient: Adjustments of the composition of the mobile phase and the gradient are acceptable provided that.
    (i) The system suitability criteria are fulfilled.
    (ii) The principal peak(s) elute(s) within $\pm 15\%$ of the retention time(s) obtained with the original conditions. This requirement does not apply when the column dimensions are changed.
    (iii) The composition of the mobile phase and the gradient are such that the first peaks are sufficiently retained and the last peaks are eluted.
- pH of the aqueous component of the mobile phase: ± 0.2 pH units, unless otherwise prescribed.
- Concentration of salts in the buffer component of a mobile phase: $\pm 10\%$

Where compliance with the system suitability criteria cannot be achieved, it is preferable to consider the dwell volume or to change the column.

Dwell volume The configuration of the equipment employed may significantly alter the resolution, retention time and relative retentions described. Should this occur, it may be due to a change in dwell volume. Monographs preferably include an isocratic step before the start of the gradient program so that an adaptation can be made to the gradient time points to take account of differences in dwell volume between the system used for analytical procedure development and that actually used. It is the user's responsibility to adapt the length of the isocratic step to the analytical equipment used. If the dwell volume used during the elaboration of the monograph is given in the monograph, the time points (t min) stated in the gradient table may be replaced by adapted time points (t_c min), calculated using the following equation.

$$t_c = t - (D - D_0)/F$$

D: Dwell volume (mL)
D_0: Dwell volume (mL) used for development of the analytical procedure
F: Flow rate (mL/min)

The isocratic step introduced for this purpose may be omitted if validation data for application of the analytical procedure without this step is available.

Detector wavelength: No adjustment permitted.

The JP Drugs are to be tested according to the provisions given in the pertinent monographs, General Notices, General Rules for Crude Drugs, General Rules for Preparations, and General Tests for their conformity to the Japanese Pharmacopoeia. (See the General Notices 5.)

Supplement I, JP XVIII   *General Tests, Processes and Apparatus* 2815

Injection volume: When the column dimensions are changed, the following equation may be used for adjusting the injection volume.

$$V_{inj2} = V_{inj1} (L_2 d_{c2}^2)/(L_1 d_{c1}^2)$$

V_{inj1}: Injection volume (μL) indicated in the monograph
V_{inj2}: Adjusted injection volume (μL)
L_1: Column length (cm) indicated in the monograph
L_2: New column length (cm)
d_{c1}: Column internal diameter (mm) indicated in the monograph
d_{c2}: New column internal diameter (mm)

This equation may not be applicable to changes from TPP columns to SPP columns.

Even in the absence of any column dimension change, the injection volume may be varied provided system suitability criteria remain within their established acceptability limits. When the injection volume is decreased, special attention is given to (limit of) detection and repeatability of the peak response(s) to be determined. An increase is permitted provided, in particular, linearity and resolution of the peak(s) to be determined remain satisfactory.

4.3. Gas chromatography
Column parameters
Stationary phase:
  Particle size: Maximum reduction of 50%. No increase permitted (packed columns).
  Film thickness: -50% to $+100\%$ (capillary columns)
Column dimensions:
  Length: -70% to $+100\%$;
  Internal diameter: $\pm 50\%$;
Column temperature: $\pm 10\%$;
Temperature program: Adjustment of temperatures is permitted as stated above. Adjustment of ramp rates and hold times of up to $\pm 20\%$ is permitted.

Flow rate: $\pm 50\%$.

The above changes are acceptable provided system suitability criteria are fulfilled, and selectivity and elution order of the specified impurities to be controlled are demonstrated to be equivalent.

Injection volume and split ratio: may be varied provided system suitability criteria remain within their established acceptability limits. When the injection volume is decreased, or the split ratio is increased, special attention is given to (limit of) detection and repeatability of the peak response(s) to be determined. An increase in injection volume or a decrease in split ratio is permitted provided, in particular, linearity and resolution of the peak(s) to be determined remain satisfactory.

Injection port temperature and transfer-line temperature in static head-space conditions: $\pm 10°C$, provided no decomposition or condensation occurs.

5. Quantitation
The following quantitation approaches may be used in general tests or monographs.

5.1. External standard method
Using a calibration function
Standard solutions with several graded amounts of a reference standard of the compound to be analyzed are prepared in a range that has been demonstrated to give a linear response, and a fixed volume of these standard solutions is injected. With the chromatograms obtained, a calibration function is prepared by plotting the peak areas or peak heights on the ordinate against the amount of reference standard on the abscissa. The calibration function is generally obtained by linear regression. Then, a sample solution is prepared according to the procedure specified in the individual monograph. The chromatography is performed under the same operating conditions as for the preparation of the calibration function, the peak area or peak height of the compound to be analyzed is measured, and the amount of the compound is read out or calculated from the calibration function.

Using one-point calibration
In an individual monograph, generally one of the standard solutions with a concentration within the linear range of the calibration function and a sample solution with a concentration close to that of the standard solution are prepared, and the chromatography is performed under fixed conditions to obtain the amount of the component by comparing the responses obtained. In this method, all procedures, such as the injection, must be carried out under constant conditions.

5.2. Internal standard method
Using a calibration function
In the internal standard method, a stable compound is chosen as an internal standard which shows a retention time close to that of the compound to be analyzed, and whose peak is well separated from all other peaks in the chromatogram.

Several standard solutions containing a fixed amount of the internal standard and graded amounts of a reference standard of the compound to be analyzed are prepared. Based on the chromatograms obtained by injection of a fixed volume of individual standard solutions, the ratio of peak area or peak height of the reference standard to that of the internal standard is calculated. A calibration function by plotting these ratios on the ordinate against the amount of the reference standard or the ratio of the amount of reference standard to that of the internal standard on the abscissa is prepared. The calibration function is generally obtained by linear regression.

Then, a sample solution containing the internal standard in the same amount as in the standard solutions used for the preparation of the calibration function is prepared according to the procedure specified in the individual monograph. The chromatography is performed under the same operating conditions as for the preparation of the calibration function. The ratio of the peak area or peak height of the compound to be analyzed to that of the internal standard is calculated, and the amount of the compound is read out or calculated from the calibration function.

The JP Drugs are to be tested according to the provisions given in the pertinent monographs, General Notices, General Rules for Crude Drugs, General Rules for Preparations, and General Tests for their conformity to the Japanese Pharmacopoeia. (See the General Notices 5.)

Using one point calibration

In an individual monograph, generally one of the standard solutions with a concentration within the linear range of the calibration function and a sample solution with a concentration close to that of the standard solution, both containing a fixed amount of the internal standard, are prepared, and the chromatography is performed under fixed conditions to determine the amount of the compound to be analyzed by comparing the ratios obtained.

5.3 Normalisation procedure

Provided linearity of the peaks has been demonstrated, individual monographs may prescribe that the percentage content of a component of the substance to be examined is calculated by determining the area of the corresponding peak as a percentage of the total area of all the peaks, excluding those due to solvents or reagents or arising from the mobile phase or the sample matrix, and those at or below the disregard limit or reporting threshold.

6. Other considerations

6.1. Detector response

The detector sensitivity is the signal output per unit concentration or unit mass of a substance in the mobile phase entering the detector. The relative detector response factor, commonly referred to as response factor, expresses the sensitivity of a detector for a given substance relative to a standard substance. The correction factor is the reciprocal of the response factor. In tests for related substances any correction factors indicated in the monograph are applied (i.e. when the response factor is outside the range 0.8-1.2).

6.2. Interfering peaks

Peaks due to solvents and reagents or arising from the mobile phase or the sample matrix are disregarded.

6.3. Measurement of peaks

Integration of the peak area of any impurity that is not completely separated from the principal peak is preferably performed by tangential skim (Fig. 2.00-9).

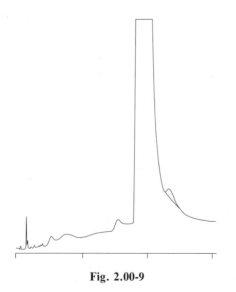

Fig. 2.00-9

6.4. Reporting threshold

When the related substances test prescribes a limit for the total of impurities or a quantitative determination of an impurity, it is important to choose an appropriate reporting threshold and appropriate conditions for the integration of the peak areas. In such tests the reporting threshold, i.e. the limit above which a peak is reported, is generally 0.05%.

Change the following as follows:

2.01 Liquid Chromatography

Liquid Chromatography is a method to develop a mixture injected into a column prepared with a suitable stationary phase by passing a liquid as a mobile phase through the column, in order to separate the mixture into its components by making use of the difference of retention capacity against the stationary phase, and to determine the components. This method can be applied to a liquid or soluble sample, and is used for identification, purity test, and quantitative determination.

1. Apparatus

Basically, the apparatus required for the liquid chromatographic procedure consists of a pumping system for the mobile phase, a sample injection port, a column, a detector and a recorder. A mobile phase component regulator, a thermostat for the column, a pumping system for reaction reagents and a chemical reaction chamber are also used, if necessary. The pumping system serves to deliver the mobile phase and the reagents into the column and connecting tube at a constant flow rate. The sample injection port is used to deliver a quantity of the sample to the apparatus with high reproducibility. The column is a tube with a smooth interior, made of inert metal, etc., in which a packing material for liquid chromatography is uniformly packed. A column with a stationary phase chemically bound on the inside wall instead of the column packed with the packing material may be used. The detector is used to detect a property of the samples which is different from that of the mobile phase, and may be an ultraviolet or visible spectrophotometer, fluorometric detector, differential refractometer, electrochemical detector, chemiluminescence detector, electric conductivity detector, mass spectrophotometer, etc. The output signal is usually proportional to the concentration of samples at amounts of less than a few μg. The recorder is used to record the output signals of the detector. As required, a data processor may be used as the recorder to record or output the chromatogram, retention times or amounts of the components. The mobile phase component regulator is used to vary the ratio of the mobile phase components in a stepwise or gradient fashion.

2. Procedure

Fix the detector, column and mobile phase to the apparatus, and adjust the flow rate and the column temperature to the values described in the operating conditions specified in the individual monograph. Inject a volume of the sample solution or the standard solution specified in the individual monograph with the sample injector into the column

Supplement I, JP XVIII   *General Tests, Processes and Apparatus*   2817

through the sample injection port. The separated components are detected by the detector, and recorded by the recorder as a chromatogram. If the components to be analyzed have no readily detectable physical properties such as absorbance or fluorescence, the detection is achieved by changing the components to suitable derivatives. Usually, the derivatization is performed as a pre- or post-column labeling.

3. Identification and purity test

When Liquid Chromatography is used for identification of a component of a sample, it is performed by confirming identity of the retention time of the component and that of an authentic specimen, or by confirming that the peak shape of the component is unchanged after mixing the sample with an authentic specimen. If a detector which is able to obtain chemical structural information of the component at the same time is used, highly specific identification can be achieved by confirming identity of the chemical structure of the component and that of an authentic specimen, in addition to the identity of their retention times.

When Liquid Chromatography is used for purity test, it is generally performed by comparing the peak area of target impurity from the sample solution with that of the main component from a standard solution, which is prepared by diluting the sample solution to a concentration corresponding to the specified limit of the impurity, or by calculating target impurity content using the peak area percentage method. Unless otherwise specified, if a sample is separated into isomers in the chromatogram, the isomer ratio is calculated by using the peak area percentage method.

The peak area percentage method is a method to calculate the proportion of the components from the ratio of the peak area of each component to the sum of the peak areas of every peak recorded in the chromatogram. In order to obtain accurate results in evaluating the proportion of the components, it is necessary to correct the area of each component based on its correction factor to the principal component.

4. Assay
4.1. Internal standard method

In the internal standard method, choose a stable compound as an internal standard which shows a retention time close to that of the compound to be assayed, and whose peak is well separated from all other peaks in the chromatogram. Prepare several kinds of standard solutions containing a fixed amount of the internal standard and several graded amounts of the authentic specimen specified in the individual monograph. Based on the chromatogram obtained by injection of a fixed volume of individual standard solutions, calculate the ratio of peak area or peak height of the authentic specimen to that of the internal standard, and prepare a calibration curve by plotting these ratios on the ordinate against the amount of the authentic specimen or the ratio of the amount of the authentic specimen to that of the internal standard on the abscissa. The calibration curve is usually obtained as a straight line passing through the origin. Then, prepare a sample solution containing the internal

standard in the same amount as in the standard solutions used for the preparation of the calibration curve according to the method specified in the individual monograph, perform the liquid chromatography under the same operating conditions as for the preparation of the calibration curve, calculate the ratio of the peak area or peak height of the objective compound to that of the internal standard, and read the amount of the compound from the calibration curve.

In an individual monograph, generally one of the standard solutions with a concentration within the linear range of the calibration curve and a sample solution with a concentration close to that of the standard solution are prepared, and the chromatography is performed with these solutions under fixed conditions to determine the amount of the objective compound.

4.2. Absolute calibration curve method

Prepare standard solutions with several graded amounts of the authentic specimen, and inject accurately a fixed volume of these standard solutions. With the chromatogram obtained, prepare a calibration curve by plotting the peak areas or peak heights on the ordinate against the amount of the authentic specimen on the abscissa. The calibration curve is generally obtained as a straight line passing through the origin. Then, prepare a sample solution according to the method specified in the individual monograph, perform the liquid chromatography under the same conditions as for the preparation of the calibration curve, measure the peak area or peak height of the objective compound, and read the amount of the compound from the calibration curve.

In an individual monograph, generally one of the standard solutions with a concentration within the linear range of the calibration curve and a sample solution with a concentration close to that of the standard solution are prepared, and the chromatography is performed with these solutions under a fixed condition to obtain the amount of the component. In this method, all procedures, such as the injection procedure, must be carried out under a strictly constant condition.

5. Method for peak measuring

Generally, the following methods are used.

5.1. Peak height measuring method

(i) Peak height method: Measure the distance between the maximum of the peak and the intersecting point of a perpendicular line from the maximum of the peak to the horizontal axis of recording paper with a tangent linking the baselines on both sides of the peak.

(ii) Automatic peak height method: Measure the signals from the detector as the peak height using a data processing system.

5.2. Peak area measuring method

(iii) Width at half-height method: Multiply the peak width at the half-height by the peak height.

(iv) Automatic integration method: Measure the signals from the detector as the peak area using a data processing system.

The JP Drugs are to be tested according to the provisions given in the pertinent monographs, General Notices, General Rules for Crude Drugs, General Rules for Preparations, and General Tests for their conformity to the Japanese Pharmacopoeia. (See the General Notices 5.)

2818   *General Tests, Processes and Apparatus*   *Supplement I, JP XVIII*

6. System suitability

System suitability testing is an integral part of test methods using chromatography, and is used to ensure that the performance of the chromatographic systems used is as suitable for the analysis of the drug as was at the time when the verification of the test method was performed using the system. System suitability testing should be carried out at every series of drug analysis. The test procedures and acceptance criteria of system suitability testing must be prescribed in the test method of drugs. The results of drug analyses are not acceptable unless the requirements of system suitability have been met.

In system suitability testing of the chromatographic systems, the evaluation of "System performance" and "System repeatability" is usually required. For quantitative purity tests, the evaluation of "Test for required detectability" may also be required. If appropriate, system suitability can also be evaluated by the parameters of system suitability prescribed in Chromatography <2.00>. However, Liquid Chromatography <2.01> and Chromatography <2.00> cannot be applied in combination.

6.1. Test for required detectability

For purity tests, when it is confirmed that the target impurity is distinctly detected at the concentration of its specification limit, it is considered verified that the system used has adequate performance to achieve its intended use.

For quantitative purity tests, "Test for required detectability" is usually required, and in order to confirm, in some degree, the linearity of response near its specification limit, the range of expected response to the injection of a certain volume of target impurity solution at the concentration of its specification limit should be prescribed. For limit test, "Test for required detectability" is not required, if the test is performed by comparing the response from sample solution with that from standard solution at the concentration of its specification limit. "Test for required detectability" is also not required, if it is confirmed that the impurity can be detected at its specification limit by the evaluation of "System repeatability" or some other procedure.

6.2. System performance

When it is confirmed that the specificity for determining the test ingredient is ensured, it is considered verified that the system used has adequate performance to achieve its intended use.

In assay, "System performance" should be defined by the resolution between the test ingredient and a target substance to be separated (a closely eluting compound is preferable), and when appropriate, by their order of elution. In purity tests, both the resolution and the order of elution between the test ingredient and a target substance to be separated (a closely eluting compound is preferable) should be prescribed. In addition, if necessary, the symmetry factor of the test ingredient should be prescribed together with them. However, if there is no suitable target substance to be separated, it is acceptable to define "System performance" using the number of theoretical plates and the symmetry factor of the test ingredient.

6.3. System repeatability

When it is confirmed that the degree of variation (precision) of the response of the test ingredient is at a level that meets the requirement of "System repeatability", it is considered verified that the system used has adequate performance to achieve its intended use.

The allowable limit of "System repeatability" is normally defined as the relative standard deviation (*RSD*) of the response of the test ingredient in replicate injections of standard solution. It is acceptable to confirm the repeatability of the system not only by replicate injections of standard solution before sample injections, but also by divided injections of standard solution before and after sample injections, or by interspersed injections of standard solution among sample injections.

In principle, total number of replicate injections should be 6. However, in the case that a long time is necessary for one analysis, such as the analysis using the gradient method, or the analysis of samples containing late eluting components, it may be acceptable to decrease the number of replicate injections by adopting new allowable limit of "System repeatability" which can guarantee a level of "System repeatability" equivalent to that at 6 replicate injections.

The allowable limit of "System repeatability" should be set at an appropriate level based on the data when suitability of the method for the evaluation of quality of the drug was verified, and the precision necessary for the quality test.

7. Point to consider on changing the operating conditions

Among the operating conditions specified in the individual monograph, inside diameter and length of the column, particle size of the packing material (pore size in the case of monolithic columns), column temperature, composition ratio of the mobile phase, composition of buffer solutions in the mobile phase, pH of the mobile phase, concentration of ion-pair forming agents in the mobile phase, ionic strength of the mobile phase, gradient program, flow rate of the mobile phase, number and timing of mobile phase composition changes in gradient program, flow rate of mobile phase in gradient program, composition and flow rate of derivatizing reagents, and reaction time and chamber temperature in chemical reaction may be partially modified after the analytical performance is appropriately verified. However, for crude drugs etc., conformance to the specifications of the system suitability may be substituted for the verification of analytical performance.

8. Terminology
The terminology used conforms to the definition in Chromatography <2.00>.

9. Note

Avoid the use of authentic specimens, internal standards, reagents or solvents containing substances that may interfere with the determination.

The JP Drugs are to be tested according to the provisions given in the pertinent monographs, General Notices, General Rules for Crude Drugs, General Rules for Preparations, and General Tests for their conformity to the Japanese Pharmacopoeia. (See the General Notices 5.)

Supplement I, JP XVIII　　　　　　　　　　　　　　*General Tests, Processes and Apparatus*　　2819

Change the following as follows:

2.02　Gas Chromatography

Gas Chromatography is a method to develop a mixture injected into a column prepared with a suitable stationary phase by passing a gas (carrier gas) as a mobile phase through the column, in order to separate the mixture into its components by making use of the difference of retention capacity against the stationary phase, and to determine the components. This method can be applied to a gaseous or vaporizable sample, and is used for identification, purity test, and quantitative determination.

1.　Apparatus

Basically, the apparatus required for the gas chromatographic procedure consists of a carrier gas-introducing port and flow regulator, a sample injection port, a column, a column oven, a detector and a recorder. A gas-introducing port and flow regulator for a combustion gas, a burning supporting gas and an accessory gas and sample injection port for headspace are also used, if necessary. The carrier gas-introducing port and flow regulator serves to deliver the carrier gas into the column at a constant flow rate, and usually consist of a pressure regulation valve, a flow rate regulation valve and a pressure gauge. The sample injection port is used to deliver a quantity of the sample to the flow line of carrier gas with high reproducibility. There are sample injection ports for packed column and for capillary column. There are both divided injection mode and non-divided injection mode to sample injection port for capillary column. The columns are usually classified as packed column or capillary column. The packed column is a tube made of inert metal, glass or synthetic resin, in which a packing material for gas chromatography is uniformly packed. The packed column with not more than 1 mm in inside diameter is also called a packed capillary column (micro packed column). A capillary column is a tube made of inert metal, glass, quartz or synthetic resin, whose inside wall is bound chemically with stationary phase for gas chromatography. The column oven has the setting capacity for a column with required length and the temperature regulation system for keeping the constant column temperature. The detector is used to detect a component separated on the column, and may be an alkaline thermal ionization detector, a flame photometry detector, mass spectrophotometer, hydrogen flame-ionization detector, an electron capture detector, a thermal conductivity detector, etc. The recorder is used to record the output signals of the detector.

2.　Procedure

Unless otherwise specified, proceed by the following method. Fix the detector, column and carrier gas to the apparatus, and adjust the flow rate and the column temperature to the values described in the operating conditions specified in the individual monograph. Inject a volume of the sample solution or the standard solution specified in the individual monograph with the sample injector into the column system through the sample injection port. The separated components are detected by the detector, and recorded by the recorder as a chromatogram.

3.　Identification and purity test

Identification of a component of a sample is performed by confirming identity of the retention time of the component and that of an authentic specimen, or by confirming that the peak shape of the component is unchanged after mixing the sample with an authentic specimen.

In general, the purity of the sample is determined by comparing the peak area of target impurity from the sample solution with that of the main component from a standard solution, which is prepared by diluting the sample solution to a concentration corresponding to the specified limit of the impurity, or by calculating target impurity content using the peak area percentage method. Unless otherwise specified, if a sample is separated into isomers in the chromatogram, the isomer ratio is calculated by using the peak area percentage method.

The peak area percentage method is a method to calculate the proportion of the components from the ratio of the peak area of each component to the sum of the peak areas of every peak recorded in the chromatogram. In order to obtain accurate results in evaluating the proportion of the components, it is necessary to correct the area of each component based on its response factor to the principal component.

4.　Assay

In general, perform the assay by using the internal standard method. The absolute calibration curve method is used when a suitable internal standard is not available. Perform the assay by using the standard addition method when the effect of the component other than the compound to be assayed on the quantitative determination is not negligible against a result of the determination.

4.1　Internal standard method

In the internal standard method, choose a stable compound as an internal standard which shows a retention time close to that of the compound to be assayed, and whose peak is well separated from all other peaks in the chromatogram. Prepare several kinds of standard solutions containing a fixed amount of the internal standard and several graded amounts of the authentic specimen specified in the individual monograph. Based on the chromatogram obtained by injection of a fixed volume of individual standard solutions, calculate the ratio of peak area or peak height of the authentic specimen to that of the internal standard, and prepare a calibration curve by plotting these ratios on the ordinate against the amount of the authentic specimen or the ratio of the amount of the authentic specimen to that of the internal standard on the abscissa. The calibration curve is usually obtained as a straight line passing through the origin. Then, prepare a sample solution containing the internal standard in the same amount as in the standard solutions used for the preparation of the calibration curve according to the method specified in the individual monograph, perform the gas chromatography under the same operating conditions as for the preparation of the calibration curve,

---

The JP Drugs are to be tested according to the provisions given in the pertinent monographs, General Notices, General Rules for Crude Drugs, General Rules for Preparations, and General Tests for their conformity to the Japanese Pharmacopoeia. (See the General Notices 5.)

2820　General Tests, Processes and Apparatus　　　　　　　　　　　　　　　　　　Supplement I, JP XVIII

calculate the ratio of the peak area or peak height of the objective compound to that of the internal standard, and read the amount of the compound from the calibration curve.

In an individual monograph, generally one of the standard solutions with a concentration within the linear range of the calibration curve and a sample solution with a concentration close to that of the standard solution are prepared, and the chromatography is performed with these solutions under fixed conditions to determine the amount of the objective compound.

4.2　Absolute calibration curve method

Prepare standard solutions with several graded amounts of the authentic specimen, and inject accurately a fixed volume of these standard solutions. With the chromatogram obtained, prepare a calibration curve by plotting the peak areas or peak heights on the ordinate against the amount of the authentic specimen on the abscissa. The calibration curve is generally obtained as a straight line passing through the origin. Then, prepare a sample solution according to the method specified in the individual monograph, perform the gas chromatography under the same conditions as for the preparation of the calibration curve, measure the peak area or peak height of the objective compound, and read the amount of the compound from the calibration curve.

In an individual monograph, generally one of the standard solutions with a concentration within the linear range of the calibration curve and a sample solution with a concentration close to that of the standard solution are prepared, and the chromatography is performed with these solutions under a fixed condition to obtain the amount of the component. In this method, all procedures, such as the injection procedure, must be carried out under a strictly constant condition.

4.3　Standard addition method

Pipet a fixed volume of more than 4 sample solutions, add exactly the standard solution so that stepwise increasing amounts of the object compound are contained in the solutions except 1 sample solution, diluted exactly each solution with and without standard solution to a definite volume, and use each solution as the sample solution. Based on the chromatogram obtained by exact injection of a fixed volume of individual sample solutions, measure the peak area or peak height of individual sample solutions. Calculate the concentration of standard objective compound added into each sample solution, plot the amounts (concentration) of added standard object compound on the abscissa and the peak area or peak height on the ordinate on the graph, extend the calibration curve obtained by linking the plots, and determine the amount of object compound to be assayed from the distance between the origin and the intersecting point of the calibration curve with the abscissa. This method is available only in the case that the calibration curve is a straight line, and passes through the origin when the absolute calibration curve method is employed. In this method, all procedures must be carried out under a strictly constant condition.

5.　Method for peak measuring

Generally, the following methods are used.

5.1　Peak height measuring method

(i)　Peak height method: Measure the distance between the maximum of the peak and the intersecting point of a perpendicular line from the maximum of the peak to the horizontal axis of recording paper with a tangent linking the baselines on either side of the peak.

(ii)　Automatic peak height method: Measure the signals from the detector as the peak height using a data processing system.

5.2　Peak area measuring method

(i)　Width at half-height method: Multiply the peak width at the half-height by the peak height.

(ii)　Automatic integration method: Measure the signals from the detector as the peak area using a data processing system.

6.　System suitability

Refer to "System suitability" described under Liquid Chromatography ⟨2.01⟩.

7.　Point to consider in changing the operating conditions

Among the operating conditions specified in the individual monograph, inside diameter and length of column, particle size of packing material, concentration or thickness of stationary phase, column temperature, temperature-rising rate, kind and flow rate of carrier gas, and split ratio may be partially modified after the analytical performance is appropriately verified. However, for crude drugs etc., conformance to the specification of the system suitability may be substituted for the verification of analytical performance. Headspace sample injection device and its operating conditions may be also modified, provided that they give equivalent or more accuracy and precision.

8.　Terminology

The terminology used conforms to the definition in Chromatography ⟨2.00⟩.

9.　Note

Avoid the use of authentic specimens, internal standards, reagents or solvents containing substances that may interfere with the determination.

Change the following as follows:

2.22　Fluorometry

Fluorometry is a method to measure the intensity of fluorescence emitted from a solution of fluorescent substance irradiated with an exciting light in a certain wavelength range. This method is also applied to the phosphorescent substances.

Fluorescence intensity F in a dilute solution is proportional to the concentration c in mol per liter of the solution and the path length l of light through the solution in centimeter.

The JP Drugs are to be tested according to the provisions given in the pertinent monographs, General Notices, General Rules for Crude Drugs, General Rules for Preparations, and General Tests for their conformity to the Japanese Pharmacopoeia. (See the General Notices 5.)

Supplement I, JP XVIII *General Tests, Processes and Apparatus* 2821

$$F = kI_0\phi\varepsilon cl$$

k: Constant
I_0: Intensity of exciting light
ϕ: Quantum yield of fluorescence or phosphorescence

Quantum yield of fluorescence or phosphorescence
= number of quanta as fluorescence or phosphorescence/number of quanta absorbed

ε: Molar extinction coefficient of the substance at the excitation wavelength

1. Apparatus

Spectrofluorometer is usually used. Generally, a xenon-lamp, laser, an alkaline halide lamp, etc. which provide stable exciting light are used as the light source. Usually, a nonfluorescent quartz cell (1 cm × 1 cm) with four transparent sides is used as the container for sample solution.

2. Procedure

Excitation spectrum is obtained by measuring fluorescence intensities of sample solution with varying excitation wavelengths at a fixed emission wavelength and drawing a curve showing the relationship between the excitation wavelength and the fluorescence intensity. Fluorescence spectrum is obtained by measuring fluorescence intensities of sample solution with varying emission wavelengths at a fixed excitation wavelength and drawing the same curve as described for the excitation spectrum. If necessary, the spectra are corrected with regard to the optical characteristics of the apparatus.

The fluorescence intensity is usually measured at the excitation and the emission wavelengths in the vicinity of excitation and emission maxima of the fluorescent substance. The fluorescence intensity is expressed as a value relative to that of a standard solution, because it is readily affected even by a slight change in the condition for the measurement.

Unless otherwise specified, the instrument is operated as follows with standard, sample, and reference solutions prepared as directed in the monograph: Fix the excitation and fluorescence wavelength scales at the designated positions, adjust the dark current to zero, put the quartz cell containing the standard solution in the light path, and adjust the instrument so that the standard solution shows the fluorescence intensity of 60% to 80% of full scale. Then perform the measurements with the cells containing the sample solution and the control solution, and read the fluorescence intensity as % under the same condition. Set the width of the wavelength properly unless otherwise specified.

3. Note

The fluorescence intensity is readily affected by the concentration, temperature and pH of the solution, and nature and purity of solvents or reagents used.

Add the following:

2.27 Near Infrared Spectrometry

Near infrared spectrometry is one of spectroscopic methods used to qualitatively and quantitatively evaluate samples from the analysis of data obtained by determining their absorption spectrum of light in the near-infrared range.

The near-infrared range lies between the visible light and infrared light, typically of wavelengths (or wave numbers) between 750 and 2500 nm (13,333 to 4000 cm^{-1}). The absorption of near-infrared light occurs due to harmonic overtones from normal vibration or combination tones in the infrared range from 2500 to 25000 nm (4000 to 400 cm^{-1}), primarily absorption of O-H, N-H, C-H and S-H that involve hydrogen atoms, in particular.

Absorption in the near-infrared range is far weaker than absorption due to normal vibration that occurs in the infrared range. Furthermore, in comparison with visible light, near-infrared light has longer wavelength, which makes it possible for the light to penetrate to a depth of several mm into solid samples including fine particles. This method is often utilized as a nondestructive analysis, as changes occurring with an absorbed light spectrum (transmitted light or reflected light) in this process provide physical and chemical information pertaining to samples.

Near-infrared spectrometry is used as a rapid and nondestructive method of analysis that replaces conventional and established analysis methods. It is necessary to perform a comparison test to evaluate this method against an existing analysis method, to verify that this method is equivalent to such existing analysis method, before using this analysis method as an evaluation test method for quality control.

Applications of this method include qualitative or quantitative evaluation of active ingredients, additives or water contents of drug substances or preparations. Furthermore, near-infrared spectrometry can also be used for the evaluation of physical conditions of substances, such as crystal forms, crystallinity, particle diameters. It is also possible to perform spectrometry on samples that are located in a remote location away from equipment main units, without sampling, by using optical fibers. It can therefore be used as an effective means to perform pharmaceutical manufacturing process control online (or in-line).

1. Equipment

Near-infrared spectrophotometers mainly include a distributed near-infrared spectrophotometer and a Fourier transform near-infrared spectrophotometer.

1.1. Distributed near-infrared spectrophotometer

This equipment is comprised of a light source section, sample section, spectrometry section, photometry section, signal processing section, data processing section, and display-record output section. Halogen lamps, tungsten lamps, light emitting diodes and other such devices that can emit high intensity near-infrared light in a stable manner are used in the light source section. The sample section is comprised

---

The JP Drugs are to be tested according to the provisions given in the pertinent monographs, General Notices, General Rules for Crude Drugs, General Rules for Preparations, and General Tests for their conformity to the Japanese Pharmacopoeia. (See the General Notices 5.)

2822 General Tests, Processes and Apparatus

of a sample cell and a sample holder. Equipment with an optical fiber section that is comprised of optical fibers and a collimator is equipped with a function for transmitting light to the sample section, which is remotely located away from the spectrophotometer main unit. Quartz is ordinarily used as material for optical fibers.

The spectrometry section is intended to extract light of required wavelength, using dispersive devices and is comprised of slits, mirrors and dispersive devices. The photometry section is comprised of detectors and amplifiers. Sensors include semiconductor detectors, as well as photomultiplier tubes. Detecting methods that use semiconductor detectors generally perform detections with single elements, but there are also occasions where array type detectors that use multiple elements are used. Such detectors are capable of simultaneously detecting multiple wavelengths (or wave numbers). The signal processing section separates signals required for measurements from output signals fed by amplifiers and then outputs such isolated signals. The signal processing methods include analog processing and digital processing.

1.2. Fourier transform near-infrared spectrophotometer

The configuration of the equipment is fundamentally the same as that of the distributed-type equipment described in Section 1.1., except for the spectrophotometry section and the signal processing section.

The spectrophotometry section is comprised of interferometers, sampling signal generators, detectors, amplifiers, A/D conversion devices, etc. The signal processing section is equipped with functions that are required for the spectrometer, as well as a function for translating an acquired interference waveform (interferogram) into an absorption spectrum by Fourier transformation.

2. Measurement method

There are three types of measurement methods that are used with near-infrared spectrometry: transmittance method, diffuse reflectance method and transmittance reflectance method. The selection of measurement methods relies on the shape of samples and applications. For example, the transmittance method or diffuse reflectance method is used for solid samples, including fine particles, and the transmittance method or transmittance reflectance method is used for liquid samples. The measurement mode, etc. of equipment are selected and set.

2.1. Transmittance method

The degree of decay for incident light intensity as the light from a light source passes through a sample, is represented as transmittance rate T (%) or absorbance A with the transmittance method.

This method is applied for taking measurements of samples that are liquids and solutions. Quartz glass cells and flow cells are used, with the layer length of 1 – 5 mm along. Furthermore, this method can also be applied for taking measurements of samples that are solids including fine particles. It is also known as the diffuse transmittance method. Selecting appropriate layer length is critical for this method, since the transmitted light intensity varies depending on

grain sizes and surface condition of samples.

2.2. Diffuse reflectance method

The ratio of reflection light intensity I emitted from a sample in a wide reflectance range and control reflection light intensity I_r emitted from the surface of a control substance is expressed as reflectance R (%) with the diffuse reflectance method. The near-infrared light penetrates to a depth of several mm into solid samples including fine particles. In that process, transmission, refraction, reflection and dispersion are repeated, and diffusion takes place, but a portion of the diffused light is emitted again from the surface of the sample and captured by a detector. The spectrum for the diffuse reflectance absorbance (A_r) can ordinarily be obtained by plotting logarithm of inverse numbers for reflectance against wavelengths (or wave numbers).

This method is applied to solid samples including fine particles, and requires a diffuse reflector such as a probe.

2.3. Transmittance reflectance method

The transmittance reflectance method is a combination of the transmittance method and reflectance method. A mirror is used to re-reflect the light that has passed through a sample in order to measure transmittance reflectance rate, T^* (%). The light path must be twice the thickness of the sample. On the other hand, the light reflected by a mirror and being introduced into a detector is used as the control light. When this method is applied to suspended samples, however, a metal plate or a ceramic reflector with a rough surface that causes diffuse reflectance is used instead of a mirror.

This is a method that is applied to solid samples, including fine particles, as well as liquids and suspended samples. The thickness of a sample must be adjusted when applying this method to a solid sample. Ordinarily adjustment is made by setting absorbance to 0.1 – 2 (transmittance of 79 – 1%), which provides the best linearity and SN ratio of a detector. A cell with appropriate layer length, according to the grain size of the fine particle, must be selected when applying the method to a fine particle sample.

3. Factors that affect spectra

Following items must be considered as factors that can affect spectra when applying near-infrared spectrometry, particularly when conducting quantitative analysis.

(i) Measurement conditions: A significant change (wavelength shift, for example) can occur when the temperature varies by a several degrees (°C). Care must be taken, particularly when a sample contains water. Also, water or residual solvent contents of a sample, as well as water (humidity) in the environment where in measurements are taken, can significantly affect absorption bands of the near-infrared range.

The thickness of a sample is a factor for spectral changes and therefore needs to be controlled at a certain thickness. Furthermore, since the condition of sample fill can potentially affect spectra when taking measurements of samples that are solids or fine particles, care must be taken with filling samples in a cell, to ensure that a certain amount is filled through a specific procedure.

The JP Drugs are to be tested according to the provisions given in the pertinent monographs, General Notices, General Rules for Crude Drugs, General Rules for Preparations, and General Tests for their conformity to the Japanese Pharmacopoeia. (See the General Notices 5.)

Supplement I, JP XVIII   *General Tests, Processes and Apparatus*   2823

Samples can potentially undergo chemical, physical or optical property changes, due to passing of time or storage after sampling. In creating calibration curves, therefore, it is necessary to pay attention that the samples for calibration curves must be prepared with adequate considerations for reducing the time to be measured, such as the measurement is carried out offline in a laboratory or online in manufacturing process (or inline).

(ii) Characteristics of samples: When a sample is physically, chemically or optically uneven, relatively large beam size must be used, multiple samples must be used, measurements must be taken at multiple points on the same samples, or a sample must be pulverized to ensure averaging of the sample. Grain size, fill condition, as well as roughness of surfaces can also affect the spectra of fine particle samples. Since variations in crystal structures (crystal polymorphism) can also affect spectra, in cases where multiple crystal forms exist, care must be taken to ensure that even standard samples for the calibration curve method have diversified distributions similar to that of samples to be analyzed.

4. Control of equipment performance
4.1. Accuracy of wavelengths (or wave numbers)

The accuracy of wavelengths (or wave numbers) of equipment is derived from the deviation of suitable substances for which peak absorption wavelengths (or wave numbers) have been defined, such as polystyrene, mixture of rare earth oxides (dysprosium, holmium and erbium; 1:1:1) or steam, from the figures indicated on the equipment. Tolerance figures in the vicinity of 3 peaks are ordinarily set in the following manner, though appropriate tolerance figures can be set depending on the intended purpose:

1200 ± 1 nm (8300 ± 8 cm^{-1})
1600 ± 1 nm (6250 ± 6 cm^{-1})
2000 ± 1.5 nm (5000 ± 4 cm^{-1})

Since the location of absorption peaks vary, depending on the substance used as reference, absorption peaks of wavelengths (or wave numbers) that are closest to the above 3 peaks are selected for suitability evaluation. A mixture of rare earth oxides, for instance, would indicate characteristic absorption peaks at 1261 nm (7930 cm^{-1}), 1681 nm (5949 cm^{-1}) and 1971 nm (5074 cm^{-1}).

The absorption peak of steam at 1368.6 nm (7306.7 cm^{-1}) can be used with a Fourier transformation type spectrophotometer, as its wave number resolution ability is high.

Other substances can also be used as the reference, so long as their adequacy for the purpose can be verified.
4.2. Spectroscopic linearity

Appropriate standard plates, such as plate-shaped polymer impregnated with varying concentrations of carbon (Carbon-doped polymer standards), can be used to evaluate spectroscopic linearity. In order to verify linearity, however, standard plates with no less than 4 levels of concentration within the reflectance of 10 – 90% must be used. When measurements are expected to be taken with absorbance of not less than 1.0, it is necessary to add standard

plates with the reflectance of either 2% or 5% or both.

In order to plot absorbance of such standard plates at locations in the vicinity of wavelengths 1200 nm (8300 cm^{-1}), 1600 nm (6250 cm^{-1}) and 2000 nm (5000 cm^{-1}) against absorbance at each wavelength (or wave number) assigned to each standard plate, ensure that the gradient of linearity and ordinate intercept obtained are ordinarily within the ranges of 1.00 ± 0.05 and 0.00 ± 0.05, respectively. Depending on the intended purpose, appropriate tolerance figures can be set.

5. Application of qualitative or quantitative analysis

Ordinarily, chemometrics methods are used for analyzing a near-infrared absorption spectrum. Conventional spectrometric methods, such as a calibration curve method, may be used as a method whenever applicable. Chemometrics ordinarily involve the quantification of chemical data, as well as numerical and statistical procedures for computerization of information. Various types of multivariate analysis are used as chemometrics for near infrared spectrometry, and are selected according to the intended purpose. Characteristics of near-infrared absorption spectrum must be emphasized and effects of complexities of spectra, as well as overlay of absorption bands must be reduced by performing mathematical preprocesses, such as primary or secondary spectral differentiation processes or normalizations, which becomes one of vital procedures in establishing analysis methods that use methodologies of chemometrics.

In near-infrared spectroscopy, sustaining and managing performance of an analysis method, once established, are critical. Continuous and systematic maintenance and inspection work are required. Furthermore, it is necessary to pay attention to whether or not appropriate evaluation procedures are available to deal with change controls or implementation of re-validation on changes made in manufacturing processes or raw materials, as well as changes arising from replacement of major components in equipment.
5.1. Qualitative analysis

Qualitative analysis is performed for each substance to be analyzed after preparing a reference library that includes inter-lot variations within the tolerance range and establishing an analysis method using chemometrics methodology. The identity of substances can be confirmed by comparison with a standard spectrum or by methods using validated chemometrics software. Also, substances can be identified by their absorbance bands.

Furthermore, multivariate analysis includes direct analysis methods that consider wavelengths (or wave numbers) and absorption as variables, such as wavelength correlation method, residual sum of squares, range sum of squares, along with factor analysis method, cluster analysis method, discriminant analysis method and SIMCA (Soft independent modeling of class analogy) that are applied after processing such as principal component analysis.

It is also possible to consider the overall near-infrared absorption spectrum as a single pattern and to identify parameters obtained by applying multivariate analysis methods or characteristic wavelength (or wave number)

The JP Drugs are to be tested according to the provisions given in the pertinent monographs, General Notices, General Rules for Crude Drugs, General Rules for Preparations, and General Tests for their conformity to the Japanese Pharmacopoeia. (See the General Notices 5.)

2824 *General Tests, Processes and Apparatus*   *Supplement I, JP XVIII*

peaks of components to be analyzed as indices for monitoring, for the purpose of manufacturing process control for drug substances or preparations.

5.2. Quantitative analysis

Quantitative analysis ordinarily uses spectra of sample groups and analysis values obtained through the existing and established analysis methods, to obtain quantitative models with methodologies of chemometrics. These are used to calculate concentrations of individual ingredients and material values of samples being measured, using conversion formulas. Chemometrics methodologies for obtaining quantitative models include multiple regression analysis method and PLS (Partial least squares) regression analysis method.

In cases where the composition of a sample is simple, concentrations of ingredients in the sample to be analyzed can be calculated by plotting a calibration curve using the absorbance of a specific wavelength (or wave number) or the correlating relationship between the parameters and concentration, using samples for preparation of calibration curves with known concentrations (calibration curve method).

Add the following:

2.28 Circular Dichroism Spectroscopy

The circular dichroism spectroscopy is a method used to analyze and determine the structure of optically active substances, discriminate active substances from enantiomers, diastereomers, etc. by using the phenomenon (circular dichroism) in which the degrees of absorption of left and right circularly polarized lights differ in the absorption wavelength region of active substances.

In this method circular dichroism is measured as the difference of absorbance of left and right circularly polarized lights as follows.

$$\Delta A = A_L - A_R$$

ΔA: Difference of absorbance of left and right circularly polarized lights
A_L: Absorbance of left circularly polarized light
A_R: Absorbance of right circularly polarized light

Also, the difference of molar absorption coefficients for left and right circularly polarized lights can be expressed as the molar circular dichroism as follows.

$$\Delta \varepsilon = \varepsilon_L - \varepsilon_R = \frac{\Delta A}{c \times l}$$

$\Delta \varepsilon$: Molar circular dichroism $[(mol/L)^{-1} \cdot cm^{-1}]$
ε_L: Molar absorption coefficient for left circularly polarized light $[(mol/L)^{-1} \cdot cm^{-1}]$
ε_R: Molar absorption coefficient for right circularly polarized light $[(mol/L)^{-1} \cdot cm^{-1}]$
c: Concentration of an optically active substance in solu-

tion (mol/L)
l: Path length (cm)

The following unit can also be used as the unit indicating circular dichroism.

Dissymmetry factor (g factor):

$$g = \frac{\Delta \varepsilon}{\varepsilon}$$

ε: Molar absorption coefficient

Molar ellipticity:

In some apparatuses, circular dichroism is expressed in units of ellipticity (°). In such a case, the molar ellipticity $[\theta]$ is calculated using the following equation.

$$[\theta] = \frac{\theta}{10 \times c \times l}$$

$[\theta]$: Molar ellipticity $(° \cdot cm^2/dmol)$
θ: Value (m°) of ellipticity calculated by apparatus
c: Concentration of an optically active substance in solution (mol/L)
l: Path length (cm)

Molar ellipticity is related with molar circular dichroism by the following equation.

$$[\theta] = 2.303 \Delta \varepsilon \frac{4500}{\pi} \approx 3300 \Delta \varepsilon$$

Molar circular dichroism and molar ellipticity are often used for analysis of peptides, proteins and nucleic acids. In this case, mean residue weight, which is the molecular mass divided by the number of monomeric residues, is used in the calculation of molar concentration (c).

Mean residue weight

$$= \frac{\text{molecular mass}}{\text{number of amino acid residues or nucleotide residues}}$$

Mean residue weight is 100 – 120 (generally 115) for peptides and proteins, and is about 330 as sodium salt for nucleic acids.

1. Apparatus

A circular dichroism spectrophotometer is used. A xenon lamp is used as the light source. Light from the light source is polarized at the time when being split by a double monochromator equipped with a crystal prism, resulting in monochromatic linearly polarized light. The slit at the exit of the monochromator eliminates extraordinary light. The monochromatic linearly polarized light is passed through a photoelastic modulator to be alternately modulated into left and right circularly polarized lights at a constant frequency and is irradiated to a sample.

After the light that has passed through a sample to be tested reaches a photomultiplier tube, the light is divided into two electrical signals and amplified. One is the direct current signal, V_{DC}, which reflects the light absorption of the sample. The other is the alternating current signal, V_{AC}, which occurs when the sample has circular dichroism and has the same frequency as the modulation frequency of the

The JP Drugs are to be tested according to the provisions given in the pertinent monographs, General Notices, General Rules for Crude Drugs, General Rules for Preparations, and General Tests for their conformity to the Japanese Pharmacopoeia. (See the General Notices 5.)

Supplement I, JP XVIII   *General Tests, Processes and Apparatus*   2825

photoelastic modulator. The phase of the direct current signal indicates the sign of the circular dichroism (+ or −), and the magnitude of the amplitude indicates the intensity of the circular dichroism. Here, V_{AC}/V_{DC} is proportional to the difference of the absorbances for left and right circular polarized lights, ΔA. Generally, the wavelength range measured by a circular dichroism spectrophotometer is about 170 to 800 nm, but some apparatuses can measure at a wider wavelength range.

2. Methods

Set temperature, wavelength, path length and sample concentration for measurement. Dissolve a sample in an appropriate solvent, place it in a cell, and measure. In the sample preparation, confirm the influence of impurities on the spectrum, the structural change of the sample depending on the concentration, the absorption of the solvent itself, and the influence of the solvent on the sample structure. Attention should be taken for the optical path length of a sample cell, especially when the optical path length is short. Furthermore, it should be noted for the absorption of light by a sample because it may reduce a signal reaching a detector.

2.1. Identification test

Specify molar circular dichroism or molar ellipticity along with the wavelength at which it is maximum. The identity of a substance can be confirmed when the molar circular dichroism or molar ellipticity at the specified maximum wavelength of the substance to be confirmed meets this specification. Or, when the spectrum of a sample is compared with the reference spectrum of the substance to be confirmed or the spectrum of the reference standard, and both spectra give the same intensity of molar circular dichroism or molar ellipticity at the same wavelength, their identity can be confirmed mutually.

2.2. Analysis of secondary structure

For peptides and proteins, specific spectra appear in the far ultra-violet region. The secondary structure of peptides and proteins can be estimated by measuring the spectrum below about 250 nm. Furthermore, it is possible to estimate the three-dimensional structure from the near ultra-violet spectrum. However, it should be noted that circular dichroism measurement observes the average property of a whole molecule. For a α-helix structure, negative maxima appear generally at 208 nm and 222 nm and a positive maximum between 191 nm and 193 nm, for a β-sheet structure, a negative maximum appears between 216 nm and 218 nm and a positive maximum between 195 nm and 200 nm, and for an irregular structure, a negative maximum appears between 195 nm and 200 nm. Methods for analyzing the proportion of secondary structures from a circular dichroism spectrum include a method using a calculation formula and a method using a database. It can also be calculated by multivariate analysis. Whenever any method is used, the method used for the calculation is specified in the test method.

3. Verification of the performance of apparatus

A wavelength-calibrated apparatus is used, and the performance of apparatus is verified using a sample with quality suitable for the measurement of circular dichroism and with known $\Delta\varepsilon$.

3.1. Accuracy of circular dichroism

Calibrate the accuracy of circular dichroism with a substance with known $\Delta\varepsilon$, such as isoandrosterone, ammonium *d*-camphorsulfonate, etc. (substances recommended by the apparatus manufacturer may be used). When using isoandrosterone, weigh exactly 10.0 mg of isoandrosterone, and dissolve in ethanol (99.5) to make exactly 10 mL. When the circular dichroism spectrum of the prepared solution is measured in the range of 280 nm to 360 nm using a cell with a path length of 10 mm, $\Delta\varepsilon$ at 304 nm is +3.3.

3.2. Linearity of modulation

Calibrate the linearity of modulation with a substance with known $\Delta\varepsilon$, such as ammonium *d*-camphorsulfonate (substances recommended by the apparatus manufacturer may be used). When using ammonium *d*-camphorsulfonate, weigh exactly 6.0 mg of ammonium *d*-camphorsulfonate and dissolve in water to make exactly 10 mL. When the circular dichroism spectrum of the prepared solution is measured in the range of 185 nm to 340 nm using a cell with a path length of 1 mm, $\Delta\varepsilon$ at 290.5 nm is +2.2 to +2.5 and $\Delta\varepsilon$ at 192.5 nm is −4.3 to −5.

Change the following as follows:

2.58 X-Ray Powder Diffraction Method

This test is harmonized with the European Pharmacopoeia and the U.S. Pharmacopeia.

The parts of the text that are not harmonized among the targeted texts for the harmonization are marked with symbols (♦ ♦), and the texts that are uniquely specified by the JP other than the targeted texts for the harmonization are marked with symbols (◇ ◇).

Information on the harmonization with the European Pharmacopoeia and the U.S. Pharmacopeia is available on the website of the Pharmaceuticals and Medical Devices Agency.

◇X-Ray Powder Diffraction Method is a method for measuring characteristic X-ray diffraction angles and intensities from randomly oriented powder crystallites irradiated by a monochromated X-ray beam.◇

Every crystalline phase of a given substance produces a characteristic X-ray diffraction pattern. Diffraction patterns can be obtained from a randomly oriented crystalline powder composed of crystallites (crystalline region within a particle) or crystal fragments of finite size. Essentially 3 types of information can be derived from a powder diffraction pattern: angular position of diffraction lines (depending on geometry and size of the unit cell); intensities of diffraction lines (depending mainly on atom type and arrangement, and preferred orientation within the sample); and diffraction line profiles (depending on instrumental resolution, crystallite size, strain and specimen thickness).

The JP Drugs are to be tested according to the provisions given in the pertinent monographs, General Notices, General Rules for Crude Drugs, General Rules for Preparations, and General Tests for their conformity to the Japanese Pharmacopoeia. (See the General Notices 5.)

Experiments giving angular positions and intensities of lines can be used for applications such as qualitative phase analysis (for example, identification of crystalline phases) and quantitative phase analysis of crystalline materials. An estimate of the amorphous and crystalline fractions[1] can also be made. The X-ray powder diffraction (XRPD) method provides an advantage over other means of analysis in that it is usually non-destructive in nature (specimen preparation is usually limited to grinding to ensure a randomly oriented sample). XRPD investigations can also be carried out under *in situ* conditions on specimens exposed to non-ambient conditions, such as low or high temperature and humidity.

1. Principle

X-ray diffraction results from the interaction between X-rays and electron clouds of atoms. Depending on the atomic arrangement, interferences arise from the elastically scattered X-rays. These interferences are constructive when the path difference between 2 diffracted X-ray waves differs by an integral number of wavelengths. This selective condition is described by the Bragg equation, also called Bragg's law (see Fig. 2.58-1)

$$2d_{hkl} \sin \theta_{hkl} = n\lambda$$

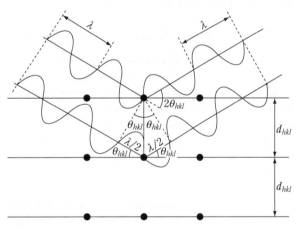

Fig. 2.58-1 Diffraction of X-rays by a crystal according to Bragg's law

The wavelength λ of the X-rays is of the same order of magnitude as the distance between successive crystal lattice planes, or d_{hkl} (also called '*d*-spacings'). θ_{hkl} is the angle between the incident ray and the family of lattice planes, and $\sin\theta_{hkl}$ is inversely proportional to the distance between successive crystal planes or *d*-spacings.

The direction and spacing of the planes with reference to the unit cell axes are defined by the Miller indices $\{hkl\}$. These indices are the reciprocals, reduced to the next-lower integer, of the intercepts that a plane makes with the unit cell axes. The unit cell dimensions are given by the spacings, *a*, *b* and *c* and the angles between them, α, β and γ. The interplanar spacing for a specified set of parallel *hkl* planes is denoted by d_{hkl}. Each such family of planes may show higher orders of diffraction where the *d* values for the related families of planes, *nh*, *nk*, *nl* are diminished by the factor $1/n$ (*n* being an integer: 2,3,4, etc.). Every set of planes throughout a crystal has a corresponding Bragg diffraction angle, θ_{hkl}, associated with it (for a specific wavelength λ).

For polycrystalline powder specimen at any angle θ_{hkl} there are always crystallites in an orientation allowing diffraction according to Bragg's law[2]. For a given X-ray wavelength, the positions of the diffraction peaks (also referred to as 'lines', 'reflections' or 'Bragg reflections') are characteristic of the crystal lattice (*d*-spacings), their theoretical intensities depend on the crystallographic unit cell content (nature and positions of atoms), and the line profiles on the perfection and extent of the crystal lattice. Under these conditions the diffraction peak has a finite intensity arising from atomic arrangement, type of atoms, thermal motion and structural imperfections, as well as from instrument characteristics. The intensity is also dependent upon many factors such as structure factor, temperature factor, polarization factor, multiplicity, Lorentz factor and microabsorption factors. The main characteristics of diffraction line profiles are 2θ position, peak height, peak area and shape (characterized by, for example, peak width or asymmetry, analytical function, empirical representation). An example of the type of powder patterns obtained for 5 different solid phases of a substance is shown in Fig. 2.58-2.

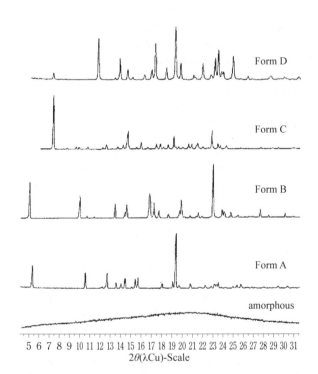

Fig. 2.58-2 X-ray powder diffraction patterns collected for 5 different solid phases of a substance (the intensities of crystalline forms A-D are normalized)

In addition to the diffraction peaks, an X-ray diffraction experiment also generates a more-or-less uniform background, upon which the peaks are superimposed. Besides specimen preparation, other factors contribute to the background, for instance the sample holder, diffuse scattering from air, the sample and/or the equipment, other instrumental parameters such as detector noise, general radiation from the X-ray tube, etc. The peak to background ratio can be increased by minimizing background and by choosing prolonged exposure times.

2. Instrument
2.1. Instrument set-up

X-ray diffraction experiments are usually performed using powder diffractometers or powder cameras. A powder diffractometer generally comprises 5 main parts: an X-ray source; incident beam optics, which may perform monochromatization, filtering, collimation and/or focusing of the beam; a goniometer; the diffracted beam optics, which may perform monochromatization, filtering, collimation and/or focusing of the beam; and a detector. Data-collection and data-processing systems are also required and are generally included with current diffraction measurement equipment.

Depending on the type of analysis to be performed (phase identification, quantitative analysis, lattice parameters determination, etc.), different XRPD instrument configurations and performance levels are required. The simplest instruments used to measure XRPD patterns are powder cameras. The replacement of photographic film as the detection method by photon detectors has led to the design of diffractometers in which the geometric arrangement of the optics is not truly focusing but parafocusing, such as in the Bragg-Brentano geometry. The Bragg-Brentano parafocusing configuration is currently the most widely used and is therefore briefly described here.

A given instrument may provide a horizontal or vertical $\theta/2\theta$ geometry or a vertical θ/θ geometry. For both geometries, the incident X-ray beam forms an angle θ with the specimen surface plane and the diffracted X-ray beam forms an angle 2θ with the direction of the incident X-ray beam (an angle θ with the specimen surface plane). One example of a basic geometric arrangement is represented in Fig. 2.58-3. The divergent beam of radiation from the X-ray tube (the so-called 'primary beam') passes through the Soller slit and a divergence slit assembly and illuminates the flat surface of the specimen. All the rays diffracted by suitably oriented crystallites in the specimen at an angle 2θ converge to a line at the receiving slit. A second set of Soller slit and a scatter slit may be placed either behind or before the receiving slit; the receiving slit is normally only used when a 0D detector is present. The axes of the line focus and of the receiving slit are at equal distances from the axis of the goniometer. The X-rays are counted by a detector, usually a scintillation counter, or a sealed-gas proportional counter. However, nowadays a position-sensitive solid-state detector or hybrid photon counting detectors are more common. The receiving slit assembly and the detector are coupled together and move tangentially to the focusing circle. For $\theta/2\theta$ scans the goniometer rotates the specimen about the same axis as that of the detector, but at half the rotational speed, in a

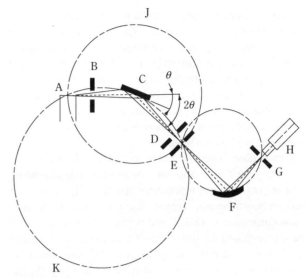

A. X-ray tube
B. Divergence slit
C. Sample
D. Anti-diffusion slit
E. Receiving slit
F. Monochromator
G. Detector receiving slit
H. Detector
J. Diffractometer circle
K. Focusing circle

Fig. 2.58-3 Geometric arrangement of the Bragg-Brentano parafocusing geometry

$\theta/2\theta$ motion. The surface of the specimen thus remains tangential to the focusing circle. The Soller slit limits the axial divergence of the beam and hence partially controls the shape of the diffracted line profile.

A diffractometer may also be used in transmission mode. The advantage with this technology is to lessen the effects due to preferred orientation. A capillary of about 0.5 – 2 mm thickness can also be used for small sample amounts.

2.2. X-ray radiation

In the laboratory, X-rays are obtained by bombarding a metal anode with electrons emitted by the thermionic effect and accelerated in a strong electric field (using a high-voltage generator). Most of the kinetic energy of the electrons is converted to heat, which limits the power of the tubes and requires efficient anode cooling. A 20- to 30-fold increase in brilliance can be obtained using rotating anodes and by using X-ray optics. Alternatively, X-ray photons may be produced in a large-scale facility (synchrotron).

The spectrum emitted by an X-ray tube operating at sufficient voltage consists of a continuous background of polychromatic radiation (Bremsstrahlung or white radiation) and additional characteristic radiation that depends on the type of anode. Normally only this characteristic radiation is used in X-ray diffraction experiments. The principal radiation sources utilized for X-ray diffraction are vacuum tubes utilizing copper, molybdenum, iron, cobalt, silver or chromium as anodes; copper and molybdenum X-rays are employed most commonly for organic substances. The choice of radiation to be used depends on the absorption

2828　General Tests, Processes and Apparatus

characteristics of the specimen and possible fluorescence by atoms present in the specimen. The wavelengths used in powder diffraction generally correspond to the K_α radiation from the anode. Consequently, it is advantageous to make the X-ray beam 'monochromatic' by eliminating all the other components of the emission spectrum. This can be partly obtained using K_β filters, i.e. metal filters selected as having an absorption edge between the K_α and K_β wavelengths emitted by the tube.

Such a filter is usually inserted between the X-ray tube and the specimen. Another, more-and-more-commonly used way to obtain a monochromatic X-ray beam is via a large monochromator crystal (usually referred to as a 'monochromator'). This crystal is placed before or behind the specimen and diffracts the different characteristic peaks of the X-ray beam (i.e. K_α and K_β) at different angles, so that only one of them may be selected to enter into the detector. It is even possible to separate $K_{\alpha 1}$ and $K_{\alpha 2}$ radiations by using a specialized monochromator. Unfortunately, the gain in getting a monochromatic beam by using a filter or a monochromator is counteracted by a loss in intensity. Another way of separating K_α and K_β wavelengths is by using curved X-rays mirrors that can simultaneously monochromate and focus or parallelize the X-ray beam.

2.3.　Radiation protection

Exposure of any part of the human body to X-rays can be injurious to health. It is therefore essential that whenever X-ray equipment is used, adequate precautions are taken to protect the operator and any other person in the vicinity. Recommended practice for radiation protection as well as limits for the levels of X-radiation exposure are those established by national legislation in each country. If there are no official regulations or recommendations in a country, the latest recommendations of the International Commission on Radiological Protection should be applied.

3.　Specimen preparation and mounting

The preparation of the powdered material and mounting of the specimen in a suitable holder are critical steps in many analytical methods, and are particularly so for XRPD analysis, since they can greatly affect the quality of the data to be collected[3]. The main sources of error due to specimen preparation and mounting are briefly discussed here for instruments in Bragg-Brentano parafocusing geometry.

3.1.　Specimen preparation

In general, the morphology of many crystalline particles tends to give a specimen that exhibits some degree of preferred orientation in the specimen holder. This is particularly evident for needle-like or plate-like crystals when size reduction yields finer needles or platelets. Preferred orientation in the specimen influences the intensities of various reflections, so that some are more intense and others are less intense, compared to what would be expected from a completely random specimen. Several techniques can be employed to improve randomness in the orientation of crystallites (and therefore to minimize preferred orientation), but further reduction of particle size is often the best and simplest approach. The optimum number of crystallites de-

pends on the diffractometer geometry, the required resolution and the specimen attenuation of the X-ray beam. In some cases, particle sizes as large as 50 μm will provide satisfactory results in phase identification. However, excessive milling (particle sizes less than approximately 0.5 μm) may cause line broadening and significant changes to the sample itself such as:

(i)　specimen contamination by particles abraded from the milling instruments (mortar, pestle, balls, etc.);

(ii)　reduced degree of crystallinity;

(iii)　solid-state transition to another polymorph;

(iv)　chemical decomposition;

(v)　introduction of internal stress;

(vi)　solid-state reactions.

Therefore, it is advisable to compare the diffraction pattern of the non-ground specimen with that corresponding to a specimen of smaller particle size (e.g. a milled specimen). If the XRPD pattern obtained is of adequate quality considering its intended use, then grinding may not be required. It should be noted that if a sample contains more than one phase and if sieving is used to isolate particles to a specific size, the initial composition may be altered.

4.　Control of the instrument performance

Goniometers and the corresponding incident and diffracted X-ray beam optics have many mechanical parts that need adjustment. The degree of alignment or misalignment directly influences the quality of the results of an XRPD investigation. Therefore, the different components of the diffractometer must be carefully adjusted (optical and mechanical systems, etc.) to minimize adequately systematic errors, while optimizing the intensities received by the detector. The search for maximum intensity and maximum resolution is always antagonistic when aligning a diffractometer. Hence, the best compromise must be sought whilst performing the alignment procedure. There are many different configurations and each supplier's equipment requires specific alignment procedures.

The overall diffractometer performance must be tested and monitored periodically using suitable certified reference materials, e.g. silicon powder or α-alumina (corundum). Depending on the type of analysis, other well-defined reference materials may also be employed, although the use of certified reference materials is preferred.

5.　Qualitative phase analysis (Identification of phases)

The identification of the phase composition of an unknown sample by XRPD is usually based on the visual or computer-assisted comparison of a portion of its XRPD pattern to the experimental or calculated pattern of a reference material. Ideally, these reference patterns are collected on well-characterized single-phase specimens. This approach makes it possible in most cases to identify a crystalline substance by its 2θ diffraction angles or d-spacings and by its relative intensities. The computer-aided comparison of the diffraction pattern of the unknown sample to the reference data can be based either on a more-or-less extended 2θ-range of the whole diffraction pattern or on a set of reduced data derived from the pattern. For example, the list

The JP Drugs are to be tested according to the provisions given in the pertinent monographs, General Notices, General Rules for Crude Drugs, General Rules for Preparations, and General Tests for their conformity to the Japanese Pharmacopoeia. (See the General Notices 5.)

Supplement I, JP XVIII

of *d*-spacings and normalized intensities I_{norm}, a so-called (d, I_{norm})-list extracted from the pattern, is the crystallographic fingerprint of the material, and can be compared to (d, I_{norm})-lists of single-phase samples compiled in databases.

For most organic crystals, when using Cu K_α radiation, it is appropriate to record the diffraction pattern in a 2θ-range from as near 0° as possible to at least 30°. The agreement in the 2θ-diffraction angles between specimen and reference is expected to be within 0.2° for the same crystal form, while relative intensities between specimen and reference may vary considerably due to preferred orientation effects. By their very nature, variable hydrates and solvates are recognized to have varying unit cell dimensions and as such shifting occurs in peak positions of the measured XRPD patterns for these materials. In these unique materials, variance in 2θ-positions of greater than 0.2° is not unexpected. As such, peak position variances such as 0.2° are not applicable to these materials. For other types of samples (e.g. inorganic salts), it may be necessary to extend the 2θ-region scanned to well beyond 30°. It is generally sufficient to scan past the 10 strongest reflections identified in single phase XRPD database files.

It is sometimes difficult or even impossible to identify phases in the following cases:

(i)   non-crystallized or amorphous substances;

(ii)   the components to be identified are present in low mass fractions of the analyte amounts (generally less than 10 per cent *m/m*);

(iii)   pronounced preferred orientation effects;

(iv)   the phase has not been filed in the database used;

(v)   formation of solid solutions;

(vi)   presence of disordered structures that alter the unit cell;

(vii)   the specimen comprises too many phases;

(viii)   presence of lattice deformations;

(ix)   structural similarity of different phases.

6.   Quantitative phase analysis

If the sample under investigation is a mixture of 2 or more known phases, of which not more than 1 is amorphous, the percentage (by volume or by mass) of each crystalline phase and of the amorphous phase can, in many cases, be determined. Quantitative phase analysis can be based on the integrated intensities, on the peak heights of several individual diffraction lines[4], or on the full pattern. These integrated intensities, peak heights or full-pattern data points are compared to the corresponding values of reference materials. These reference materials shall be single-phase or a mixture of known phases. The difficulties encountered during quantitative analysis are due to specimen preparation (the accuracy and precision of the results require in particular homogeneity of all phases and a suitable particle size distribution in each phase) and to matrix effects. Amounts of crystalline phases as small as 10 per cent may usually be determined in solid matrices, and in favorable cases amounts of crystalline phases less than 10 per cent may be determined.

General Tests, Processes and Apparatus   2829

6.1.   Polymorphic samples

For a sample composed of 2 polymorphic phases a and b, the following expression may be used to quantify the fraction F_a of phase a:

$$F_a = \frac{1}{1 + K\,(I_b/I_a)}$$

The fraction is derived by measuring the intensity ratio between the 2 phases, knowing the value of the constant K. K is the ratio of the absolute intensities of the 2 pure polymorphic phases I_{oa}/I_{ob}. Its value can be determined by measuring standard samples.

6.2.   Methods using a standard

The most commonly used methods for quantitative analysis are:

– the 'external standard method';

– the 'internal standard method';

– the 'spiking method' (often also called the 'standard addition method').

The 'external standard method' is the most general method and consists of comparing the X-ray diffraction pattern of the mixture, or the respective line intensities, with those measured in a reference mixture or with the theoretical intensities of a structural model, if it is fully known.

To limit errors due to matrix effects, an internal reference material with crystallite size and X-ray absorption coefficient comparable to those of the components of the sample, and with a diffraction pattern that does not overlap at all that of the sample to be analyzed, can be used. A known quantity of this reference material is added to the sample to be analyzed and to each of the reference mixtures. Under these conditions, a linear relationship between line intensity and concentration exists. This application, called the 'internal standard method', requires a precise measurement of diffraction intensities.

In the 'spiking method' (or 'standard addition method'), some of the pure phase a is added to the mixture containing the unknown concentration of the phase a. Multiple additions are made to prepare an intensity-versus-concentration plot in which the negative *x* intercept is the concentration of the phase a in the original sample.

7.   Estimate of the amorphous and crystalline fractions

In a mixture of crystalline and amorphous phases, the crystalline and amorphous fractions can be estimated in several ways. The choice of the method used depends on the nature of the sample:

(i)   if the sample consists of crystalline fractions and an amorphous fraction of different chemical compositions, the amounts of each of the individual crystalline phases may be estimated using appropriate standard substances as described above; the amorphous fraction is then deduced indirectly by subtraction;

(ii)   if the sample consists of one amorphous and one crystalline fraction, either as a 1-phase or a 2-phase mixture, with the same elemental composition, the amount of the crystalline phase ('the degree of crystallinity') can be estimated by measuring 3 areas of the diffractogram:

The JP Drugs are to be tested according to the provisions given in the pertinent monographs, General Notices, General Rules for Crude Drugs, General Rules for Preparations, and General Tests for their conformity to the Japanese Pharmacopoeia. (See the General Notices 5.)

2830　*General Tests, Processes and Apparatus*　　　*Supplement I, JP XVIII*

A: Sum of the area of all the peaks arising from diffraction of the crystalline fraction of the sample:

B: Area under the diffractogram generated by the sample (excluding area *A*);

C: Area of the background noise (due to air scattering, fluorescence, equipment, etc.)

When these areas have been measured, the degree of crystallinity can be roughly estimated using the following formula:

$$\%\text{crystallinity} = 100A/(A + B - C)$$

It is noteworthy that this method does not yield absolute degree-of-crystallinity values and hence is generally used for comparative purposes only. More sophisticated methods are also available, such as the Ruland method.

8.　Single crystal structure

In general, the determination of crystal structures is performed from X-ray diffraction data obtained using single crystals. However, crystal structure analysis of organic crystals is a challenging task, since the lattice parameters are comparatively large, the symmetry is low and the scattering properties are normally very low. For any given crystalline form of a substance, knowledge of the crystal structure allows the calculation of the corresponding XRPD pattern, thereby providing a 'preferred-orientation-free' reference XRPD pattern, which may be used for phase identification.

(1) There are many other applications of the X-ray powder diffraction technique that can be applied to crystalline pharmaceutical substances, such as determination of crystal structures, refinement of crystal structures, determination of crystallographic purity of crystalline phases, characterization of crystallographic texture, etc. These applications are not described in this chapter.

(2) An 'ideal' powder for diffraction experiments consists of a large number of small, randomly oriented spherical particles (coherently diffracting crystalline domains). If this number is sufficiently large, there are always enough crystallites in any diffracting orientation to give reproducible diffraction patterns.

(3) Similarly, changes in the specimen can occur during data collection in the case of a nonequilibrium specimen (temperature, humidity).

(4) If the crystal structures of all components are known, the Rietveld method can be used to quantify them with good accuracy. If the crystal structures of the components are not known, the Pawley or least squares methods can be used.

3.04　Particle Size Determination

Change the 2.1. Procedure and below as follows:

2.1.　Procedure
2.1.1　Test Sieves

Unless otherwise specified in the monograph, use those sieves listed in the Table 3.04-1 as recommended in the particular region.

Sieves are selected to cover the entire range of particle sizes present in the test specimen. A nest of sieves having a $\sqrt{2}$ progression of the area of the sieve openings is recommended. The nest of sieves is assembled with the coarsest screen at the top and the finest at the bottom. Use micrometers or millimeters in denoting test sieve openings. [Note—Sieve numbers are provided in the table for conversion purposes only.] Test sieves are made from stainless steel or, less preferably, from brass or other suitable nonreactive wire.

2.1.1.1.　Calibration of test sieves

Calibration and recalibration of test sieves is in accordance with the most current edition of ISO 3310-1[2]. Sieves should be carefully examined for gross distortions and fractures, especially at their screen frame joints, before use. Sieves may be calibrated optically to estimate the average opening size, and opening variability, of the sieve mesh. Alternatively, for the evaluation of the effective opening of test sieves in the size range of 212 to 850 μm, Standard Glass Spheres are available. Unless otherwise specified in the individual monograph, perform the sieve analysis at controlled room temperature and at ambient relative humidity.

2.1.1.2.　Cleaning Test Sieves

Ideally, test sieves should be cleaned using only an air jet or a liquid stream. If some apertures remain blocked by test particles, careful gentle brushing may be used as a last resort.

2.1.2.　Test Specimen

If the test specimen weight is not given in the monograph for a particular material, use a test specimen having a weight between 25 and 100 g, depending on the bulk density of the material, and test sieves having a diameter of 200 mm or 203 mm (8 inch). For sieves of 75 mm or 76 mm (3-inch diameter) the amount of material that can be accommodated is approximately 1/7th of which can be accommodated on a 200 mm or 203 mm sieve. Determine the most appropriate weight for a given material by test sieving accurately weighed specimens of different weights, such as 25, 50, and 100 g, for the same time period on a mechanical shaker. [Note—If the test results are similar for the 25-g and 50-g specimens, but the 100-g specimen shows a lower percentage through the finest sieve, the 100-g specimen size is too large.] Where only a specimen of 10 to 25 g is available, smaller diameter test sieves conforming to the same mesh specifications may be substituted, but the endpoint must be re-determined. The use of test samples having a smaller mass (e.g. down to 5 g) may be needed. For materials with

The JP Drugs are to be tested according to the provisions given in the pertinent monographs, General Notices, General Rules for Crude Drugs, General Rules for Preparations, and General Tests for their conformity to the Japanese Pharmacopoeia. (See the General Notices 5.)

Table 3.04-1 Sizes of standard sieve series in range of interest

ISO Nominal Aperture			US Sieve No.	Recommended USP Sieves (microns)	European Sieve No.	Japan Sieve No.
Principal sizes R 20/3	Supplementary sizes R 20	R 40/3				
11.20 mm	11.20 mm	11.20 mm			11200	
	10.00 mm					
		9.50 mm				
	9.00 mm					
8.00 mm	8.00 mm	8.00 mm				
	7.10 mm					
		6.70 mm				
	6.30 mm					
5.60 mm	5.60 mm	5.60 mm			5600	3.5
	5.00 mm					
		4.75 mm				4
	4.50 mm					
4.00 mm	4.00 mm	4.00 mm	5	4000	4000	4.7
	3.55 mm					
		3.35 mm	6			5.5
	3.15 mm					
2.80 mm	2.80 mm	2.80 mm	7	2800	2800	6.5
	2.50 mm					
		2.36 mm	8			7.5
	2.24 mm					
2.00 mm	2.00 mm	2.00 mm	10	2000	2000	8.6
	1.80 mm					
		1.70 mm	12			10
	1.60 mm					
1.40 mm	1.40 mm	1.40 mm	14	1400	1400	12
	1.25 mm					
		1.18 mm	16			14
	1.12 mm					
1.00 mm	1.00 mm	1.00 mm	18	1000	1000	16
	900 µm					
		850 µm	20			18
	800 µm					
710 µm	710 µm	710 µm	25	710	710	22
	630 µm					
		600 µm	30			26
	560 µm					
500 µm	500 µm	500 µm	35	500	500	30
	450 µm					
		425 µm	40			36
	400 µm					
355 µm	355 µm	355 µm	45	355	355	42
	315 µm					
		300 µm	50			50
	280 µm					
250 µm	250 µm	250 µm	60	250	250	60
	224 µm					
		212 µm	70			70
	200 µm					
180 µm	180 µm	180 µm	80	180	180	83
	160 µm					
		150 µm	100			100
	140 µm					
125 µm	125 µm	125 µm	120	125	125	119
	112 µm					
		106 µm	140			140
	100 µm					
90 µm	90 µm	90 µm	170	90	90	166
	80 µm					
		75 µm	200			200
	71 µm					
63 µm	63 µm	63 µm	230	63	63	235
	56 µm					
		53 µm	270			282
	50 µm					
45 µm	45 µm	45 µm	325	45	45	330
	40 µm					
		38 µm			38	391

The JP Drugs are to be tested according to the provisions given in the pertinent monographs, General Notices, General Rules for Crude Drugs, General Rules for Preparations, and General Tests for their conformity to the Japanese Pharmacopoeia. (See the General Notices 5.)

2832 *General Tests, Processes and Apparatus*

low apparent particle density, or for materials mainly comprising particles with a highly iso-diametrical shape, specimen weights below 5 g for a 200 mm or 203 mm sieve may be necessary to avoid excessive blocking of the sieve. During validation of a particular sieve analysis method, it is expected that the problem of sieve blocking will have been addressed.

If the test material is prone to picking up or losing significant amounts of water with varying humidity, the test must be carried out in an appropriately controlled environment. Similarly, if the test material is known to develop an electrostatic charge, careful observation must be made to ensure that such charging is not influencing the analysis. An antistatic agent, such as colloidal silicon dioxide and/or aluminum oxide, may be added at a 0.5 percent (m/m) level to minimize this effect. If both of the above effects cannot be eliminated, an alternative particle-sizing technique must be selected.

2.1.3. Agitation Methods

Several different sieve and powder agitation devices are commercially available, all of which may be used to perform sieve analyses. However, the different methods of agitation may give different results for sieve analyses and endpoint determinations because of the different types and magnitude of the forces acting on the individual particles under test. Methods using mechanical agitation or electromagnetic agitation, and that can induce either a vertical oscillation or a horizontal circular motion, or tapping or a combination of both tapping and horizontal circular motion are available. Entrainment of the particles in an air stream may also be used. The results must indicate which agitation method was used and the agitation parameters used (if they can be varied), since changes in the agitation conditions will give different results for the sieve analysis and endpoint determinations, and may be sufficiently different to give a failing result under some circumstances.

2.1.4. Endpoint Determination

The test sieving analysis is complete when the weight on any of the test sieves does not change by more than 5% or 0.1 g (10% in the case of 75 mm or 76 mm sieves) of the previous weight on that sieve. If less than 5% of the total specimen weight is present on a given sieve, the endpoint for that sieve is increased to a weight change of not more than 20% of the previous weight on that sieve.

If more than 50% of the total specimen weight is found on any one sieve, unless this is indicated in the monograph, the test should be repeated, but with the addition to the sieve nest of a more coarse sieve intermediate between that carrying the excessive weight and the next coarsest sieve in the original nest, i.e., addition of the ISO series sieve omitted from the nest of sieves.

2.2. Sieving Methods

2.2.1. Mechanical Agitation (Dry Sieving Method)

Tare each test sieve to the nearest 0.1 g. Place an accurately weighed quantity of test specimen on the top (coarsest) sieve, and replace the lid. Agitate the nest of sieves for 5 minutes. Then carefully remove each from the nest without loss of material. Reweigh each sieve, and determine the weight of material on each sieve. Determine the weight of material in the collecting pan in a similar manner. Reassemble the nest of sieves, and agitate for 5 minutes. Remove and weigh each sieve as previously described. Repeat these steps until the endpoint criteria are met (*see Endpoint Determination under Test Sieves*). Upon completion of the analysis, reconcile the weights of material. Total losses must not exceed 5% of the weight of the original test specimen.

Repeat the analysis with a fresh specimen, but using a single sieving time equal to that of the combined times used above. Confirm that this sieving time conforms to the requirements for endpoint determination. When this endpoint has been validated for a specific material, then a single fixed time of sieving may be used for future analyses, providing the particle size distribution falls within normal variation.

If there is evidence that the particles retained on any sieve are aggregates rather than single particles, the use of mechanical dry sieving is unlikely to give good reproducibility, a different particle size analysis method should be used.

2.2.2. Air Entrainment Methods (Air Jet and Sonic Shifter Sieving)

Different types of commercial equipment that use a moving air current are available for sieving. A system that uses a single sieve at a time is referred to as *air jet* sieving. It uses the same general sieving methodology as that described under the *Dry Sieving Method*, but with a standardized air jet replacing the normal agitation mechanism. It requires sequential analyses on individual sieves starting with the finest sieve to obtain a particle size distribution. Air jet sieving often includes the use of finer test sieves than used in ordinary dry sieving. This technique is more suitable where only oversize or undersize fractions are needed.

In the *sonic sifting* method, a nest of sieves is used, and the test specimen is carried in a vertically oscillating column of air that lifts the specimen and then carries it back against the mesh openings at a given number of pulses per minute. It may be necessary to lower the sample amount to 5 g, when sonic sifting is employed.

The air jet sieving and sonic sieving methods may be useful for powders or granules when mechanical sieving techniques are incapable of giving a meaningful analysis.

These methods are highly dependent upon proper dispersion of the powder in the air current. This requirement may be hard to achieve if the method is used at the lower end of the sieving range (i.e., below 75 μm), when the particles tend to be more cohesive, and especially if there is any tendency for the material to develop an electrostatic charge. For the above reasons endpoint determination is particularly critical, and it is very important to confirm that the oversize material comprises single particles and is not composed of aggregates.

2.3. Interpretation

The raw data must include the weight of test specimen, the total sieving time, and the precise sieving methodology and the set values for any variable parameters, in addition to the weights retained on the individual sieves and in the pan. It may be convenient to convert the raw data into a cu-

---

The JP Drugs are to be tested according to the provisions given in the pertinent monographs, General Notices, General Rules for Crude Drugs, General Rules for Preparations, and General Tests for their conformity to the Japanese Pharmacopoeia. (See the General Notices 5.)

Supplement I, JP XVIII General Tests, Processes and Apparatus 2833

mulative weight distribution, and if it is desired to express the distribution in terms of a cumulative weight undersize, the range of sieves used should include a sieve through which all the material passes. If there is evidence on any of the test sieves that the material remaining on it is composed of aggregates formed during the sieving process, the analysis is invalid.

[1]Additional information on particle size measurement, sample size, and data analysis is available, for example, in ISO 9276.
[2]International Organization for Standardization (ISO) Specification ISO 3310-1: Test sieves-Technical requirements and testing—Part 1: Test sieves of metal wire cloth.

9.01   Reference Standards

Add the following to Section (1):

Anastrozole RS

Budesonide RS

Temozolomide RS

Delete the following from section (2), and add them to section (1):

Amikacin Sulfate RS

Cefaclor RS

Cefalexin RS

Clindamycin Phosphate RS

Doxorubicin Hydrochloride RS

Delete the following:

Nartograstim RS

9.41   Reagents, Test Solutions

Add the following:

1,4-Diaminobutane $C_4H_{12}N_2$ White to slightly pale yellow powder or masses, or colorless to pale yellow clear liquid.

Lead tetraacetate $Pb(CH_3COO)_4$ White to pale brown powder. Melting point: about 176°C (with decomposition).

Lead tetraacetate-fluorescein sodium TS To 5 mL of a solution of lead tetraacetate in acetic acid (100) (3 in 100) and 2.5 mL of a solution of fluorescein sodium in ethanol (99.5) (1 in 100) add dichloromethane to make 100 mL. Pre-

pare before use.

Nootkatone for thin-layer chromatography $C_{15}H_{22}O$ White to pale yellow, crystals or crystalline powder. Very soluble in methanol, in ethanol (99.5) and in hexane, and practically insoluble in water.
Identification—Determine the infrared absorption spectrum of nootkatone for thin-layer chromatography as directed in the potassium bromide disk method as directed under Infrared Spectrophotometry <2.25>: it exhibits absorption at the wave numbers of about 2950 cm^{-1}, 1670 cm^{-1}, and 898 cm^{-1}.
Purity Related substances—Dissolve 2 mg of nootkatone for thin-layer chromatography in 2 mL of hexane, and use this solution as the sample solution. Pipet 1 mL of the sample solution, add hexane to make exactly 20 mL, and use this solution as the standard solution. Perform the test with these solutions as directed under Thin-Layer Chromatography <2.03>. Perform the test with 10 μL each of the sample solution and standard solution as directed in the Identification under Bitter Cardamon: the spots other than the principal spot with an Rf value of about 0.35 obtained from the sample solution are not more intense than the spot from the standard solution.

Phosphate buffer solution (pH 3.2) To 900 mL of a solution of sodium dihydrogen phosphate dihydrate (1 in 250) add 100 mL of diluted phosphoric acid (1 in 400), and adjust to pH 3.2 with phosphoric acid or sodium hydroxide TS.

Potassium phosphate trihydrate $K_3PO_4.3H_2O$ White, crystalline powder or powder. Freely soluble in water. The pH of a solution of potassium phosphate trihydrate (1 in 100) is between 11.5 and 12.5.
Identification—(1) A solution of potassium phosphate trihydrate (1 in 20) responds to Qualitative Tests <1.09> (3) for potassium salt.
(2) A solution of potassium phosphate trihydrate (1 in 20) responds to Qualitative Tests <1.09> (1) for phosphate.

Temozolomide $C_6H_6N_6O_2$ [Same as the namesake monograph]

Change the following as follows:

Amygdalin for assay $C_{20}H_{27}NO_{11}$ Amygdalin for thin-layer chromatography. It meets the requirement of the following amygdalin for assay 1 or amygdalin for assay 2 (Purity value by quantitative NMR). The former is used after drying in a desiccator (silica gel) for 24 hours, and the latter is used with correction for its amount based on the result obtained in the Assay 2.
1) Amygdalin for assay 1
Absorbance <2.24> $E_{1cm}^{1\%}$ (263 nm): 5.2 – 5.8 [20 mg calculated on the anhydrous basis, methanol, 20 mL; separately determine the water <2.48> (5 mg, coulometric titration)].
Purity Related substances—Dissolve 5 mg of amygdalin for assay 1 in 10 mL of the mobile phase, and use this solu-

The JP Drugs are to be tested according to the provisions given in the pertinent monographs, General Notices, General Rules for Crude Drugs, General Rules for Preparations, and General Tests for their conformity to the Japanese Pharmacopoeia. (See the General Notices 5.)

2834 *General Tests, Processes and Apparatus*

tion as the sample solution. Pipet 1 mL of the sample solution, add the mobile phase to make exactly 100 mL, and use this solution as the standard solution. Perform the test with exactly 10 µL each of the sample solution and standard solution as directed under Liquid Chromatography <2.01> according to the following conditions, and determine each peak area by the automatic integration method: the total area of the peaks other than amygdalin from the sample solution is not larger than the peak area of amygdalin from the standard solution.

Operating conditions

Detector, column, column temperature, mobile phase and flow rate: Proceed as directed in the operating conditions in the Assay (3) under Keishibukuryogan Extract.

Time span of measurement: About 3 times as long as the retention time of amygdalin.

System suitability

Test for required detectability: Pipet 1 mL of the standard solution, and add the mobile phase to make exactly 20 mL. Confirm that the peak area of amygdalin obtained with 10 µL of this solution is equivalent to 3.5 to 6.5% of that with 10 µL of the standard solution.

System performance: When the procedure is run with 10 µL of the standard solution under the above operating conditions, the number of theoretical plates and the symmetry factor of the peak of amygdalin are not less than 5000 and not more than 1.5, respectively.

System repeatability: When the test is repeated 6 times with 10 µL of the standard solution under the above operating conditions, the relative standard deviation of the peak area of amygdalin is not more than 1.5%.

2) Amygdalin for assay 2 (Purity value by quantitative NMR)

Unity of peak—Dissolve 1 mg of amygdalin for assay 2 in 5 mL of diluted methanol (1 in 2), and use this solution as the sample solution. Perform the test with 10 µL of the sample solution as directed under Liquid Chromatography <2.01> according to the following conditions, and compare the absorption spectra of at least 3 points including the top of amygdalin peak and around the two middle peak heights of before and after the top: no difference in form is observed among their spectra.

Operating conditions

Column, column temperature, mobile phase and flow rate: Proceed as directed in the operating conditions in the Assay (3) under Keishibukuryogan Extract.

Detector: A photodiode array detector (wavelength: 210 nm, measuring range of spectrum: 200 – 400 nm).

System suitability

System performance: When the procedure is run with 10 µL of the sample solution under the above operating conditions, the number of theoretical plates and the symmetry factor of the peak of amygdalin are not less than 5000 and not more than 1.5, respectively.

Assay—Weigh accurately 5 mg of amygdalin for assay 2 and 1 mg of DSS-d_6 for nuclear magnetic resonance spectroscopy using an ultramicrobalance, dissolve in 1 mL of deuterated dimethylsulfoxide for nuclear magnetic reso-

Supplement I, JP XVIII

nance spectroscopy, and use this solution as the sample solution. Transfer the sample solution into an NMR tube 5 mm in outer diameter, and measure ^{1}H-NMR as directed under Nuclear Magnetic Resonance Spectroscopy <2.21> and Crude Drugs Test <5.01> according to the following conditions, using DSS-d_6 for nuclear magnetic resonance spectroscopy as the reference standard for qNMR. Calculate the resonance intensity A (equivalent to 1 hydrogen) of the signal around δ 6.03 ppm assuming the signal of the reference standard for qNMR as δ 0 ppm.

$$\text{Amount (\%) of amygdalin } (C_{20}H_{27}NO_{11})$$
$$= M_S \times I \times P/(M \times N) \times 2.0388$$

M: Amount (mg) of amygdalin for assay 2 taken

M_S: Amount (mg) of DSS-d_6 for nuclear magnetic resonance spectroscopy taken

I: Signal resonance intensity A based on the signal resonance intensity of DSS-d_6 for nuclear magnetic resonance spectroscopy as 9.000

N: Number of the hydrogen derived from A

P: Purity (%) of DSS-d_6 for nuclear magnetic resonance spectroscopy

Operating conditions

Apparatus: A nuclear magnetic resonance spectrometer having ^{1}H resonance frequency of not less than 400 MHz.

Target nucleus: ^{1}H.

Digital resolution: 0.25 Hz or lower.

Measuring spectrum range: 20 ppm or upper, including between -5 ppm and 15 ppm.

Spinning: off.

Pulse angle: 90°.

^{13}C decoupling: on.

Delay time: Repeating pulse waiting time not less than 60 seconds.

Integrating times: 8 or more times.

Dummy scanning: 2 or more times.

Measuring temperature: A constant temperature between 20°C and 30°C.

System suitability

Test for required detectability: When the procedure is run with the sample solution under the above operating conditions, the SN ratio of the signal of around δ 6.03 ppm is not less than 100.

System performance: When the procedure is run with the sample solution under the above operating conditions, the signal of around δ 6.03 ppm is not overlapped with any signal of obvious foreign substances.

System repeatability: When the test is repeated 6 times with the sample solution under the above operating conditions, the relative standard deviation of the ratio of the resonance intensity A to that of the reference standard for qNMR is not more than 1.0%.

Anti-urokinase serum Antiserum obtained from rabbit immunized with Urokinase, which meets the following performance test. Storage at -20°C or lower.

Performance test—Dissolve 1.0 g of agar in 100 mL of boric acid-sodium hydroxide buffer solution (pH 8.4) by

The JP Drugs are to be tested according to the provisions given in the pertinent monographs, General Notices, General Rules for Crude Drugs, General Rules for Preparations, and General Tests for their conformity to the Japanese Pharmacopoeia. (See the General Notices 5.)

Supplement I, JP XVIII

warming, and pour the solution into a Petri dish to make a depth of about 2 mm. After cooling, bore three of a pair-well 2.5 mm in diameter with a space of 6 mm each other. In one of the wells of each pair-well, place 10 μL of antiurokinase serum, and in each another well, place 10 μL of a solution of Urokinase containing 30,000 Units per mL in isotonic sodium chloride solution, 10 μL of human serum and 10 μL of human urine, respectively, and allow to stand overnight: one or two clear precipitin lines appear between anti-urokinase serum and urokinase, and not appears between anti-urokinase serum and human serum or human urine.

Arbutin for assay $C_{12}H_{16}O_7$ Arbutin for thin-layer chromatography. It meets the requirement of the following arbutin for assay 1 or arbutin for assay 2 (Purity value by quantitative NMR). The former is used after drying (in vacuum, silica gel, 12 hours). The latter is used after allowing to stand in a desiccator, whose humidity is adjusted between 57% and 60% RH at 20 to 25°C with sodium bromide-saturated solution, for 24 hours and weighed at 20 to 25°C under 45 to 60% RH, and corrected for its amount based on the result obtained in the Assay 2.

1) Arbutin for assay 1

Absorbance ⟨2.24⟩ $E_{1\,cm}^{1\%}$ (280 nm): 70 – 76 [4 mg, previously dried in a desiccator (in vacuum, silica gel) for 12 hours, water, 100 mL].

Purity Related substances—Dissolve 1 mg of arbutin for assay 1 in 2.5 mL of water, and use this solution as the sample solution. Pipet 1 mL of the sample solution, add water to make exactly 100 mL, and use this solution as the standard solution. Perform the test with exactly 10 μL each of the sample solution and standard solution as directed under Liquid Chromatography ⟨2.01⟩ according to the following conditions, and determine each peak area of the both solutions by the automatic integration method: the total area of the peaks other than arbutin from the sample solution is not larger than the peak area of arbutin from the standard solution.

Operating conditions

Detector: An ultraviolet absorption photometer (wavelength: 280 nm).

Column: A stainless steel column 4.6 mm in inside diameter and 15 cm in length, packed with octadecylsilanized silica gel for liquid chromatography (5 μm in particle diameter).

Column temperature: A constant temperature of about 20°C.

Mobile phase: A mixture of water, methanol and 0.1 mol/L hydrochloric acid TS (94:5:1).

Flow rate: Adjust so that the retention time of arbutin is about 6 minutes.

Time span of measurement: About 3 times as long as the retention time of arbutin, beginning after the solvent peak.

System suitability

Test for required detectability: Pipet 1 mL of the standard solution, and add water to make exactly 20 mL. Confirm that the peak area of arbutin obtained with 10 μL of

this solution is equivalent to 3.5 to 6.5% of that with 10 μL of the standard solution.

System performance: Dissolve 1 mg each of arbutin for assay 1, hydroquinone and gallic acid monohydrate in 2 mL of water. When the procedure is run with 10 μL of this solution under the above operating conditions, arbutin, hydroquinone and gallic acid are eluted in this order, and each resolution between these peaks is not less than 1.5, respectively.

System repeatability: When the test is repeated 6 times with 10 μL of the standard solution under the above operating conditions, the relative standard deviation of the peak area of arbutin is not more than 1.5%.

2) Arbutin for assay 2 (Purity value by quantitative NMR)

Unity of peak—Dissolve 1 mg of arbutin for assay 2 in 2.5 mL of water, and use this solution as the sample solution. Perform the test with 10 μL of the sample solution as directed under Liquid Chromatography ⟨2.01⟩ according to the following conditions, and compare the absorption spectra of at least 3 points including the top of arbutin peak and around the two middle peak heights of before and after the top: no difference in form is observed between their spectra.

Operating conditions

Detector: A photodiode array detector (wavelength: 280 nm, measuring range of spectrum: 220 – 400 nm).

Column: A stainless steel column 4.6 mm in inside diameter and 15 cm in length, packed with octadecylsilanized silica gel for liquid chromatography (5 μm in particle diameter).

Column temperature: A constant temperature of about 20°C.

Mobile phase: A mixture of water, methanol and 0.1 mol/L hydrochloric acid TS (94:5:1).

Flow rate: Adjust so that the retention time of arbutin is about 6 minutes.

System suitability

System performance: Dissolve 1 mg each of arbutin for assay 2, hydroquinone and gallic acid monohydrate in 2 mL of water. When the procedure is run with 10 μL of this solution under the above operating conditions, arbutin, hydroquinone and gallic acid are eluted in this order, and each resolution between these peaks is not less than 1.5, respectively.

Assay—Weigh accurately 1 mg of 1,4-BTMSB-d_4 for nuclear magnetic resonance spectroscopy and 5 mg of arbutin for assay 2, previously allowed to stand in a desiccator, whose humidity is adjusted to 57 to 60% RH at 20 to 25°C with sodium bromide-saturated solution, for 24 hours, at 20 to 25°C under 45 to 60% RH, using an ultramicrobalance, dissolve both in 1 mL of deuterated methanol for nuclear magnetic resonance spectroscopy, and use this solution as the sample solution. Transfer the sample solution into an NMR tube 5 mm in outer diameter, and measure ^{1}H-NMR as directed under Nuclear Magnetic Resonance Spectroscopy ⟨2.21⟩ and Crude Drugs Test ⟨5.01⟩ according to the following conditions, using 1,4-BTMSB-d_4 for nuclear magnetic resonance spectroscopy as the reference standard

The JP Drugs are to be tested according to the provisions given in the pertinent monographs, General Notices, General Rules for Crude Drugs, General Rules for Preparations, and General Tests for their conformity to the Japanese Pharmacopoeia. (See the General Notices 5.)

for qNMR. Calculate the resonance intensities, A_1 (equivalent to 2 hydrogen) and A_2 (equivalent to 2 hydrogen), of the signals around δ 6.44 ppm and δ 6.71 ppm assuming the signal of the reference standard for qNMR as δ 0 ppm.

$$\text{Amount (\%) of arbutin (C}_{12}\text{H}_{16}\text{O}_7)$$
$$= M_S \times I \times P/(M \times N) \times 1.2020$$

M: Amount (mg) of arbutin for assay 2 taken

M_S: Amount (mg) of 1,4-BTMSB-d_4 for nuclear magnetic resonance spectroscopy taken

I: Sum of the signal resonance intensities, A_1 and A_2, based on the signal resonance intensity of 1,4-BTMSB-d_4 for nuclear magnetic resonance spectroscopy as 18.000

N: Sum of number of the hydrogen derived from A_1 and A_2

P: Purity (%) of 1,4-BTMSB-d_4 for nuclear magnetic resonance spectroscopy

Operating conditions

Apparatus: A nuclear magnetic resonance spectrometer having ^{1}H resonance frequency of not less than 400 MHz.

Target nucleus: ^{1}H.

Digital resolution: 0.25 Hz or lower.

Measuring spectrum range: 20 ppm or upper, including between -5 ppm and 15 ppm.

Spinning: off.

Pulse angle: 90°.

^{13}C decoupling: on.

Delay time: Repeating pulse waiting time not less than 60 seconds.

Integrating times: 8 or more times.

Dummy scanning: 2 or more times.

Measuring temperature: A constant temperature between 20°C and 30°C.

System suitability

Test for required detectability: When the procedure is run with the sample solution under the above operating conditions, the SN ratios of the signals of around δ 6.44 ppm and δ 6.71 ppm are not less than 100.

System performance: When the procedure is run with the sample solution under the above operating conditions, the signal of around δ 6.44 ppm and δ 6.71 ppm are not overlapped with any signal of obvious foreign substance, and the ratio of the resonance intensities, A_1/A_2, is between 0.99 and 1.01.

System repeatability: When the test is repeated 6 times with the sample solution under the above operating conditions, the relative standard deviation of the ratio of the resonance intensity, A_1 or A_2, to that of the reference standard for qNMR is not more than 1.0%.

Benzyl parahydroxybenzoate $C_{14}H_{12}O_3$ White, fine crystals or crystalline powder. Freely soluble in ethanol (95), and very slightly soluble in water.

Melting point <2.60>: 109 – 114°C

Content: not less than 99.0%. Assay—Weigh accurately about 1 g of benzyl parahydroxybenzoate, add exactly 20 mL of 1 mol/L sodium hydroxide VS, heat at about 70°C for 1 hour, and immediately cool in ice. Titrate <2.50> the excess sodium hydroxide with 0.5 mol/L sulfuric acid VS up to the second equivalent point (potentiometric titration). Perform a blank determination in the same manner.

Each mL of 1 mol/L sodium hydroxide VS
= 228.2 mg of $C_{14}H_{12}O_3$

Dehydrocorydaline nitrate for assay $C_{22}H_{24}N_2O_7$ Dehydrocorydaline nitrate for thin-layer chromatography. It meets the requirement of the following dehydrocorydaline nitrate for assay 1 or dehydrocorydaline nitrate for assay 2 (Purity value by quantitative NMR). The former is used after drying in a desiccator (silica gel) for 1 hours, and the latter is used with correction for its amount based on the result obtained in the Assay 2.

1) Dehydrocorydaline nitrate for assay 1

Absorbance <2.24> $E_{1\,\text{cm}}^{1\%}$ (333 nm): 577 – 642 (3 mg, water, 500 mL). Use the sample dried in a desiccator (silica gel) for not less than 1 hour for the test.

Purity Related substances—Dissolve 5.0 mg of dehydrocorydaline nitrate for assay 1 in 10 mL of the mobile phase, and use this solution as the sample solution. Pipet 1 mL of the sample solution, add the mobile phase to make exactly 100 mL, and use this solution as the standard solution. Perform the test with exactly 5 μL each of the sample solution and standard solution as directed under Liquid Chromatography <2.01> according to the following conditions, and determine each peak area by the automatic integration method: the total area of the peaks other than dehydrocorydaline obtained from the sample solution is not larger than the peak area of dehydrocorydaline from the standard solution.

Operating conditions

Column, column temperature, mobile phase, and flow rate: Proceed as directed in the operating conditions in the Assay under Corydalis Tuber.

Detector: An ultraviolet absorption photometer (wavelength: 230 nm).

Time span of measurement: About 3 times as long as the retention time of dehydrocorydaline, beginning after the peak of nitric acid.

System suitability

Test for required detectability: Pipet 1 mL of the standard solution, and add the mobile phase to make exactly 20 mL. Confirm that the peak area of dehydrocorydaline obtained with 5 μL of this solution is equivalent to 3.5 to 6.5% of that with 5 μL of the standard solution.

System performance: Dissolve 1 mg each of dehydrocorydaline nitrate for assay 1 and berberine chloride hydrate in 20 mL of a mixture of water and acetonitrile (20:9). When the procedure is run with 5 μL of this solution under the above operating conditions, berberine and dehydrocorydaline are eluted in this order with the resolution between these peaks being not less than 1.5.

System repeatability: When the test is repeated 6 times with 5 μL of the standard solution under the above operating conditions, the relative standard deviation of the peak area of dehydrocorydaline is not more than 1.5%.

The JP Drugs are to be tested according to the provisions given in the pertinent monographs, General Notices, General Rules for Crude Drugs, General Rules for Preparations, and General Tests for their conformity to the Japanese Pharmacopoeia. (See the General Notices 5.)

Supplement I, JP XVIII *General Tests, Processes and Apparatus* 2837

2) Dehydrocorydaline nitrate for assay 2 (Purity value by quantitative NMR)

Unity of peak—Dissolve 1 mg of dehydrocorydaline nitrate for assay 2 in 2 mL of a mixture of methanol and dilute hydrochloric acid (3:1), and use this solution as the sample solution. Perform the test with 5 μL of the sample solution as directed under Liquid Chromatography <2.01> according to the following conditions, and compare the absorption spectra of at least 3 points including the top of dehydrocorydaline peak and around the two middle peak heights of before and after the top: no difference in form is observed among their spectra.

Operating conditions

Column, column temperature, mobile phase, and flow rate: Proceed as directed in the operating conditions in the Assay under Corydalis Tuber.

Detector: A photodiode array detector (wavelength: 230 nm, spectrum range of measurement: 220 – 400 nm).

System suitability

System performance: Dissolve 1 mg each of dehydrocorydaline nitrate for assay 2 and berberine chloride hydrate in 20 mL of a mixture of water and acetonitrile (20:9). When the procedure is run with 5 μL of this solution under the above operating conditions, berberine and dehydrocorydaline are eluted in this order with the resolution between these peaks being not less than 1.5.

Assay—Weigh accurately 5 mg of dehydrocorydaline nitrate for assay 2 and 1 mg of DDS-d_6 for nuclear magnetic resonance spectroscopy using an ultramicrobalance, dissolve both in 1 mL of deuterated dimethylsulfoxide for nuclear magnetic resonance spectroscopy, and use this solution as the sample solution. Transfer the sample solution into an NMR tube 5 mm in outer diameter, and measure ^{1}H-NMR as directed under Nuclear Magnetic Resonance Spectroscopy <2.21> and Crude Drugs Test <5.01> according to the following conditions, using DDS-d_6 for nuclear magnetic resonance spectroscopy as the reference standard for qNMR. Calculate the resonance intensity, A (equivalent to 1 hydrogen) of the signal around δ 7.42 ppm assuming the signal of the reference standard for qNMR as δ 0 ppm.

Amount (%) of dehydrocorydaline nitrate ($C_{22}H_{24}N_2O_7$)
$$= M_S \times I \times P/(M \times N) \times 1.9096$$

M: Amount (mg) of dehydrocorydaline nitrate for assay 2 taken

M_S: Amount (mg) of DDS-d_6 for nuclear magnetic resonance spectroscopy taken

I: Signal resonance intensity A based on the signal resonance intensity of DDS-d_6 for nuclear magnetic resonance spectroscopy as 9.000

N: Number of the hydrogen derived from A

P: Purity (%) of DDS-d_6 for nuclear magnetic resonance spectroscopy

Operating conditions

Apparatus: A nuclear magnetic resonance spectrometer having ^{1}H resonance frequency of not less than 400 MHz.

Target nucleus: ^{1}H.

Digital resolution: 0.25 Hz or lower.

Measuring spectrum range: 20 ppm or upper, including between -5 ppm and 15 ppm.

Spinning: off.

Pulse angle: 90°.

^{13}C decoupling: on.

Delay time: Repeating pulse waiting time not less than 60 seconds.

Integrating times: 8 or more times.

Dummy scanning: 2 or more times.

Measuring temperature: A constant temperature between 20°C and 30°C.

System suitability

Test for required detectability: When the procedure is run with the sample solution under the above operating conditions, the SN ratio of the signal around δ 7.42 ppm is not less than 100.

System performance: When the procedure is run with the sample solution under the above operating conditions, the signal around δ 7.42 ppm is not overlapped with any signal of obvious foreign substances.

System repeatability: When the test is repeated 6 times with the sample solution under the above operating conditions, the relative standard deviation of the ratio of the resonance intensity A to that of the reference standard for qNMR is not more than 1.0%.

Dehydrocorydaline nitrate for thin-layer chromatography $C_{22}H_{24}N_2O_7$ Yellow, crystals or crystalline powder. Sparingly soluble in methanol, and slightly soluble in water and in ethanol (99.5). Melting point: about 240°C (with decomposition).

Purity Related substances—Dissolve 5.0 mg of dehydrocorydaline nitrate for thin-layer chromatography in 1 mL of a mixture of water and methanol (1:1), and use this solution as the sample solution. Pipet 0.5 mL of the sample solution, add a mixture of water and methanol (1:1) to make exactly 50 mL, and use this solution as the standard solution. Perform the test with these solutions as directed under Thin-layer Chromatography <2.03>. Spot 5 μL each of the sample solution and standard solution on a plate of silica gel for thin-layer chromatography. Develop immediately with a mixture of methanol, a solution of ammonium acetate (3 in 10) and acetic acid (100) (20:1:1) to a distance of about 10 cm, and air-dry the plate. Spray evenly Dragendorff's TS on the plate, air-dry the plate, and then spray evenly sodium nitrite TS: the spot other than the principal spot obtained from the sample solution is not more intense than the spot from the standard solution.

Diphenyl sulfone for assay $C_{12}H_{10}O_2S$ White, crystals or crystalline powder. It dissolves in dimethylsulfoxide.

It is used after correcting with the amount of diphenyl sulfone obtained in the Assay.

Identification—Proceed as directed in the Assay: it exhibits a triplet-like signal equivalent to 4 protons around δ 7.65 ppm, a triplet-like signal equivalent to 2 protons around δ 7.73 ppm, and a doublet-like signal equivalent to 4 protons around δ 7.99 ppm.

The JP Drugs are to be tested according to the provisions given in the pertinent monographs, General Notices, General Rules for Crude Drugs, General Rules for Preparations, and General Tests for their conformity to the Japanese Pharmacopoeia. (See the General Notices 5.)

General Tests, Processes and Apparatus

Unity of peak—Dissolve 10 mg of diphenyl sulfone for assay in 100 mL of methanol. To 10 mL of this solution add methanol to make 100 mL, and use this solution as the sample solution. Perform the test with 10 μL of the sample solution as directed under Liquid Chromatography <2.01> according to the following conditions, and compare the absorption spectra of at least 3 points including the top of diphenyl sulfone peak and around the two middle peak heights of before and after the top: no difference in form is observed between their spectra.

Operating conditions

Column, column temperature, mobile phase, and flow rate: Proceed as directed in the operating conditions in the Assay under Perilla Herb.

Detector: A photodiode array detector (wavelength: 234 nm, spectrum range of measurement: 220 – 400 nm).

System suitability

System performance: Dissolve 1 mg each of (E)-asarone and perillaldehyde for thin-layer chromatography in the sample solution to make 50 mL. When the procedure is run with 10 μL of this solution under the above operating conditions, diphenyl sulfone, perillaldehyde and (E)-asarone are eluted in this order with the resolutions between these peaks being not less than 1.5.

The unity of peak is unnecessary if the content (%) of diphenyl sulfone ($C_{12}H_{10}O_2S$) is between 99.5% and 100.5%.

Assay—Weigh accurately 5 mg of diphenyl sulfone for assay and 1 mg of DSS-d_6 for nuclear magnetic resonance spectroscopy using an ultramicrobalance, dissolve in 2 mL of deuterated dimethylsulfoxide for nuclear magnetic resonance spectroscopy, and use this solution as the sample solution. Transfer the sample solution into an NMR tube 5 mm in outer diameter, measure ^{1}H-NMR as directed under Nuclear Magnetic Resonance Spectroscopy <2.21> and Crude Drugs Test <5.01> according to the following conditions, using DSS-d_6 for nuclear magnetic resonance spectroscopy as the reference standard for qNMR. Calculate the resonance intensities, A_1 (equivalent to 6 hydrogens) and A_2 (equivalent to 4 hydrogens), of the signals around δ 7.64 – 7.74 ppm and δ 7.98 – 8.01 ppm assuming the signal of the reference standard for qNMR as δ 0 ppm.

$$\text{Amount (\%) of diphenyl sulfone } (C_{12}H_{10}O_2S)$$
$$= M_S \times I \times P/(M \times N) \times 0.9729$$

M: Amount (mg) of diphenyl sulfone for assay taken

M_S: Amount (mg) of DSS-d_6 for nuclear magnetic resonance spectroscopy taken

I: Sum of the signal resonance intensities, A_1 and A_2, based on the signal resonance intensity of DSS-d_6 for nuclear magnetic resonance spectroscopy as 9.000

N: Sum of numbers of the hydrogen derived from A_1 and A_2

P: Purity (%) of DSS-d_6 for nuclear magnetic resonance spectroscopy

Operating conditions

Apparatus: An apparatus of nuclear magnetic resonance spectrum measurement having ^{1}H resonance frequency of not less than 400 MHz.

Target nucleus: ^{1}H.

Digital resolution: 0.25 Hz or lower.

Measuring spectrum range: 20 ppm or upper, including between −5 ppm and 15 ppm.

Spinning: off.

Pulse angle: 90°.

^{13}C decoupling: on.

Delay time: Repeating pulse waiting time not less than 60 seconds.

Integrating times: 8 or more times.

Dummy scanning: 2 or more times.

Measuring temperature: A constant temperature between 20°C and 30°C.

System suitability

Test for required detectability: When the procedure is run with the sample solution under the above operating conditions, the SN ratio of each signal around δ 7.64 – 7.74 ppm and δ 7.98 – 8.01 ppm is not less than 100.

System performance: When the procedure is run with the sample solution under the above operating conditions, the signals around δ 7.64 – 7.74 ppm and δ 7.98 – 8.01 ppm are not overlapped with any signal of obvious foreign substance, and the ratio of the resonance intensities, $(A_1/6)/(A_2/4)$, of each signal around δ 7.64 – 7.74 ppm and δ 7.98 – 8.01 ppm is between 0.99 and 1.01, respectively.

System repeatability: When the test is repeated 6 times with the sample solution under the above operating conditions, the relative standard deviation of the ratio of the resonance intensity, A_1 or A_2, to that of the reference standard for qNMR are not more than 1.0%.

[6]-Gingerol for assay $C_{17}H_{26}O_4$ [6]-Gingerol for thin-layer chromatography. It meets the following additional requirements. It is used with correction for its amount based on the result obtained in the Assay.

Unity of peak—Dissolve 5 mg of [6]-gingerol for assay in 5 mL of methanol, and use this solution as the sample solution. Perform the test with 10 μL of the sample solution as directed under Liquid Chromatography <2.01> according to the following conditions, and compare the absorption spectra of at least 3 points including the top of [6]-gingerol peak and around the two middle peak heights of before and after the top: no difference in form is observed among their spectra.

Operating conditions

Column, column temperature, mobile phase, and flow rate: Proceed as directed in the operating conditions in the Assay (3) under Hangekobokuto Extract.

Detector: A photodiode array detector (wavelength: 282 nm, measuring range of spectrum: 220 – 400 nm).

System suitability

System performance: When the procedure is run with 10 μL of the sample solution under the above operating conditions, the number of theoretical plates and the symmetry factor of the peak of [6]-gingerol are not less than 5000 and not more than 1.5, respectively.

The JP Drugs are to be tested according to the provisions given in the pertinent monographs, General Notices, General Rules for Crude Drugs, General Rules for Preparations, and General Tests for their conformity to the Japanese Pharmacopoeia. (See the General Notices 5.)

Supplement I, JP XVIII | *General Tests, Processes and Apparatus* 2839

Assay—Weigh accurately 5 mg of [6]-gingerol for assay and 1 mg of 1,4-BTMSB-d_4 for nuclear magnetic resonance spectroscopy using an ultramicrobalance, dissolve both in 1 mL of deuterated methanol for nuclear magnetic resonance spectroscopy, and use this solution as the sample solution. Transfer the sample solution into an NMR tube 5 mm in outer diameter, and measure ^{1}H-NMR as directed under Nuclear Magnetic Resonance Spectroscopy <2.21> and Crude Drugs Test <5.01> according to the following conditions, using 1,4-BTMSB-d_4 for nuclear magnetic resonance spectroscopy as the reference standard for qNMR. Calculate the resonance intensities, A_1 (equivalent to 3 hydrogens) and A_2 (equivalent to 1 hydrogen), of the signals around δ 3.56 ppm and δ 6.52 ppm assuming the signal of the reference standard for qNMR as δ 0 ppm.

$$\text{Amount (\%) of [6]-gingerol } (C_{17}H_{26}O_4)$$
$$= M_S \times I \times P/(M \times N) \times 1.2997$$

M: Amount (mg) of [6]-gingerol for assay taken

M_S: Amount (mg) of 1,4-BTMSB-d_4 for nuclear magnetic resonance spectroscopy taken

I: Sum of the signal resonance intensities, A_1 and A_2, based on the signal resonance intensity of 1,4-BTMSB-d_4 for nuclear magnetic resonance spectroscopy as 18.000

N: Sum of the numbers of the hydrogen derived from A_1 and A_2

P: Purity (%) of 1,4-BTMSB-d_4 for nuclear magnetic resonance spectroscopy

Operating conditions

Apparatus: A nuclear magnetic resonance spectrometer having ^{1}H resonance frequency of not less than 400 MHz.

Target nucleus: ^{1}H.

Digital resolution: 0.25 Hz or lower.

Measuring spectrum range: 20 ppm or upper, including between -5 ppm and 15 ppm.

Spinning: off.

Pulse angle: 90°.

^{13}C decoupling: on.

Delay time: Repeating pulse waiting time not less than 60 seconds.

Integrating times: 8 or more times.

Dummy scanning: 2 or more times.

Measuring temperature: A constant temperature between 20°C and 30°C.

System suitability

Test for required detectability: When the procedure is run with the sample solution under the above operating conditions, the SN ratio of each signal around δ 3.56 ppm and δ 6.52 ppm is not less than 100.

System performance: When the procedure is run with the sample solution under the above operating conditions, the signals around δ 3.56 ppm and δ 6.52 ppm are not overlapped with any signal of obvious foreign substance, and the ratio of the resonance intensities, $(A_1/3)/A_2$, of each signal around δ 3.56 ppm and δ 6.52 ppm is between 0.99 and 1.01.

System repeatability: When the test is repeated 6 times with the sample solution under the above operating conditions, the relative standard deviation of the ratio of the resonance intensity, A_1 or A_2, to that of the reference standard for qNMR is not more than 1.0%.

Hirsutine for assay $C_{22}H_{28}N_2O_3$ Hirsutine for thin-layer chromatography. It meets the requirement of the following hirsutine for assay 1 or hirsutine for assay 2 (Purity value by quantitative NMR). Hirsutine for assay 2 is used with correction for its amount based on the result obtained in the Assay 2.

1) Hirsutine for assay 1

Absorbance <2.24>: $E_{1\,cm}^{1\%}$ (245 nm): 354 – 389 (5 mg calculated on the anhydrous basis, a mixture of methanol and dilute acetic acid (7:3), 500 mL).

Purity Related substances—Dissolve 5 mg of hirsutine for assay 1 in 100 mL of a mixture of methanol and dilute acetic acid (7:3), use this solution as the sample solution. Pipet 1 mL of the sample solution, add a mixture of methanol and dilute acetic acid (7:3) to make exactly 50 mL, and use this solution as the standard solution. Perform the test with exactly 20 μL each of the sample solution and standard solution as directed under Liquid-chromatography <2.01> according to the following conditions. Determine each peak area by the automatic integration method: the total area of the peaks other than hirsutine obtained from the sample solution is not larger than the peak area of hirsutine from the standard solution.

Operating conditions

Detector, column, column temperature, mobile phase, and flow rate: Proceed as directed in the operating conditions in the Assay under Uncaria Hook.

Time span of measurement: About 1.5 times as long as the retention time of hirsutine, beginning after the solvent peak.

System suitability

Test for required detectability: Pipet 1 mL of the standard solution, add a mixture of methanol and dilute acetic acid (7:3) to make exactly 20 mL. Confirm that the peak area of hirsutine obtained with 20 μL of this solution is equivalent to 3.5 to 6.5% of that with 20 μL of the standard solution.

System performance: Dissolve 1 mg of rhynchophylline for assay in 20 mL of a mixture of methanol and dilute acetic acid (7:3). To 5 mL of this solution add 1 mL of ammonia solution (28), and warm at about 50°C for 2 hours or heat under a reflux condenser for 10 minutes. After cooling, to 1 mL of the reaction solution add a mixture of methanol and dilute acetic acid (7:3) to make 5 mL. When the procedure is run with 20 μL of this solution under the above operating conditions, the peak of isorhynchophylline is observed in addition to the peak of rhynchophylline, and the resolution between these peaks is not less than 1.5.

System repeatability: When the test is repeated 6 times with 20 μL of the standard solution under the above operating conditions, the relative standard deviation of the peak area of hirsutine is not more than 1.5%.

The JP Drugs are to be tested according to the provisions given in the pertinent monographs, General Notices, General Rules for Crude Drugs, General Rules for Preparations, and General Tests for their conformity to the Japanese Pharmacopoeia. (See the General Notices 5.)

2840 General Tests, Processes and Apparatus

2) Hirsutine for assay 2 (Purity value by quantitative NMR)

Unity of peak—Dissolve 1 mg of hirsutine for assay 2 in 20 mL of a mixture of methanol and dilute acetic acid (7:3), and use this solution as the sample solution. Perform the test with 20 μL of the sample solution as directed under Liquid Chromatography <2.01> according to the following conditions, and compare the absorption spectra of at least 3 points including the top of hirsutine peak and around the two middle peak heights of before and after the top: no difference in form is observed among their spectra.
Operating conditions

Column, column temperature, mobile phase, and flow rate: Proceed as directed in the operating conditions in the Assay under Uncaria Hook.

Detector: A photodiode array detector (wavelength: 245 nm, spectrum range of measurement: 220 – 400 nm).
System suitability

System performance: Dissolve 1 mg of rhynchophylline for assay in 20 mL of a mixture of methanol and dilute acetic acid (7:3). To 5 mL of this solution add 1 mL of ammonia solution (28), and warm at about 50°C for 2 hours or heat under a reflux condenser for 10 minutes. After cooling, to 1 mL of the reaction solution add a mixture of methanol and dilute acetic acid (7:3) to make 5 mL. When the procedure is run with 20 μL of this solution under the above operating conditions, the peak of isorhynchophylline is observed in addition to the peak of rhynchophylline, and the resolution between these peaks is not less than 1.5.

Assay—Weigh accurately 5 mg of hirsutine for assay 2 and 1 mg of 1,4-BTMSB-d_4 for nuclear magnetic resonance spectroscopy using an ultramicrobalance, dissolve both in 1 mL of deuterated acetone for nuclear magnetic resonance spectroscopy, and use this solution as the sample solution. Transfer the sample solution into an NMR tube 5 mm in outer diameter, and measure ^{1}H-NMR as directed under Nuclear Magnetic Resonance Spectroscopy <2.21> and Crude Drugs Test <5.01> according to the following conditions, using 1,4-BTMSB-d_4 for nuclear magnetic resonance spectroscopy as the reference standard for qNMR. Calculate the resonance intensity A (equivalent to 2 hydrogens) of the signal around δ 6.70 – δ 6.79 ppm assuming the signal of the reference standard for qNMR as δ 0 ppm.

$$\text{Amount (\%) of hirsutine } (C_{22}H_{28}N_2O_3)$$
$$= M_S \times I \times P/(M \times N) \times 1.6268$$

M: Amount (mg) of hirsutine for assay 2 taken

M_S: Amount (mg) of 1,4-BTMSB-d_4 for nuclear magnetic resonance spectroscopy taken

I: Signal resonance intensity A based on the signal resonance intensity of 1,4-BTMSB-d_4 for nuclear magnetic resonance spectroscopy as 18.000

N: Number of the hydrogen derived from A

P: Purity (%) of 1,4-BTMSB-d_4 for nuclear magnetic resonance spectroscopy

Operating conditions

Apparatus: A nuclear magnetic resonance spectrometer having ^{1}H resonance frequency of not less than 400 MHz.

Target nucleus: ^{1}H.

Digital resolution: 0.25 Hz or lower.

Measuring spectrum range: 20 ppm or upper, including between -5 ppm and 15 ppm.

Spinning: off.

Pulse angle: 90°.

^{13}C decoupling: on.

Delay time: Repeating pulse waiting time not less than 60 seconds.

Integrating times: 8 or more times.

Dummy scanning: 2 or more times.

Measuring temperature: A constant temperature between 20°C and 30°C.
System suitability

Test for required detectability: When the procedure is run with the sample solution under the above operating conditions, the SN ratio of the signal around δ 6.70 – δ 6.79 ppm is not less than 100.

System performance: When the procedure is run with the sample solution under the above operating conditions, the signal around δ 6.70 – δ 6.79 ppm is not overlapped with any signal of obvious foreign substances.

System repeatability: When the test is repeated 6 times with the sample solution under the above operating conditions, the relative standard deviation of the ratio of the resonance intensity A to that of the reference standard for qNMR is not more than 1.0%.

Loganin for assay $C_{17}H_{26}O_{10}$ Loganin for thin-layer chromatography. It meets the following additional requirements. It is used with correction for its amount based on the result obtained in the Assay.

Unity of peak—Dissolve 2 mg of loganin for assay in 5 mL of the mobile phase, and use this solution as the sample solution. Perform the test with 10 μL of the sample solution as directed under Liquid Chromatography <2.01> according to the following conditions, and compare the absorption spectra of at least 3 points including the top of loganin peak and around the two middle peak heights of before and after the top: no difference in form is observed among their spectra.
Operating conditions

Column, column temperature, mobile phase, and flow rate: Proceed as directed in the operating conditions in the Assay (1) under Goshajinkigan Extract.

Detector: A photodiode array detector (wavelength: 238 nm, spectrum range of measurement: 220 – 400 nm).
System suitability

System performance: When the procedure is run with 10 μL of the sample solution under the above operating conditions, the number of theoretical plates and the symmetry factor of the peak of loganin are not less than 5000 and not more than 1.5, respectively.

Assay—Weigh accurately 5 mg of loganin for assay and 1 mg of 1,4-BTMSB-d_4 for nuclear magnetic resonance spectroscopy using an ultramicrobalance, dissolve in 1 mL of deuterated methanol for nuclear magnetic resonance spec-

The JP Drugs are to be tested according to the provisions given in the pertinent monographs, General Notices, General Rules for Crude Drugs, General Rules for Preparations, and General Tests for their conformity to the Japanese Pharmacopoeia. (See the General Notices 5.)

Supplement I, JP XVIII

troscopy, and use this solution as the sample solution. Transfer the sample solution into an NMR tube 5 mm in outer diameter, and measure ^{1}H-NMR as directed under Nuclear Magnetic Resonance Spectroscopy <2.21> and Crude Drugs Test <5.01> according to the following conditions, using 1,4-BTMSB-d_4 for nuclear magnetic resonance spectroscopy as the reference standard for qNMR. Calculate the resonance intensity A (equivalent to 1 hydrogen) of the signal around δ 7.14 ppm assuming the signal of the reference standard for qNMR as δ 0 ppm.

$$\text{Amount (\%) of loganin } (C_{17}H_{26}O_{10})$$
$$= M_S \times I \times P/(M \times N) \times 1.7235$$

M: Amount (mg) of loganin for assay taken

M_S: Amount (mg) of 1,4-BTMSB-d_4 for nuclear magnetic resonance spectroscopy taken

I: Signal resonance intensity A based on the signal resonance intensity of 1,4-BTMSB-d_4 for nuclear magnetic resonance spectroscopy as 18.000

N: Number of the hydrogen derived from A

P: Purity (%) of 1,4-BTMSB-d_4 for nuclear magnetic resonance spectroscopy

Operating conditions

Apparatus: A nuclear magnetic resonance spectrometer having ^{1}H resonance frequency of not less than 400 MHz.

Target nucleus: ^{1}H.

Digital resolution: 0.25 Hz or lower.

Measuring spectrum range: 20 ppm or upper, including between -5 ppm and 15 ppm.

Spinning: off.

Pulse angle: 90°.

^{13}C decoupling: on.

Delay time: Repeating pulse waiting time not less than 60 seconds.

Integrating times: 8 or more times.

Dummy scanning: 2 or more times.

Measuring temperature: A constant temperature between 20°C and 30°C.

System suitability

Test for required detectability: When the procedure is run with the sample solution under the above operating conditions, the SN ratio of each signal around δ 5.02 ppm and δ 7.14 ppm is not less than 100.

System performance: When the procedure is run with the sample solution under the above operating conditions, the two signals around δ 5.02 ppm and δ 7.14 ppm are not overlapped with any signal of obvious foreign substance. Furthermore, when determined the resonance intensities A_1 and A, both equivalent to 1 hydrogen, of each signal around δ 5.02 ppm and δ 7.14 ppm, the ratio of them, A_1/A, is between 0.99 and 1.01.

System repeatability: When the test is repeated 6 times with the sample solution under the above operating conditions, the relative standard deviation of the ratio of the resonance intensity A to that of the reference standard for qNMR is not more than 1.0%.

Plantago seed for thin-layer chromatography [Same as

the monograph Plantago Seed meeting the following additional specifications.]

Identification (1) To 1 g of pulverized plantago seed for thin-layer chromatography add 3 mL of methanol, and warm on a water bath for 3 minutes. After cooling, centrifuge, and use the supernatant liquid as the sample solution. Perform the test with the sample solution as directed under Thin-layer Chromatography <2.03>. Spot 10 μL of the sample solution on a plate of silica gel for thin-layer chromatography. Develop the plate with a mixture of acetone, ethyl acetate, water and acetic acid (100) (10:10:3:1) to a distance of about 10 cm, and air-dry the plate. Splay evenly 4-methoxybenzaldehyde-sulfuric acid TS on the plate, heat the plate at 105°C for 10 minutes: spots equivalent to those described below appear.

Rf value	Color and shape of the spot
Around 0	A strong spot, very dark blue
Around 0.08	A very dark blue spot
Around 0.1 – 0.2	A leading spot, very dark blue
Around 0.25	A strong spot, deep blue (corresponding to plantagoguanidinic acid)
Around 0.35	A strong spot, dark grayish blue (corresponding to geniposidic acid)
Around 0.45	A weak spot, grayish yellowish green
Around 0.50	A strong spot, deep yellow-green (corresponding to verbascoside)
Around 0.6	A weak spot, light blue
Around 0.85	A deep blue spot
Around 0.9 – 0.95	A tailing spot, grayish blue

(2) Proceed with the sample solution obtained in (1) as directed in the method under (1), except using a mixture of ethyl acetate, water and formic acid (6:1:1) as developing solvent: spots equivalent to those described below appear.

Rf value	Color and shape of the spot
Around 0	A yellow-greenish dark gray spot
Around 0.05	A weak spot, dark grayish yellow-green
Around 0.2	A weak spot, dark green
Around 0.25	A strong spot, dark reddish purple (corresponding to geniposidic acid)
Around 0.35	A weak spot, bright blue
Around 0.4 – 0.45	A weak tailing spot, dull greenish blue
Around 0.45	A strong spot, deep yellow-green (corresponding to verbascoside)
Around 0.5	A strong spot, deep blue (corresponding to plantagoguanidinic acid)
Around 0.95	A strong spot, dark grayish blue-green
Around 0.97	A dark grayish blue-green spot

Rhynchophylline for assay $C_{22}H_{28}N_2O_4$ Rhynchophylline for thin-layer chromatography. It meets the require-

The JP Drugs are to be tested according to the provisions given in the pertinent monographs, General Notices, General Rules for Crude Drugs, General Rules for Preparations, and General Tests for their conformity to the Japanese Pharmacopoeia. (See the General Notices 5.)

2842   *General Tests, Processes and Apparatus*   *Supplement I, JP XVIII*

ment of the following rhynchophylline for assay 1 or rhynchophylline for assay 2 (Purity value by quantitative NMR). Rhynchophylline for assay 2 is used with correction for its amount based on the result obtained in the Assay 2.

1) Rhynchophylline for assay 1

Absorbance <2.24>: $E_{1 cm}^{1\%}$ (245 nm): 473 – 502 (5 mg, a mixture of methanol and dilute acetic acid (7:3), 500 mL).

Purity Related substances—Dissolve 5 mg of rhynchophylline for assay 1 in 100 mL of a mixture of methanol and dilute acetic acid (7:3), and use this solution as the sample solution. Pipet 1 mL of the sample solution, add a mixture of methanol and dilute acetic acid (7:3) to make exactly 100 mL, and use this solution as the standard solution. Perform the test with exactly 20 µL each of the sample solution and standard solution as directed under Liquid-chromatography <2.01> according to the following conditions. Determine the peak area of each solution by the automatic integration method: the total area of the peaks other than rhynchophylline obtained from the sample solution is not larger than the peak area of rhynchophylline from the standard solution.

Operating conditions

Detector, column, column temperature, mobile phase, and flow rate: Proceed as directed in the operating conditions in the Assay under Uncaria Hook.

Time span of measurement: About 4 times as long as the retention time of rhynchophylline, beginning after the solvent peak.

System suitability

Test for required detectability: Pipet 1 mL of the standard solution, add a mixture of methanol and dilute acetic acid (7:3) to make exactly 20 mL. Confirm that the peak area of rhynchophylline obtained with 20 µL of this solution is equivalent to 3.5 to 6.5% of that with 20 µL of the standard solution.

System performance: To 5 mL of the sample solution add 1 mL of ammonia solution (28), and warm at about 50°C for 2 hours or heat under a reflux condenser for 10 minutes. After cooling, to 1 mL of the reaction solution add a mixture of methanol and dilute acetic acid (7:3) to make 5 mL. When the procedure is run with 20 µL of this solution under the above operating conditions, the peak of isorhynchophylline is observed in addition to the peak of rhynchophylline, and the resolution between these peaks is not less than 1.5.

System repeatability: When the test is repeated 6 times with 20 µL of the standard solution under the above operating conditions, the relative standard deviation of the peak area of rhynchophylline is not more than 1.5%.

2) Rhynchophylline for assay 2 (Purity value by quantitative NMR)

Unity of peak—Dissolve 1 mg of rhynchophylline for assay 2 in 100 mL of a mixture of methanol and dilute acetic acid (7:3), and use this solution as the sample solution. Perform the test with 20 µL of the sample solution as directed under Liquid Chromatography <2.01> according to the following conditions, and compare the absorption spectra of at least 3 points including the top of rhynchophylline peak and

around the two middle peak heights of before and after the top: no difference in form is observed among their spectra.

Operating conditions

Column, column temperature, mobile phase, and flow rate: Proceed as directed in the operating conditions in the Assay under Uncaria Hook.

Detector: A photodiode array detector (wavelength: 245 nm, spectrum range of measurement: 220 – 400 nm).

System suitability

System performance: Dissolve 1 mg of rhynchophylline for assay 2 in 20 mL of a mixture of methanol and dilute acetic acid (7:3). To 5 mL of this solution add 1 mL of ammonia solution (28), and warm at about 50°C for 2 hours or heat under a reflux condenser for 10 minutes. After cooling, to 1 mL of the reaction solution add a mixture of methanol and dilute acetic acid (7:3) to make 5 mL. When the procedure is run with 20 µL of this solution under the above operating conditions, the peak of isorhynchophylline is observed in addition to the peak of rhynchophylline, and the resolution between these peaks is not less than 1.5.

Assay—Weigh accurately 5 mg of rhynchophylline for assay 2 and 1 mg of 1,4-BTMSB-d_4 for nuclear magnetic resonance spectroscopy using an ultramicrobalance, dissolve both in 1 mL of deuterated acetone for nuclear magnetic resonance spectroscopy, and use this solution as the sample solution. Transfer the sample solution into an NMR tube 5 mm in outer diameter, and measure ^{1}H-NMR as directed under Nuclear Magnetic Resonance Spectroscopy <2.21> and Crude Drugs Test <5.01> according to the following conditions, using 1,4-BTMSB-d_4 for nuclear magnetic resonance spectroscopy as the reference standard for qNMR. Calculate the resonance intensities, A_1 (equivalent to 1 hydrogen) and A_2 (equivalent to 1 hydrogen), of the signals around δ 6.60 ppm and δ 6.73 ppm assuming the signal of the reference standard for qNMR as δ 0 ppm.

$$\text{Amount (\%) of rhynchophylline } (C_{22}H_{28}N_2O_4)$$
$$= M_S \times I \times P/(M \times N) \times 1.6974$$

M: Amount (mg) of rhynchophylline for assay 2 taken

M_S: Amount (mg) of 1,4-BTMSB-d_4 for nuclear magnetic resonance spectroscopy taken

I: Sum of the signal resonance intensities, A_1 and A_2, based on the signal resonance intensity of 1,4-BTMSB-d_4 for nuclear magnetic resonance spectroscopy as 18.000

N: Sum of the numbers of the hydrogen derived from A_1 and A_2

P: Purity (%) of 1,4-BTMSB-d_4 for nuclear magnetic resonance spectroscopy

Operating conditions

Apparatus: A nuclear magnetic resonance spectrometer having ^{1}H resonance frequency of not less than 400 MHz.

Target nucleus: ^{1}H.

Digital resolution: 0.25 Hz or lower.

Measuring spectrum range: 20 ppm or upper, including between −5 ppm and 15 ppm.

Spinning: off.

The JP Drugs are to be tested according to the provisions given in the pertinent monographs, General Notices, General Rules for Crude Drugs, General Rules for Preparations, and General Tests for their conformity to the Japanese Pharmacopoeia. (See the General Notices 5.)

Pulse angle: 90°.

^{13}C decoupling: on.

Delay time: Repeating pulse waiting time not less than 60 seconds.

Integrating times: 8 or more times.

Dummy scanning: 2 or more times.

Measuring temperature: A constant temperature between 20°C and 30°C.

System suitability

Test for required detectability: When the procedure is run with the sample solution under the above operating conditions, the SN ratio of the signal around δ 6.60 ppm and δ 6.73 ppm is not less than 100.

System performance: When the procedure is run with the sample solution under the above operating conditions, the signals around δ 6.60 ppm and δ 6.73 ppm are not overlapped with any signal of obvious foreign substances, and the ratio of the resonance intensities, A_1/A_2, of the signals around δ 6.60 ppm and δ 6.73 ppm is between 0.99 and 1.01.

System repeatability: When the test is repeated 6 times with the sample solution under the above operating conditions, the relative standard deviation of the ratios of the resonance intensities, A_1 and A_2, to that of the reference standard for qNMR are not more than 1.0%.

[6]-Shogaol for assay $C_{17}H_{24}O_3$ [6]-Shogaol for thin-layer chromatography. It meets the following additional requirements . It is used with correction for its amount based on the result obtained in the Assay.

Unity of peak—Dissolve 5 mg of [6]-shogaol for assay in 10 mL of a mixture of acetonitrile and water (2:1), and use this solution as the sample solution. Perform the test with 10 μL of the sample solution as directed under Liquid Chromatography <2.01> according to the following conditions, and compare the absorption spectra of at least 3 points including the top of [6]-shogaol peak and around the two middle peak heights of before and after the top: no difference in form is observed among their spectra.

Operating conditions

Column, column temperature, mobile phase, and flow rate: Proceed as directed in the operating conditions in the Assay (2) under Mukoi-Daikenchuto Extract.

Detector: A photodiode array detector (wavelength: 225 nm, spectrum range of measurement: 220 – 400 nm).

System suitability

System performance: When the procedure is run with 10 μL of the sample solution under the above operating conditions, the number of theoretical plates and the symmetry factor of the peak of [6]-shogaol are not less than 5000 and not more than 1.5, respectively.

Assay—Weigh accurately 5 mg of [6]-shogaol for assay and 1 mg of 1,4-BTMSB-d_4 for nuclear magnetic resonance spectroscopy using an ultramicrobalance, dissolve in 1 mL of deuterated methanol for nuclear magnetic resonance spectroscopy, and use this solution as the sample solution. Transfer the sample solution into an NMR tube 5 mm in outer diameter, and measure ^{1}H-NMR as directed under

Nuclear Magnetic Resonance Spectroscopy <2.21> and Crude Drugs Test <5.01> according to the following conditions, using 1,4-BTMSB-d_4 for nuclear magnetic resonance spectroscopy as the reference standard for qNMR. Calculate the resonance intensity A (equivalent to 3 hydrogens) of the signal around δ 3.57 ppm assuming the signal of the reference standard for qNMR as δ 0 ppm.

$$\text{Amount (\%) of [6]-shogaol } (C_{17}H_{24}O_3)$$
$$= M_S \times I \times P/(M \times N) \times 1.2202$$

M: Amount (mg) of [6]-shogaol for assay taken

M_S: Amount (mg) of 1,4-BTMSB-d_4 for nuclear magnetic resonance spectroscopy taken

I: Signal resonance intensity A based on the signal resonance intensity of 1,4-BTMSB-d_4 for nuclear magnetic resonance spectroscopy as 18.000

N: Number of the hydrogen derived from A

P: Purity (%) of 1,4-BTMSB-d_4 for nuclear magnetic resonance spectroscopy

Operating conditions

Apparatus: A nuclear magnetic resonance spectrometer having ^{1}H resonance frequency of not less than 400 MHz.

Target nucleus: ^{1}H.

Digital resolution: 0.25 Hz or lower.

Measuring spectrum range: 20 ppm or upper, including between − 5 ppm and 15 ppm.

Spinning: off.

Pulse angle: 90°.

^{13}C decoupling: on.

Delay time: Repeating pulse waiting time not less than 60 seconds.

Integrating times: 8 or more times.

Dummy scanning: 2 or more times.

Measuring temperature: A constant temperature between 20°C and 30°C.

System suitability

Test for required detectability: When the procedure is run with the sample solution under the above operating conditions, the SN ratio of each signal around δ 3.57 ppm and δ 6.37 – 6.43 ppm is not less than 100.

System performance: When the procedure is run with the sample solution under the above operating conditions, the two signals around δ 3.57 ppm and δ 6.37 – 6.43 ppm are not overlapped with any signal of obvious foreign substance. Furthermore, when determined the resonance intensities, A (equivalent to 3 hydrogens) and A_1 (equivalent to 2 hydrogens) of each signal around δ 3.57 ppm and δ 6.37 – 6.43 ppm, the ratio of the resonance intensities, $(A/3)/(A_1/2)$, of each signal around δ 3.57 ppm and δ 6.37 – 6.43 ppm is between 0.99 and 1.01.

System repeatability: When the test is repeated 6 times with the sample solution under the above operating conditions, the relative standard deviation of the ratio of the resonance intensity A to that of the reference standard for qNMR is not more than 1.0%.

Sindbis virus RNA virus of *Togaviridae*, proliferated by chick embryo cell primary culture or chick embryo fibrob-

---

The JP Drugs are to be tested according to the provisions given in the pertinent monographs, General Notices, General Rules for Crude Drugs, General Rules for Preparations, and General Tests for their conformity to the Japanese Pharmacopoeia. (See the General Notices 5.)

2844　*General Tests, Processes and Apparatus*

last-derived cell line (ATCC CRL-12203, etc.) culture. Determine the number of plaques on the cell culture, and use the virus with not less than 1×10^8 PFU/mL.

Delete the following:

Blocking TS for nartograstim test

Bovine serum albumin TS for nartograstim test

Buffer solution for nartograstim sample

Freund's complete adjuvant

Molecular mass marker for nartograstim test

Polyacrylamide gel for nartograstim

Potency measuring medium for nartograstim test

Rabbit anti-nartograstim antibody

Rabbit anti-nartograstim antibody TS

Reduction buffer solution for nartograstim sample

Subculture medium for nartograstim

Washing fluid for nartograstim test

9.42　Solid Supports/Column Packings for Chromatography

Add the following:

Octadecylsilyl and octylsilyl groups bound to porous silica gel for liquid chromatography　A porous silica gel bound with octadecylsilyl and octylsilyl groups, prepared for liquid chromatography.

Polyamine silica gel for liquid chromatography　Prepared for liquid chromatography.

The JP Drugs are to be tested according to the provisions given in the pertinent monographs, General Notices, General Rules for Crude Drugs, General Rules for Preparations, and General Tests for their conformity to the Japanese Pharmacopoeia. (See the General Notices 5.)

Official Monographs

Remove the following items from the Purity and move up the after item number sequentially:

Official Monographs	Purity Tests to be removed
Acebutolol Hydrochloride	Heavy metals, Arsenic
Acemetacin	Heavy metals
Acetaminophen	Heavy metals, Arsenic
Acetazolamide	Heavy metals
Acetic Acid	Heavy metals
Glacial Acetic Acid	Heavy metals
Acetohexamide	Heavy metals
Acetylcholine Chloride for Injection	Heavy metals
Acetylcysteine	Heavy metals
Aciclovir	Heavy metals
Aclarubicin Hydrochloride	Heavy metals
Acrinol Hydrate	Heavy metals
Adrenaline	Heavy metals
Afloqualone	Heavy metals
Alacepril	Heavy metals
L-Alanine	Heavy metals
Aldioxa	Heavy metals
Alendronate Sodium Hydrate	Heavy metals
Alimemazine Tartrate	Heavy metals, Arsenic
Allopurinol	Heavy metals, Arsenic
Alprazolam	Heavy metals
Alprenolol Hydrochloride	Heavy metals, Arsenic
Alprostadil Injection	Heavy metals
Dried Aluminum Hydroxide Gel	Heavy metals, Arsenic
Aluminum Monostearate	Heavy metals
Aluminum Potassium Sulfate Hydrate	Heavy metals, Arsenic
Natural Aluminum Silicate	Heavy metals, Arsenic
Synthetic Aluminum Silicate	Heavy metals, Arsenic
Amantadine Hydrochloride	Heavy metals, Arsenic
Ambenonium Chloride	Heavy metals
Amidotrizoic Acid	Heavy metals, Arsenic
Amikacin Sulfate	Heavy metals

The JP Drugs are to be tested according to the provisions given in the pertinent monographs, General Notices, General Rules for Crude Drugs, General Rules for Preparations, and General Tests for their conformity to the Japanese Pharmacopoeia. (See the General Notices 5.)

2846　　*Official Monographs*

Official Monographs	Purity Tests to be removed
Aminophylline Hydrate	Heavy metals
Amiodarone Hydrochloride	Heavy metals
Amitriptyline Hydrochloride	Heavy metals
Amlexanox	Heavy metals
Amlodipine Besilate	Heavy metals
Ammonia Water	Heavy metals
Amobarbital	Heavy metals
Amosulalol Hydrochloride	Heavy metals
Amoxapine	Heavy metals
Amoxicillin Hydrate	Heavy metals, Arsenic
Anhydrous Ampicillin	Heavy metals, Arsenic
Ampicillin Hydrate	Heavy metals, Arsenic
Ampicillin Sodium	Heavy metals, Arsenic
Ampiroxicam	Heavy metals
Antipyrine	Heavy metals
Aprindine Hydrochloride	Heavy metals
Arbekacin Sulfate	Heavy metals
Argatroban Hydrate	Heavy metals, Arsenic
L-Arginine	Heavy metals
L-Arginine Hydrochloride	Heavy metals, Arsenic
Arotinolol Hydrochloride	Heavy metals
Ascorbic Acid	Heavy metals
L-Aspartic Acid	Heavy metals
Aspirin	Heavy metals
Aspoxicillin Hydrate	Heavy metals, Arsenic
Atenolol	Heavy metals
Atorvastatin Calcium Hydrate	Heavy metals
Auranofin	Heavy metals, Arsenic
Azathioprine	Heavy metals, Arsenic
Azelastine Hydrochloride	Heavy metals, Arsenic
Azelnidipine	Heavy metals
Azithromycin Hydrate	Heavy metals
Azosemide	Heavy metals
Aztreonam	Heavy metals
Bacampicillin Hydrochloride	Heavy metals, Arsenic
Bacitracin	Heavy metals
Baclofen	Heavy metals, Arsenic

The JP Drugs are to be tested according to the provisions given in the pertinent monographs, General Notices, General Rules for Crude Drugs, General Rules for Preparations, and General Tests for their conformity to the Japanese Pharmacopoeia. (See the General Notices 5.)

Supplement I, JP XVIII   *Official Monographs*   2847

Official Monographs	Purity Tests to be removed
Bamethan Sulfate	Heavy metals, Arsenic
Barbital	Heavy metals
Barium Sulfate	Heavy metals, Arsenic
Beclometasone Dipropionate	Heavy metals
Bekanamycin Sulfate	Heavy metals, Arsenic
Benidipine Hydrochloride	Heavy metals
Benserazide Hydrochloride	Heavy metals
Benzbromarone	Heavy metals
Benzoic Acid	Heavy metals
Benzylpenicillin Benzathine Hydrate	Heavy metals, Arsenic
Benzylpenicillin Potassium	Heavy metals, Arsenic
Bepotastine Besilate	Heavy metals
Berberine Chloride Hydrate	Heavy metals
Betahistine Mesilate	Heavy metals
Betamethasone	Heavy metals
Betamethasone Dipropionate	Heavy metals
Betamipron	Heavy metals
Betaxolol Hydrochloride	Heavy metals, Arsenic
Bethanechol Chloride	Heavy metals
Bezafibrate	Heavy metals
Bicalutamide	Heavy metals
Bifonazole	Heavy metals
Biotin	Heavy metals, Arsenic
Biperiden Hydrochloride	Heavy metals, Arsenic
Bisacodyl	Heavy metals
Bismuth Subgallate	Arsenic, Copper, Lead, Silver
Bisoprolol Fumarate	Heavy metals
Bleomycin Hydrochloride	Copper
Bleomycin Sulfate	Copper
Boric Acid	Heavy metals, Arsenic
Bromazepam	Heavy metals
Bromfenac Sodium Hydrate	Heavy metals
Bromhexine Hydrochloride	Heavy metals
Bromocriptine Mesilate	Heavy metals
Bromovalerylurea	Heavy metals, Arsenic
Brotizolam	Heavy metals
Bucillamine	Heavy metals, Arsenic

The JP Drugs are to be tested according to the provisions given in the pertinent monographs, General Notices, General Rules for Crude Drugs, General Rules for Preparations, and General Tests for their conformity to the Japanese Pharmacopoeia. (See the General Notices 5.)

Official Monographs	Purity Tests to be removed
Bucumolol Hydrochloride	Heavy metals, Arsenic
Bufetolol Hydrochloride	Heavy metals
Buformin Hydrochloride	Heavy metals, Arsenic
Bumetanide	Heavy metals, Arsenic
Bunazosin Hydrochloride	Heavy metals
Bupivacaine Hydrochloride Hydrate	Heavy metals
Bupranolol Hydrochloride	Heavy metals, Arsenic
Buprenorphine Hydrochloride	Heavy metals
Busulfan	Heavy metals
Butenafine Hydrochloride	Heavy metals
Butropium Bromide	Heavy metals
Butyl Parahydroxybenzoate	Heavy metals
Cabergoline	Heavy metals
Cadralazine	Heavy metals
Anhydrous Caffeine	Heavy metals
Caffeine Hydrate	Heavy metals
Caffeine and Sodium Benzoate	Heavy metals, Arsenic
Precipitated Calcium Carbonate	Heavy metals, Arsenic, Barium
Calcium Chloride Hydrate	Heavy metals, Arsenic, Barium
Calcium Folinate Hydrate	Heavy metals
Calcium Gluconate Hydrate	Heavy metals, Arsenic
Calcium Hydroxide	Heavy metals, Arsenic
Calcium Lactate Hydrate	Heavy metals, Arsenic
Calcium Levofolinate Hydrate	Heavy metals, Platinum
Calcium Pantothenate	Heavy metals
Calcium Paraaminosalicylate Hydrate	Heavy metals, Arsenic
Anhydrous Dibasic Calcium Phosphate	Heavy metals
Dibasic Calcium Phosphate Hydrate	Heavy metals
Monobasic Calcium Phosphate Hydrate	Heavy metals
Calcium Polystyrene Sulfonate	Heavy metals, Arsenic
Calcium Sodium Edetate Hydrate	Heavy metals
Calcium Stearate	Heavy metals
Camostat Mesilate	Heavy metals, Arsenic
Candesartan Cilexetil	Heavy metals
Captopril	Heavy metals, Arsenic
Carbamazepine	Heavy metals
Carbazochrome Sodium Sulfonate Hydrate	Heavy metals

The JP Drugs are to be tested according to the provisions given in the pertinent monographs, General Notices, General Rules for Crude Drugs, General Rules for Preparations, and General Tests for their conformity to the Japanese Pharmacopoeia. (See the General Notices 5.)

Supplement I, JP XVIII   *Official Monographs*   2849

Official Monographs	Purity Tests to be removed
Carbidopa Hydrate	Heavy metals
L-Carbocisteine	Heavy metals, Arsenic
Carmellose	Heavy metals
Carmellose Calcium	Heavy metals
Carmellose Sodium	Heavy metals, Arsenic
Croscarmellose Sodium	Heavy metals
Carmofur	Heavy metals
Carteolol Hydrochloride	Heavy metals, Arsenic
Carumonam Sodium	Heavy metals, Arsenic
Carvedilol	Heavy metals
Cefaclor	Heavy metals, Arsenic
Cefadroxil	Heavy metals
Cefalexin	Heavy metals, Arsenic
Cefalotin Sodium	Heavy metals, Arsenic
Cefatrizine Propylene Glycolate	Heavy metals, Arsenic
Cefazolin Sodium	Heavy metals, Arsenic
Cefazolin Sodium Hydrate	Heavy metals
Cefbuperazone Sodium	Heavy metals, Arsenic
Cefcapene Pivoxil Hydrochloride Hydrate	Heavy metals
Cefdinir	Heavy metals
Cefditoren Pivoxil	Heavy metals
Cefepime Dihydrochloride Hydrate	Heavy metals
Cefmenoxime Hydrochloride	Heavy metals, Arsenic
Cefmetazole Sodium	Heavy metals, Arsenic
Cefminox Sodium Hydrate	Heavy metals, Arsenic
Cefodizime Sodium	Heavy metals, Arsenic
Cefoperazone Sodium	Heavy metals, Arsenic
Cefotaxime Sodium	Heavy metals, Arsenic
Cefotetan	Heavy metals
Cefotiam Hexetil Hydrochloride	Heavy metals, Arsenic
Cefotiam Hydrochloride	Heavy metals, Arsenic
Cefozopran Hydrochloride	Heavy metals, Arsenic
Cefpiramide Sodium	Heavy metals
Cefpirome Sulfate	Heavy metals, Arsenic
Cefpodoxime Proxetil	Heavy metals
Cefroxadine Hydrate	Heavy metals
Cefsulodin Sodium	Heavy metals, Arsenic

The JP Drugs are to be tested according to the provisions given in the pertinent monographs, General Notices, General Rules for Crude Drugs, General Rules for Preparations, and General Tests for their conformity to the Japanese Pharmacopoeia. (See the General Notices 5.)

Official Monographs	Purity Tests to be removed
Ceftazidime Hydrate	Heavy metals
Cefteram Pivoxil	Heavy metals
Ceftibuten Hydrate	Heavy metals
Ceftizoxime Sodium	Heavy metals, Arsenic
Ceftriaxone Sodium Hydrate	Heavy metals, Arsenic
Cefuroxime Axetil	Heavy metals
Celecoxib	Heavy metals
Cellacefate	Heavy metals
Microcrystalline Cellulose	Heavy metals
Powdered Cellulose	Heavy metals
Cetirizine Hydrochloride	Heavy metals
Cetotiamine Hydrochloride Hydrate	Heavy metals
Cetraxate Hydrochloride	Heavy metals, Arsenic
Chenodeoxycholic Acid	Heavy metals, Barium
Chloramphenicol	Heavy metals
Chloramphenicol Palmitate	Heavy metals, Arsenic
Chloramphenicol Sodium Succinate	Heavy metals
Chlordiazepoxide	Heavy metals
Chlorhexidine Hydrochloride	Heavy metals, Arsenic
Chlormadinone Acetate	Heavy metals, Arsenic
Chlorphenesin Carbamate	Heavy metals, Arsenic
Chlorpheniramine Maleate	Heavy metals
d-Chlorpheniramine Maleate	Heavy metals
Chlorpromazine Hydrochloride	Heavy metals
Chlorpropamide	Heavy metals
Cibenzoline Succinate	Heavy metals, Arsenic
Ciclacillin	Heavy metals, Arsenic
Ciclosporin	Heavy metals
Cilastatin Sodium	Heavy metals, Arsenic
Cilazapril Hydrate	Heavy metals
Cilnidipine	Heavy metals
Cilostazol	Heavy metals
Cimetidine	Heavy metals, Arsenic
Cinoxacin	Heavy metals
Ciprofloxacin	Heavy metals
Ciprofloxacin Hydrochloride Hydrate	Heavy metals
Citicoline	Heavy metals, Arsenic

The JP Drugs are to be tested according to the provisions given in the pertinent monographs, General Notices, General Rules for Crude Drugs, General Rules for Preparations, and General Tests for their conformity to the Japanese Pharmacopoeia. (See the General Notices 5.)

Official Monographs	Purity Tests to be removed
Anhydrous Citric Acid	Heavy metals
Citric Acid Hydrate	Heavy metals
Clarithromycin	Heavy metals
Clebopride Malate	Heavy metals
Clemastine Fumarate	Heavy metals, Arsenic
Clindamycin Hydrochloride	Heavy metals
Clindamycin Phosphate	Heavy metals, Arsenic
Clinofibrate	Heavy metals, Arsenic
Clobetasol Propionate	Heavy metals
Clocapramine Hydrochloride Hydrate	Heavy metals
Clofedanol Hydrochloride	Heavy metals
Clofibrate	Heavy metals, Arsenic
Clomifene Citrate	Heavy metals
Clomipramine Hydrochloride	Heavy metals, Arsenic
Clonazepam	Heavy metals
Clonidine Hydrochloride	Heavy metals, Arsenic
Cloperastine Fendizoate	Heavy metals
Cloperastine Hydrochloride	Heavy metals
Clopidogrel Sulfate	Heavy metals
Clorazepate Dipotassium	Heavy metals, Arsenic
Clotiazepam	Heavy metals, Arsenic
Clotrimazole	Heavy metals, Arsenic
Cloxacillin Sodium Hydrate	Heavy metals, Arsenic
Cloxazolam	Heavy metals, Arsenic
Colestimide	Heavy metals
Colistin Sodium Methanesulfonate	Heavy metals, Arsenic
Copovidone	Heavy metals
Croconazole Hydrochloride	Heavy metals
Crospovidone	Heavy metals
Cyanamide	Heavy metals
Cyclopentolate Hydrochloride	Heavy metals
Cyclophosphamide Hydrate	Heavy metals
Cycloserine	Heavy metals
Cyproheptadine Hydrochloride Hydrate	Heavy metals
L-Cysteine	Heavy metals
L-Cysteine Hydrochloride Hydrate	Heavy metals
L-Cystine	Heavy metals

The JP Drugs are to be tested according to the provisions given in the pertinent monographs, General Notices, General Rules for Crude Drugs, General Rules for Preparations, and General Tests for their conformity to the Japanese Pharmacopoeia. (See the General Notices 5.)

2852　*Official Monographs*　　　　　　　　　　　　　　　　　　*Supplement I, JP XVIII*

Official Monographs	Purity Tests to be removed
Cytarabine	Heavy metals
Danazol	Heavy metals
Dantrolene Sodium Hydrate	Heavy metals
Daunorubicin Hydrochloride	Heavy metals
Deferoxamine Mesilate	Heavy metals, Arsenic
Dehydrocholic Acid	Heavy metals, Barium
Purified Dehydrocholic Acid	Heavy metals, Barium
Dehydrocholic Acid Injection	Heavy metals
Demethylchlortetracycline Hydrochloride	Heavy metals
Dexamethasone	Heavy metals
Dextran 40	Heavy metals, Arsenic
Dextran 70	Heavy metals, Arsenic
Dextran Sulfate Sodium Sulfur 5	Heavy metals, Arsenic
Dextran Sulfate Sodium Sulfur 18	Heavy metals, Arsenic
Dextrin	Heavy metals
Dextromethorphan Hydrobromide Hydrate	Heavy metals
Diazepam	Heavy metals
Dibekacin Sulfate	Heavy metals
Dibucaine Hydrochloride	Heavy metals
Diclofenac Sodium	Heavy metals, Arsenic
Diethylcarbamazine Citrate	Heavy metals
Difenidol Hydrochloride	Heavy metals, Arsenic
Diflorasone Diacetate	Heavy metals
Diflucortolone Valerate	Heavy metals
Dihydroergotoxine Mesilate	Heavy metals
Dilazep Hydrochloride Hydrate	Heavy metals, Arsenic
Diltiazem Hydrochloride	Heavy metals, Arsenic
Dimemorfan Phosphate	Heavy metals, Arsenic
Dimercaprol	Heavy metals
Dimorpholamine	Heavy metals
Diphenhydramine	Heavy metals
Diphenhydramine Hydrochloride	Heavy metals
Diphenhydramine Tannate	Heavy metals
Dipyridamole	Heavy metals, Arsenic
Disopyramide	Heavy metals, Arsenic
Distigmine Bromide	Heavy metals
Disulfiram	Heavy metals, Arsenic

The JP Drugs are to be tested according to the provisions given in the pertinent monographs, General Notices, General Rules for Crude Drugs, General Rules for Preparations, and General Tests for their conformity to the Japanese Pharmacopoeia. (See the General Notices 5.)

Supplement I, JP XVIII   *Official Monographs*   2853

Official Monographs	Purity Tests to be removed
Dobutamine Hydrochloride	Heavy metals
Docetaxel Hydrate	Heavy metals
Domperidone	Heavy metals
Donepezil Hydrochloride	Heavy metals
Dopamine Hydrochloride	Heavy metals, Arsenic
Doripenem Hydrate	Heavy metals
Dorzolamide Hydrochloride	Heavy metals
Doxapram Hydrochloride Hydrate	Heavy metals, Arsenic
Doxazosin Mesilate	Heavy metals
Doxifluridine	Heavy metals
Doxycycline Hydrochloride Hydrate	Heavy metals
Droperidol	Heavy metals
Droxidopa	Heavy metals, Arsenic
Dydrogesterone	Heavy metals
Ebastine	Heavy metals
Ecabet Sodium Hydrate	Heavy metals
Ecothiopate Iodide	Heavy metals
Edaravone	Heavy metals
Edrophonium Chloride	Heavy metals, Arsenic
Emedastine Fumarate	Heavy metals
Emorfazone	Heavy metals, Arsenic
Enalapril Maleate	Heavy metals
Enoxacin Hydrate	Heavy metals, Arsenic
Entacapone	Heavy metals
Enviomycin Sulfate	Heavy metals, Arsenic
Epalrestat	Heavy metals
Eperisone Hydrochloride	Heavy metals
Ephedrine Hydrochloride	Heavy metals
Epirizole	Heavy metals, Arsenic
Epirubicin Hydrochloride	Heavy metals
Eplerenone	Heavy metals
Eribulin Mesilate	Heavy metals
Erythromycin	Heavy metals
Estazolam	Heavy metals, Arsenic
Estriol	Heavy metals
Etacrynic Acid	Heavy metals, Arsenic
Ethambutol Hydrochloride	Heavy metals, Arsenic

The JP Drugs are to be tested according to the provisions given in the pertinent monographs, General Notices, General Rules for Crude Drugs, General Rules for Preparations, and General Tests for their conformity to the Japanese Pharmacopoeia. (See the General Notices 5.)

Official Monographs	Purity Tests to be removed
Ethenzamide	Heavy metals, Arsenic
Ethionamide	Heavy metals, Arsenic
Ethosuximide	Heavy metals, Arsenic
Ethyl Aminobenzoate	Heavy metals
Ethylcellulose	Heavy metals
Ethyl L-Cysteine Hydrochloride	Heavy metals
Ethylenediamine	Heavy metals
Ethyl Icosapentate	Heavy metals, Arsenic
Ethyl Loflazepate	Heavy metals, Arsenic
Ethyl Parahydroxybenzoate	Heavy metals
Etidronate Disodium	Heavy metals, Arsenic
Etilefrine Hydrochloride	Heavy metals
Etizolam	Heavy metals
Etodolac	Heavy metals
Etoposide	Heavy metals
Famotidine	Heavy metals
Faropenem Sodium Hydrate	Heavy metals
Felbinac	Heavy metals
Felodipine	Heavy metals
Fenbufen	Heavy metals, Arsenic
Fenofibrate	Heavy metals
Fentanyl Citrate	Heavy metals
Ferrous Sulfate Hydrate	Heavy metals, Arsenic
Fexofenadine Hydrochloride	Heavy metals
Flavin Adenine Dinucleotide Sodium	Heavy metals, Arsenic
Flavoxate Hydrochloride	Heavy metals, Arsenic
Flecainide Acetate	Heavy metals
Flomoxef Sodium	Heavy metals, Arsenic
Flopropione	Heavy metals
Fluconazole	Heavy metals
Flucytosine	Heavy metals, Arsenic
Fludiazepam	Heavy metals
Fludrocortisone Acetate	Heavy metals
Flunitrazepam	Heavy metals
Fluorometholone	Heavy metals
Fluorouracil	Heavy metals, Arsenic
Fluphenazine Enanthate	Heavy metals

The JP Drugs are to be tested according to the provisions given in the pertinent monographs, General Notices, General Rules for Crude Drugs, General Rules for Preparations, and General Tests for their conformity to the Japanese Pharmacopoeia. (See the General Notices 5.)

Supplement I, JP XVIII *Official Monographs* 2855

Official Monographs	Purity Tests to be removed
Flurazepam Hydrochloride	Heavy metals
Flurbiprofen	Heavy metals
Flutamide	Heavy metals
Flutoprazepam	Heavy metals
Fluvoxamine Maleate	Heavy metals
Formoterol Fumarate Hydrate	Heavy metals
Fosfomycin Calcium Hydrate	Heavy metals, Arsenic
Fosfomycin Sodium	Heavy metals, Arsenic
Fradiomycin Sulfate	Heavy metals, Arsenic
Fructose	Heavy metals, Arsenic
Fructose Injection	Heavy metals, Arsenic
Fudosteine	Heavy metals, Arsenic
Furosemide	Heavy metals
Fursultiamine Hydrochloride	Heavy metals
Gabexate Mesilate	Heavy metals, Arsenic
β-Galactosidase (Aspergillus)	Heavy metals, Arsenic
β-Galactosidase (Penicillium)	Heavy metals, Arsenic
Gatifloxacin Hydrate	Heavy metals
Gefarnate	Heavy metals
Gefitinib	Heavy metals
Gelatin	Heavy metals, Arsenic
Purified Gelatin	Heavy metals, Arsenic
Gentamicin Sulfate	Heavy metals
Glibenclamide	Heavy metals
Gliclazide	Heavy metals
Glimepiride	Heavy metals
Glucose	Heavy metals
Glucose Hydrate	Heavy metals
Purified Glucose	Heavy metals
L-Glutamic Acid	Heavy metals
L-Glutamine	Heavy metals
Glutathione	Heavy metals, Arsenic
Glycerin	Heavy metals
Concentrated Glycerin	Heavy metals
Glycine	Heavy metals, Arsenic
Guaifenesin	Heavy metals, Arsenic
Guanabenz Acetate	Heavy metals

The JP Drugs are to be tested according to the provisions given in the pertinent monographs, General Notices, General Rules for Crude Drugs, General Rules for Preparations, and General Tests for their conformity to the Japanese Pharmacopoeia. (See the General Notices 5.)

2856   *Official Monographs*   *Supplement I, JP XVIII*

Official Monographs	Purity Tests to be removed
Guanethidine Sulfate	Heavy metals
Haloperidol	Heavy metals
Haloxazolam	Heavy metals, Arsenic
Heparin Calcium	Heavy metals, Barium
Heparin Sodium	Barium
Heparin Sodium Injection	Barium
L-Histidine	Heavy metals
L-Histidine Hydrochloride Hydrate	Heavy metals
Homochlorcyclizine Hydrochloride	Heavy metals
Hydralazine Hydrochloride	Heavy metals
Hydrochloric Acid	Heavy metals, Arsenic, Mercury
Dilute Hydrochloric Acid	Heavy metals, Arsenic, Mercury
Hydrochlorothiazide	Heavy metals
Hydrocortisone Butyrate	Heavy metals
Hydrocortisone Sodium Phosphate	Heavy metals, Arsenic
Hydrocotarnine Hydrochloride Hydrate	Heavy metals
Hydrogenated Oil	Heavy metals
Hydroxyethylcellulose	Heavy metals
Hydroxypropylcellulose	Heavy metals
Low Substituted Hydroxypropylcellulose	Heavy metals
Hydroxyzine Hydrochloride	Heavy metals
Hydroxyzine Pamoate	Heavy metals, Arsenic
Hymecromone	Heavy metals, Arsenic
Hypromellose	Heavy metals
Hypromellose Acetate Succinate	Heavy metals
Hypromellose Phthalate	Heavy metals
Ibudilast	Heavy metals
Ibuprofen	Heavy metals, Arsenic
Ibuprofen Piconol	Heavy metals
Idarubicin Hydrochloride	Silver
Idoxuridine	Heavy metals
Ifenprodil Tartrate	Heavy metals
Imidapril Hydrochloride	Heavy metals
Imipenem Hydrate	Heavy metals, Arsenic
Indapamide	Heavy metals
Indenolol Hydrochloride	Heavy metals, Arsenic
Indigocarmine	Arsenic

The JP Drugs are to be tested according to the provisions given in the pertinent monographs, General Notices, General Rules for Crude Drugs, General Rules for Preparations, and General Tests for their conformity to the Japanese Pharmacopoeia. (See the General Notices 5.)

Official Monographs	Purity Tests to be removed
Indometacin	Heavy metals, Arsenic
Iohexol	Heavy metals
Iopamidol	Heavy metals
Iotalamic Acid	Heavy metals, Arsenic
Iotroxic Acid	Heavy metals
Ipratropium Bromide Hydrate	Heavy metals, Arsenic
Ipriflavone	Heavy metals, Arsenic
Irbesartan	Heavy metals
Irinotecan Hydrochloride Hydrate	Heavy metals
Irsogladine Maleate	Heavy metals
Isepamicin Sulfate	Heavy metals
L-Isoleucine	Heavy metals, Arsenic
Isomalt Hydrate	Heavy metals
Isoniazid	Heavy metals, Arsenic
l-Isoprenaline Hydrochloride	Heavy metals
Isopropylantipyrine	Heavy metals, Arsenic
Isosorbide	Heavy metals, Arsenic
Isosorbide Dinitrate	Heavy metals
Isosorbide Mononitrate 70%/Lactose 30%	Heavy metals
Isoxsuprine Hydrochloride	Heavy metals
Itraconazole	Heavy metals
Josamycin	Heavy metals
Josamycin Propionate	Heavy metals
Kainic Acid Hydrate	Heavy metals, Arsenic
Kanamycin Monosulfate	Heavy metals, Arsenic
Kanamycin Sulfate	Heavy metals, Arsenic
Ketamine Hydrochloride	Heavy metals, Arsenic
Ketoconazole	Heavy metals
Ketoprofen	Heavy metals
Ketotifen Fumarate	Heavy metals
Kitasamycin Tartrate	Heavy metals
Labetalol Hydrochloride	Heavy metals
Lactic Acid	Heavy metals
L-Lactic Acid	Heavy metals
Anhydrous Lactose	Heavy metals
Lactose Hydrate	Heavy metals
Lactulose	Heavy metals, Arsenic

The JP Drugs are to be tested according to the provisions given in the pertinent monographs, General Notices, General Rules for Crude Drugs, General Rules for Preparations, and General Tests for their conformity to the Japanese Pharmacopoeia. (See the General Notices 5.)

2858 *Official Monographs* *Supplement I, JP XVIII*

Official Monographs	Purity Tests to be removed
Lafutidine	Heavy metals
Lanoconazole	Heavy metals
Lansoprazole	Heavy metals, Arsenic
Latamoxef Sodium	Heavy metals, Arsenic
Lenampicillin Hydrochloride	Heavy metals, Arsenic
L-Leucine	Heavy metals, Arsenic
Levallorphan Tartrate	Heavy metals
Levodopa	Heavy metals, Arsenic
Levofloxacin Hydrate	Heavy metals
Levomepromazine Maleate	Heavy metals
Lidocaine	Heavy metals
Lincomycin Hydrochloride Hydrate	Heavy metals
Lisinopril Hydrate	Heavy metals
Lithium Carbonate	Heavy metals, Arsenic, Barium
Lobenzarit Sodium	Heavy metals, Arsenic
Lorazepam	Heavy metals, Arsenic
Losartan Potassium	Heavy metals
Loxoprofen Sodium Hydrate	Heavy metals
L-Lysine Acetate	Heavy metals
L-Lysine Hydrochloride	Heavy metals, Arsenic
Lysozyme Hydrochloride	Heavy metals
Magnesium Aluminosilicate	Heavy metals
Magnesium Aluminometasilicate	Heavy metals
Magnesium Carbonate	Heavy metals, Arsenic
Magnesium Oxide	Heavy metals
Magnesium Stearate	Heavy metals
Magnesium Sulfate Hydrate	Heavy metals, Arsenic
Maltose Hydrate	Heavy metals, Arsenic
Manidipine Hydrochloride	Heavy metals, Arsenic
D-Mannitol	Heavy metals
Maprotiline Hydrochloride	Heavy metals
Meclofenoxate Hydrochloride	Heavy metals, Arsenic
Medazepam	Heavy metals, Arsenic
Medicinal Carbon	Heavy metals, Arsenic
Medicinal Soap	Heavy metals
Medroxyprogesterone Acetate	Heavy metals
Mefenamic Acid	Heavy metals, Arsenic

The JP Drugs are to be tested according to the provisions given in the pertinent monographs, General Notices, General Rules for Crude Drugs, General Rules for Preparations, and General Tests for their conformity to the Japanese Pharmacopoeia. (See the General Notices 5.)

Supplement I, JP XVIII   *Official Monographs*   2859

Official Monographs	Purity Tests to be removed
Mefloquine Hydrochloride	Heavy metals, Arsenic
Mefruside	Heavy metals, Arsenic
Meglumine	Heavy metals
Melphalan	Heavy metals, Arsenic
Menatetrenone	Heavy metals
Mepenzolate Bromide	Heavy metals, Arsenic
Mepitiostane	Heavy metals
Mepivacaine Hydrochloride	Heavy metals
Mequitazine	Heavy metals
Mercaptopurine Hydrate	Heavy metals
Meropenem Hydrate	Heavy metals
Mesalazine	Heavy metals
Mestranol	Heavy metals, Arsenic
Metenolone Acetate	Heavy metals
Metenolone Enanthate	Heavy metals
Metformin Hydrochloride	Heavy metals
L-Methionine	Heavy metals, Arsenic
Methoxsalen	Heavy metals, Arsenic
Methylcellulose	Heavy metals
Methyldopa Hydrate	Heavy metals, Arsenic
dl-Methylephedrine Hydrochloride	Heavy metals
Methyl Parahydroxybenzoate	Heavy metals
Methylprednisolone Succinate	Heavy metals, Arsenic
Methyl Salicylate	Heavy metals
Meticrane	Heavy metals, Arsenic
Metildigoxin	Arsenic
Metoclopramide	Heavy metals, Arsenic
Metoprolol Tartrate	Heavy metals
Metronidazole	Heavy metals
Metyrapone	Heavy metals, Arsenic
Mexiletine Hydrochloride	Heavy metals
Miconazole	Heavy metals, Arsenic
Miconazole Nitrate	Heavy metals, Arsenic
Micronomicin Sulfate	Heavy metals
Midecamycin	Heavy metals
Midecamycin Acetate	Heavy metals
Miglitol	Heavy metals

The JP Drugs are to be tested according to the provisions given in the pertinent monographs, General Notices, General Rules for Crude Drugs, General Rules for Preparations, and General Tests for their conformity to the Japanese Pharmacopoeia. (See the General Notices 5.)

Official Monographs	Purity Tests to be removed
Migrenin	Heavy metals
Minocycline Hydrochloride	Heavy metals
Mitiglinide Calcium Hydrate	Heavy metals
Mizoribine	Heavy metals
Montelukast Sodium	Heavy metals
Mosapride Citrate Hydrate	Heavy metals
Mupirocin Calcium Hydrate	Inorganic salt
Nabumetone	Heavy metals
Nadolol	Heavy metals
Nafamostat Mesilate	Heavy metals
Naftopidil	Heavy metals
Nalidixic Acid	Heavy metals
Naphazoline Nitrate	Heavy metals
Naproxen	Heavy metals, Arsenic
Nateglinide	Heavy metals
Nicardipine Hydrochloride	Heavy metals
Nicergoline	Heavy metals
Niceritrol	Heavy metals, Arsenic
Nicomol	Heavy metals, Arsenic
Nicorandil	Heavy metals
Nicotinamide	Heavy metals
Nicotinic Acid	Heavy metals
Nifedipine	Heavy metals, Arsenic
Nilvadipine	Heavy metals
Nitrazepam	Heavy metals, Arsenic
Nitrendipine	Heavy metals
Nizatidine	Heavy metals
Norfloxacin	Heavy metals, Arsenic
Norgestrel	Heavy metals
Nortriptyline Hydrochloride	Heavy metals, Arsenic
Noscapine	Heavy metals
Nystatin	Heavy metals
Ofloxacin	Heavy metals
Olmesartan Medoxomil	Heavy metals
Olopatadine Hydrochloride	Heavy metals
Omeprazole	Heavy metals
Orciprenaline Sulfate	Heavy metals

The JP Drugs are to be tested according to the provisions given in the pertinent monographs, General Notices, General Rules for Crude Drugs, General Rules for Preparations, and General Tests for their conformity to the Japanese Pharmacopoeia. (See the General Notices 5.)

Supplement I, JP XVIII *Official Monographs* 2861

Official Monographs	Purity Tests to be removed
Oxapium Iodide	Heavy metals
Oxaprozin	Heavy metals, Arsenic
Oxazolam	Heavy metals, Arsenic
Oxethazaine	Heavy metals
Oxprenolol Hydrochloride	Heavy metals, Arsenic
Oxybuprocaine Hydrochloride	Heavy metals
Oxydol	Heavy metals, Arsenic
Oxytetracycline Hydrochloride	Heavy metals
Ozagrel Sodium	Heavy metals
Panipenem	Heavy metals
Pantethine	Heavy metals, Arsenic
Paraffin	Heavy metals
Liquid Paraffin	Heavy metals
Light Liquid Paraffin	Heavy metals
Parnaparin Sodium	Heavy metals
Paroxetine Hydrochloride Hydrate	Heavy metals
Pazufloxacin Mesilate	Heavy metals
Pemirolast Potassium	Heavy metals
Penbutolol Sulfate	Heavy metals, Arsenic
Pentazocine	Heavy metals, Arsenic
Pentobarbital Calcium	Heavy metals
Pentoxyverine Citrate	Heavy metals, Arsenic
Peplomycin Sulfate	Copper
Perphenazine	Heavy metals
Perphenazine Maleate	Heavy metals, Arsenic
White Petrolatum	Heavy metals, Arsenic
Yellow Petrolatum	Heavy metals, Arsenic
Phenethicillin Potassium	Heavy metals, Arsenic
Phenobarbital	Heavy metals
L-Phenylalanine	Heavy metals, Arsenic
Phenylbutazone	Heavy metals, Arsenic
Phenytoin	Heavy metals
Phenytoin Sodium for Injection	Heavy metals
Phytonadione	Heavy metals
Pilsicainide Hydrochloride Hydrate	Heavy metals
Pimaricin	Heavy metals
Pimozide	Heavy metals, Arsenic

The JP Drugs are to be tested according to the provisions given in the pertinent monographs, General Notices, General Rules for Crude Drugs, General Rules for Preparations, and General Tests for their conformity to the Japanese Pharmacopoeia. (See the General Notices 5.)

Official Monographs	Purity Tests to be removed
Pindolol	Heavy metals, Arsenic
Pioglitazone Hydrochloride	Heavy metals
Pipemidic Acid Hydrate	Heavy metals, Arsenic
Piperacillin Hydrate	Heavy metals
Piperacillin Sodium	Heavy metals, Arsenic
Piperazine Adipate	Heavy metals
Piperazine Phosphate Hydrate	Heavy metals, Arsenic
Pirarubicin	Heavy metals
Pirenoxine	Heavy metals
Pirenzepine Hydrochloride Hydrate	Heavy metals
Piroxicam	Heavy metals
Pitavastatin Calcium Hydrate	Heavy metals
Pivmecillinam Hydrochloride	Heavy metals, Arsenic
Polaprezinc	Lead
Polymixin B Sulfate	Heavy metals
Polyoxyl 40 Stearate	Heavy metals
Polysorbate 80	Heavy metals
Potassium Bromide	Heavy metals, Arsenic, Barium
Potassium Canrenoate	Heavy metals, Arsenic
Potassium Carbonate	Heavy metals, Arsenic
Potassium Chloride	Heavy metals, Arsenic
Potassium Clavulanate	Heavy metals, Arsenic
Potassium Hydroxide	Heavy metals
Potassium Iodide	Heavy metals, Arsenic, Barium
Potassium Permanganate	Arsenic
Potassium Sulfate	Heavy metals, Arsenic
Povidone	Heavy metals
Povidone-Iodine	Heavy metals, Arsenic
Pranlukast Hydrate	Heavy metals, Arsenic
Pranoprofen	Heavy metals
Prasterone Sodium Sulfate Hydrate	Heavy metals
Pravastatin Sodium	Heavy metals
Prazepam	Heavy metals, Arsenic
Prazosin Hydrochloride	Heavy metals
Prednisolone	Selenium
Prednisolone Sodium Phosphate	Heavy metals
Primidone	Heavy metals

The JP Drugs are to be tested according to the provisions given in the pertinent monographs, General Notices, General Rules for Crude Drugs, General Rules for Preparations, and General Tests for their conformity to the Japanese Pharmacopoeia. (See the General Notices 5.)

Supplement I, JP XVIII   *Official Monographs*   2863

Official Monographs	Purity Tests to be removed
Probenecid	Heavy metals, Arsenic
Probucol	Heavy metals
Procainamide Hydrochloride	Heavy metals, Arsenic
Procaine Hydrochloride	Heavy metals
Procarbazine Hydrochloride	Heavy metals
Procaterol Hydrochloride Hydrate	Heavy metals
Prochlorperazine Maleate	Heavy metals
Proglumide	Heavy metals, Arsenic
L-Proline	Heavy metals
Promethazine Hydrochloride	Heavy metals
Propafenone Hydrochloride	Heavy metals
Propiverine Hydrochloride	Heavy metals
Propranolol Hydrochloride	Heavy metals
Propylene Glycol	Heavy metals
Propyl Parahydroxybenzoate	Heavy metals
Prothionamide	Heavy metals, Arsenic
Protirelin	Heavy metals
Protirelin Tartrate Hydrate	Heavy metals, Arsenic
Pullulan	Heavy metals
Pyrantel Pamoate	Heavy metals, Arsenic
Pyrazinamide	Heavy metals
Pyridostigmine Bromide	Heavy metals, Arsenic
Pyridoxal Phosphate Hydrate	Heavy metals, Arsenic
Pyridoxine Hydrochloride	Heavy metals
Quetiapine Fumarate	Heavy metals
Quinapril Hydrochloride	Heavy metals
Quinine Ethyl Carbonate	Heavy metals
Quinine Sulfate Hydrate	Heavy metals
Rabeprazole Sodium	Heavy metals
Ranitidine Hydrochloride	Heavy metals, Arsenic
Rebamipide	Heavy metals
Ribavirin	Heavy metals, Arsenic
Riboflavin Butyrate	Heavy metals
Ribostamycin Sulfate	Heavy metals, Arsenic
Rifampicin	Heavy metals, Arsenic
Rilmazafone Hydrochloride Hydrate	Heavy metals
Ringer's Solution	Heavy metals, Arsenic

The JP Drugs are to be tested according to the provisions given in the pertinent monographs, General Notices, General Rules for Crude Drugs, General Rules for Preparations, and General Tests for their conformity to the Japanese Pharmacopoeia. (See the General Notices 5.)

Official Monographs	Purity Tests to be removed
Risperidone	Heavy metals
Ritodrine Hydrochloride	Heavy metals
Rosuvastatin Calcium	Heavy metals
Roxatidine Acetate Hydrochloride	Heavy metals
Roxithromycin	Heavy metals
Saccharin	Heavy metals
Saccharin Sodium Hydrate	Heavy metals
Salazosulfapyridine	Heavy metals, Arsenic
Salbutamol Sulfate	Heavy metals
Salicylic Acid	Heavy metals
Sarpogrelate Hydrochloride	Heavy metals, Arsenic
Scopolamine Butylbromide	Heavy metals
L-Serine	Heavy metals
Purified Shellac	Heavy metals
White Shellac	Heavy metals
Light Anhydrous Silicic Acid	Heavy metals
Silodosin	Heavy metals
Silver Nitrate	Copper and Lead in the Purity (2) (Change the test name from ''Bismuth, copper and lead'' to ''Bismuth'')
Simvastatin	Heavy metals
Sitagliptin Phosphate Hydrate	Heavy metals
Sivelestat Sodium Hydrate	Heavy metals
Sodium Acetate Hydrate	Heavy metals, Arsenic
Sodium Aurothiomalate	Heavy metals, Arsenic
Sodium Benzoate	Heavy metals, Arsenic
Sodium Bicarbonate	Heavy metals, Arsenic
Sodium Bisulfite	Heavy metals
Sodium Borate	Heavy metals, Arsenic
Sodium Bromide	Heavy metals, Arsenic, Barium
Dried Sodium Carbonate	Heavy metals
Sodium Carbonate Hydrate	Heavy metals
Sodium Chloride	Heavy metals
Isotonic Sodium Chloride Solution	Heavy metals, Arsenic
Sodium Citrate Hydrate	Heavy metals, Arsenic
Sodium Cromoglicate	Heavy metals
Disodium Edetate Hydrate	Heavy metals, Arsenic
Sodium Fusidate	Heavy metals

The JP Drugs are to be tested according to the provisions given in the pertinent monographs, General Notices, General Rules for Crude Drugs, General Rules for Preparations, and General Tests for their conformity to the Japanese Pharmacopoeia. (See the General Notices 5.)

Supplement I, JP XVIII   *Official Monographs*   2865

Official Monographs	Purity Tests to be removed
Purified Sodium Hyaluronate	Heavy metals
Sodium Hydroxide	Heavy metals, Mercury
Sodium Iodide	Heavy metals
Sodium L-Lactate Solution	Heavy metals, Arsenic
Sodium L-Lactate Ringer's Solution	Heavy metals
Dibasic Sodium Phosphate Hydrate	Heavy metals
Sodium Picosulfate Hydrate	Heavy metals, Arsenic
Sodium Polystyrene Sulfonate	Heavy metals, Arsenic
Sodium Pyrosulfite	Heavy metals
Sodium Risedronate Hydrate	Heavy metals, Arsenic
Sodium Salicylate	Heavy metals, Arsenic
Sodium Starch Glycolate	Heavy metals
Dried Sodium Sulfite	Heavy metals
Sodium Thiosulfate Hydrate	Heavy metals, Arsenic
Sodium Valproate	Heavy metals
Sorbitan Sesquioleate	Heavy metals
D-Sorbitol	Heavy metals, Arsenic, Nickel
D-Sorbitol Solution	Heavy metals, Arsenic, Nickel
Spiramycin Acetate	Heavy metals
Stearic Acid	Heavy metals
Streptomycin Sulfate	Heavy metals, Arsenic
Sucralfate Hydrate	Heavy metals, Arsenic
White Soft Sugar	Heavy metals
Sulbactam Sodium	Heavy metals
Sulbenicillin Sodium	Heavy metals, Arsenic
Sulfamethizole	Heavy metals, Arsenic
Sulfamethoxazole	Heavy metals, Arsenic
Sulfamonomethoxine Hydrate	Heavy metals, Arsenic
Sulfisoxazole	Heavy metals
Sulfobromophthalein Sodium	Heavy metals, Arsenic
Sulfur	Arsenic
Sulindac	Heavy metals, Arsenic
Sulpiride	Heavy metals
Sulpyrine Hydrate	Heavy metals
Sultamicillin Tosilate Hydrate	Heavy metals
Sultiame	Heavy metals, Arsenic
Tacrolimus Hydrate	Heavy metals

The JP Drugs are to be tested according to the provisions given in the pertinent monographs, General Notices, General Rules for Crude Drugs, General Rules for Preparations, and General Tests for their conformity to the Japanese Pharmacopoeia. (See the General Notices 5.)

2866   *Official Monographs*   *Supplement I, JP XVIII*

Official Monographs	Purity Tests to be removed
Talampicillin Hydrochloride	Heavy metals, Arsenic
Taltirelin Hydrate	Heavy metals
Tamoxifen Citrate	Heavy metals
Tamsulosin Hydrochloride	Heavy metals
Tartaric Acid	Heavy metals, Arsenic
Taurine	Heavy metals
Tazobactam	Heavy metals
Tegafur	Heavy metals, Arsenic
Teicoplanin	Heavy metals, Arsenic
Telmisartan	Heavy metals
Temocapril Hydrochloride	Heavy metals
Teprenone	Heavy metals
Terbinafine Hydrochloride	Heavy metals
Terbutaline Sulfate	Heavy metals, Arsenic
Tetracaine Hydrochloride	Heavy metals
Tetracycline Hydrochloride	Heavy metals
Theophylline	Heavy metals, Arsenic
Thiamazole	Heavy metals, Arsenic, Selenium
Thiamine Chloride Hydrochloride	Heavy metals
Thiamine Nitrate	Heavy metals
Thiamylal Sodium	Heavy metals
Thiopental Sodium	Heavy metals
Thiopental Sodium for Injection	Heavy metals
Thioridazine Hydrochloride	Heavy metals, Arsenic
L-Threonine	Heavy metals, Arsenic
Tiapride Hydrochloride	Heavy metals
Tiaramide Hydrochloride	Heavy metals, Arsenic
Ticlopidine Hydrochloride	Heavy metals, Arsenic
Timepidium Bromide Hydrate	Heavy metals
Timolol Maleate	Heavy metals
Tinidazole	Heavy metals, Arsenic
Tipepidine Hibenzate	Heavy metals, Arsenic
Tizanidine Hydrochloride	Heavy metals
Tobramycin	Heavy metals
Tocopherol	Heavy metals
Tocopherol Acetate	Heavy metals
Tocopherol Nicotinate	Heavy metals, Arsenic

The JP Drugs are to be tested according to the provisions given in the pertinent monographs, General Notices, General Rules for Crude Drugs, General Rules for Preparations, and General Tests for their conformity to the Japanese Pharmacopoeia. (See the General Notices 5.)

Official Monographs	Purity Tests to be removed
Todralazine Hydrochloride Hydrate	Heavy metals, Arsenic
Tofisopam	Heavy metals, Arsenic
Tolbutamide	Heavy metals
Tolnaftate	Heavy metals
Tolperisone Hydrochloride	Heavy metals
Tosufloxacin Tosilate Hydrate	Heavy metals, Arsenic
Tramadol Hydrochloride	Heavy metals
Tranexamic Acid	Heavy metals, Arsenic
Tranilast	Heavy metals
Trapidil	Heavy metals, Arsenic
Trehalose Hydrate	Heavy metals
Trepibutone	Heavy metals
Triamcinolone	Heavy metals
Triamcinolone Acetonide	Heavy metals
Triamterene	Heavy metals, Arsenic
Triazolam	Heavy metals
Trichlormethiazide	Heavy metals, Arsenic
Triclofos Sodium	Heavy metals, Arsenic
Trientine Hydrochloride	Heavy metals
Trihexyphenidyl Hydrochloride	Heavy metals
Trimebutine Maleate	Heavy metals, Arsenic
Trimetazidine Hydrochloride	Heavy metals
Trimethadione	Heavy metals
Trimetoquinol Hydrochloride Hydrate	Heavy metals
Tropicamide	Heavy metals
Troxipide	Heavy metals
L-Tryptophan	Heavy metals, Arsenic
Tulobuterol	Heavy metals
Tulobuterol Hydrochloride	Heavy metals
L-Tyrosine	Heavy metals
Ubenimex	Heavy metals
Ubidecarenone	Heavy metals
Ulinastatin	Heavy metals
Urapidil	Heavy metals
Urea	Heavy metals
Urokinase	Heavy metals
Ursodeoxycholic Acid	Heavy metals, Barium

The JP Drugs are to be tested according to the provisions given in the pertinent monographs, General Notices, General Rules for Crude Drugs, General Rules for Preparations, and General Tests for their conformity to the Japanese Pharmacopoeia. (See the General Notices 5.)

Official Monographs	Purity Tests to be removed
Valaciclovir Hydrochloride	Heavy metals, Palladium
L-Valine	Heavy metals, Arsenic
Valsartan	Heavy metals
Vancomycin Hydrochloride	Heavy metals
Verapamil Hydrochloride	Heavy metals, Arsenic
Voglibose	Heavy metals
Voriconazole	Heavy metals
Warfarin Potassium	Heavy metals
Wine	Arsenic
Xylitol	Heavy metals, Arsenic, Nickel
Zaltoprofen	Heavy metals, Arsenic
Zidovudine	Heavy metals
Zinc Chloride	Heavy metals, Arsenic
Zinc Oxide	Lead, Arsenic
Zinc Sulfate Hydrate	Heavy metals, Arsenic
Zolpidem Tartrate	Heavy metals
Zonisamide	Heavy metals
Zopiclone	Heavy metals

Amphotericin B for Injection

注射用アムホテリシン B

Change the description of Uniformity of dosage units as follows:

Uniformity of dosage units ⟨*6.02*⟩ It meets the requirement of the Mass variation test (*T*: Being specified separately when the drug is granted approval based on the Law.).

Amphotericin B Tablets

アムホテリシン B 錠

Change the description of Uniformity of dosage units as follows:

Uniformity of dosage units ⟨*6.02*⟩ It meets the requirement of the Mass variation test (*T*: Being specified separately when the drug is granted approval based on the Law.).

Ampicillin Sodium and Sulbactam Sodium for Injection

注射用アンピシリンナトリウム・スルバクタムナトリウム

Change the description of Uniformity of dosage units as follows:

Uniformity of dosage units ⟨*6.02*⟩ Perform the test according to the following method: it meets the requirement of the Content uniformity test (*T*: Being specified separately when the drug is granted approval based on the Law.).

Dissolve 1 Ampicillin Sodium and Sulbactam Sodium for Injection in the mobile phase to make exactly V mL so that each mL contains 5 mg (potency) of ampicillin ($C_{16}H_{19}N_3O_4S$). Pipet 5 mL of this solution, add exactly 5 mL of the internal standard solution, then add the mobile phase to make 50 mL, and use this solution as the sample solution. Then, proceed as directed in the Assay.

Amount [mg (potency)] of ampicillin ($C_{16}H_{19}N_3O_4S$)
$= M_{S1} \times Q_{Ta}/Q_{Sa} \times V/10$

Amount [mg (potency)] of sulbactam ($C_8H_{11}NO_5S$)
$= M_{S2} \times Q_{Tb}/Q_{Sb} \times V/10$

The JP Drugs are to be tested according to the provisions given in the pertinent monographs, General Notices, General Rules for Crude Drugs, General Rules for Preparations, and General Tests for their conformity to the Japanese Pharmacopoeia. (See the General Notices 5.)

Supplement I, JP XVIII

M_{S1}: Amount [mg (potency)] of Ampicillin RS taken
M_{S2}: Amount [mg (potency)] of Sulbactam RS taken

Internal standard solution—A solution of parahydroxybenzoic acid in the mobile phase (1 in 1000).

Add the following:

Anastrozole

アナストロゾール

$C_{17}H_{19}N_5$: 293.37
2,2'-[5-(1*H*-1,2,4-Triazol-1-ylmethyl)benzene-1,3-diyl]bis(2-methylpropanenitrile)
[*120511-73-1*]

Anastrozole contains not less than 98.0% and not more than 102.0% of anastrozole ($C_{17}H_{19}N_5$).

Description Anastrozole occurs as a white, crystalline powder or powder.

It is very soluble in acetonitrile, freely soluble in methanol and in ethanol (99.5), and very slightly soluble in water.

It shows crystal polymorphism.

Identification (1) Determine the absorption spectrum of a solution of Anastrozole in methanol (1 in 50,000) as directed under Ultraviolet-visible Spectrophotometry <2.24>, and compare the spectrum with the Reference Spectrum or the spectrum of a solution of Anastrozole RS prepared in the same manner as the sample solution: both spectra exhibit similar intensities of absorption at the same wavelengths.

(2) Determine the infrared absorption spectrum of Anastrozole as directed in the potassium bromide disk method under Infrared Spectrophotometry <2.25>, and compare the spectrum with the Reference Spectrum or the spectrum of Anastrozole RS: both spectra exhibit similar intensities of absorption at the same wave numbers.

Purity Related substances—Weigh accurately about 50 mg of Anastrozole, add 10 mL of acetonitrile for liquid chromatography, sonicate to dissolve, add the mobile phase A to make exactly 25 mL, and use this solution as the sample solution. Separately, weigh accurately about 50 mg of Anastrozole RS, add 10 mL of acetonitrile for liquid chromatography, sonicate to dissolve, and add the mobile phase A to make exactly 25 mL. Pipet 1 mL of this solution, add the mobile phase A to make exactly 100 mL, and use this solution as the standard solution. Perform the test with exactly 10 μL each of the sample solution and standard solution as directed under Liquid Chromatography <2.01> according to the following conditions. Determine the peak area, A_T, of

each related substance from the sample solution, and the peak area, A_S, of anastrozole from the standard solution by the automatic integration method, and calculate the amounts of related substances by the following equation: the amounts of the related substances A and B, having the relative retention time of about 0.63 and about 2.2 to anastrozole, obtained from the sample solution are not more than 0.2%, respectively, each of other related substances is not more than 0.1%, and the total amount of other related substances is not more than 0.2%. Furthermore, the total amount of the related substances is not more than 0.5%.

$$\text{Amount (\%) of related substance} = M_S/M_T \times A_T/A_S$$

M_S: Amount (mg) of Anastrozole RS taken
M_T: Amount (mg) of Anastrozole taken

Operating conditions—

Detector, column, column temperature, mobile phases A and B, flowing of mobile phase and flow rate: Proceed as directed in the operating conditions in the Assay.

Time span of measurement: For 40 minutes after injection of the sample solution.

System suitability—

Test for required detectability: Pipet 1 mL of the standard solution, and add the mobile phase A to make exactly 20 mL. Confirm that the peak area of anastrozole obtained with 10 μL of this solution is equivalent to 3 to 7% of that with 10 μL of the standard solution.

System performance: When the procedure is run with 10 μL of the standard solution under the above operating conditions, the number of theoretical plates and the symmetry factor of the peak of anastrozole are not less than 1500 and not more than 1.4, respectively.

System repeatability: When the test is repeated 6 times with 10 μL of the standard solution under the above operating conditions, the relative standard deviation of the peak area of anastrozole is not more than 2.0%.

Water <2.48> Not more than 0.3% (50 mg, coulometric titration).

Residue on ignition <2.44> Not more than 0.1% (1 g).

Assay Weigh accurately about 25 mg each of Anastrozole and Anastrozole RS, to each add 20 mL of acetonitrile for liquid chromatography, sonicate to dissolve, add the mobile phase A to make exactly 50 mL, and use these solutions as the sample solution and the standard solution, respectively. Perform the test with exactly 10 μL each of the sample solution and standard solution as directed under Liquid Chromatography <2.01> according to the following conditions, and determine the peak areas, A_T and A_S, of anastrozole in each solution.

$$\text{Amount (mg) of anastrozole } (C_{17}H_{19}N_5) = M_S \times A_T/A_S$$

M_S: Amount (mg) of Anastrozole RS taken

The JP Drugs are to be tested according to the provisions given in the pertinent monographs, General Notices, General Rules for Crude Drugs, General Rules for Preparations, and General Tests for their conformity to the Japanese Pharmacopoeia. (See the General Notices 5.)

2870 Official Monographs

Operating conditions—

Detector: An ultraviolet absorption photometer (wavelength: 215 nm).

Column: A stainless steel column 3.2 mm in inside diameter and 10 cm in length, packed with octadecylsilyl and octylsilyl groups bound to porous silica gel for liquid chromatography (5 μm in particle diameter).

Column temperature: A constant temperature of about 25°C.

Mobile phase A: A mixture of water, methanol for liquid chromatography, acetonitrile for liquid chromatography and trifluoroacetic acid (1200:600:200:1).

Mobile phase B: A mixture of methanol for liquid chromatography, water, acetonitrile for liquid chromatography and trifluoroacetic acid (900:800:300:1).

Flowing of mobile phase: Control the gradient by mixing the mobile phases A and B as directed in the following table.

Time after injection of sample (min)	Mobile phase A (vol%)	Mobile phase B (vol%)
0 – 10	100	0
10 – 40	100 → 0	0 → 100

Flow rate: 0.75 mL per minute (the retention time of anastrozole is about 6 minutes).

System suitability—

System performance: When the procedure is run with 10 μL of the standard solution under the above operating conditions, the number of theoretical plates and the symmetry factor of the peak of anastrozole are not less than 1200 and not more than 1.4, respectively.

System repeatability: When the test is repeated 6 times with 10 μL of the standard solution under the above operating conditions, the relative standard deviation of the peak area of anastrozole is not more than 1.0%.

Containers and storage   Containers—Well-closed containers.

Others
Related substance A:
2-[3-(1-Cyanoethyl)-5-(1H-1,2,4-triazol-1-ylmethyl)phenyl]-2-methylpropanenitrile

Related substance B:
2,3-Bis[3-(2-cyanopropan-2-yl)-5-(1H-1,2,4-triazol-1-ylmethyl)phenyl]-2-methylpropanenitrile

Add the following:

Anastrozole Tablets

アナストロゾール錠

Anastrozole Tablets contain not less than 95.0% and not more than 105.0% of the labeled amount of anastrozole ($C_{17}H_{19}N_5$: 293.37).

Method of preparation   Prepare as directed under Tablets, with Anastrozole.

Identification   To a quantity of powdered Anastrozole Tablets, equivalent to 8 mg of Anastrozole, add 10 mL of diethyl ether, sonicate, and filter through a membrane filter with a pore size not exceeding 0.45 μm. To the filtrate add 0.40 g of potassium bromide for infrared spectrophotometry, and evaporate the diethyl ether. Determine the infrared absorption spectrum of the residue as directed in the potassium bromide disk method under Infrared Spectrophotometry <2.25>: it exhibits absorption at the wave numbers of about 3100 cm^{-1}, 2980 cm^{-1}, 2240 cm^{-1}, 1606 cm^{-1}, 1502 cm^{-1}, 1359 cm^{-1}, 1206 cm^{-1}, 1139 cm^{-1}, 876 cm^{-1}, 763 cm^{-1}, 713 cm^{-1} and 680 cm^{-1}.

Uniformity of dosage units <6.02>   Perform the test according to the following method: it meets the requirement of the Content uniformity test.

To 1 tablet of Anastrozole Tablets add 8 mL of a mixture of water, acetonitrile for liquid chromatography and trifluoroacetic acid (1000:1000:1), sonicate, and shake thoroughly until the tablet is completely disintegrated. Add a mixture of water, acetonitrile for liquid chromatography and trifluoroacetic acid (1000:1000:1) to make exactly V mL so that each mL contains about 0.1 mg of anastrozole ($C_{17}H_{19}N_5$). Filter this solution through a membrane filter with a pore size not exceeding 0.45 μm, discard 3 mL of the first filtrate, and use the subsequent filtrate as the sample solution. Then, proceed as directed in the Assay.

Amount (mg) of anastrozole ($C_{17}H_{19}N_5$)
$$= M_S \times A_T/A_S \times V/500$$

M_S: Amount (mg) of Anastrozole RS taken

The JP Drugs are to be tested according to the provisions given in the pertinent monographs, General Notices, General Rules for Crude Drugs, General Rules for Preparations, and General Tests for their conformity to the Japanese Pharmacopoeia. (See the General Notices 5.)

Supplement I, JP XVIII *Official Monographs* 2871

Dissolution <6.10> When the test is performed at 50 revolutions per minute according to the Paddle method, using 1000 mL of water as the dissolution medium, the dissolution rate in 15 minutes of Anastrozole Tablets is not less than 80%.

Start the test with 1 tablet of Anastrozole Tablets, withdraw not less than 10 mL of the medium at the specified minute after starting the test, and filter through a membrane filter with a pore size not exceeding 0.45 μm. Discard not less than 3 mL of the first filtrate, pipet V mL of the subsequent filtrate, add water to make exactly V' mL so that each mL contains about 1.0 μg of anastrozole ($C_{17}H_{19}N_5$), and use this solution as the sample solution. Separately, weigh accurately about 50 mg of Anastrozole RS, add 20 mL of acetonitrile for liquid chromatography, sonicate, and add water to make exactly 250 mL. Pipet 5 mL of this solution, add water to make exactly 100 mL. Pipet 10 mL of this solution, add water to make exactly 100 mL, and use this solution as the standard solution. Perform the test with exactly 100 μL each of the sample solution and standard solution as directed under Liquid Chromatography <2.01> according to the following conditions, and determine the peak areas, A_T and A_S, of anastrozole in each solution.

Dissolution rate (%) with respect to the labeled amount of anastrozole ($C_{17}H_{19}N_5$)
$$= M_S \times A_T/A_S \times V'/V \times 1/C \times 2$$

M_S: Amount (mg) of Anastrozole RS taken
C: Labeled amount (mg) of anastrozole ($C_{17}H_{19}N_5$) in 1 tablet

Operating conditions—
Detector, column and column temperature: Proceed as directed in the operating conditions in the Assay under Anastrozole.
Mobile phase: A mixture of water, acetonitrile for liquid chromatography and trifluoroacetic acid (700:300:1).
Flow rate: Adjust so that the retention time of anastrozole is about 7 minutes.
System suitability—
System performance: To 15 mg of methyl parahydroxybenzoate and 50 mg of Anastrozole RS, add 20 mL of acetonitrile for liquid chromatography, sonicate, and add water to make 250 mL. To 5 mL of this solution add water to make 100 mL. To 10 mL of this solution add water to make 100 mL, and use this solution as the solution for system suitability test. When the procedure is run with 100 μL of the solution for system suitability test under the above operating conditions, methyl parahydroxybenzoate and anastrozole are eluted in this order with the resolution between these peaks being not less than 4.
System repeatability: When the test is repeated 6 times with 100 μL of the solution for system suitability test under the above operating conditions, the relative standard deviation of the peak area of anastrozole is not more than 1.5%.

Assay Weigh accurately the mass of not less than 20 tablets of Anastrozole Tablets, and powder. Weigh accu-

rately a portion of the powder, equivalent to about 10 mg of anastrozole ($C_{17}H_{19}N_5$), add 80 mL of a mixture of water, acetonitrile for liquid chromatography and trifluoroacetic acid (1000:1000:1), sonicate to dissolve, and add a mixture of water, acetonitrile for liquid chromatography and trifluoroacetic acid (1000:1000:1) to make exactly 100 mL. Filter this solution through a membrane filter with a pore size not exceeding 0.45 μm, discard 3 mL of the first filtrate, and use the subsequent filtrate as the sample solution. Separately, weigh accurately about 50 mg of Anastrozole RS, add 50 mL of a mixture of water, acetonitrile for liquid chromatography and trifluoroacetic acid (1000:1000:1), sonicate to dissolve, and add a mixture of water, acetonitrile for liquid chromatography and trifluoroacetic acid (1000:1000:1) to make exactly 100 mL. Pipet 10 mL of this solution, add a mixture of water, acetonitrile for liquid chromatography and trifluoroacetic acid (1000:1000:1) to make exactly 50 mL, and use this solution as the standard solution. Perform the test with exactly 10 μL each of the sample solution and standard solution as directed under Liquid Chromatography <2.01> according to the following conditions, and determine the peak areas, A_T and A_S, of anastrozole in each solution.

Amount (mg) of anastrozole ($C_{17}H_{19}N_5$)
$$= M_S \times A_T/A_S \times 1/5$$

MS: Amount (mg) of Anastrozole RS taken

Operating conditions—
Detector, column and column temperature: Proceed as directed in the operating conditions in the Assay under Anastrozole.
Mobile phase: A mixture of water, methanol for liquid chromatography, acetonitrile for liquid chromatography and trifluoroacetic acid (7000:2000:1000:7).
Flow rate: Adjust so that the retention time of anastrozole is about 15 minutes.
System suitability—
System performance: To 30 mg of ethyl parahydroxybenzoate and 50 mg of Anastrozole RS, add 50 mL of a mixture of water, acetonitrile for liquid chromatography and trifluoroacetic acid (1000:1000:1), sonicate to dissolve, and add a mixture of water, acetonitrile for liquid chromatography and trifluoroacetic acid (1000:1000:1) to make 100 mL. To 10 mL of this solution add a mixture of water, acetonitrile for liquid chromatography and trifluoroacetic acid (1000:1000:1) to make 50 mL, and use this solution as the solution for system suitability test. When the procedure is run with 10 μL of the solution for system suitability test under the above operating conditions, ethyl parahydroxybenzoate and anastrozole are eluted in this order with the resolution between these peaks being not less than 4.
System repeatability: When the test is repeated 6 times with 10 μL of the solution for system suitability test under the above operating conditions, the relative standard deviation of the peak area of anastrozole is not more than 1.5%.

Containers and storage Containers—Tight containers.

The JP Drugs are to be tested according to the provisions given in the pertinent monographs, General Notices, General Rules for Crude Drugs, General Rules for Preparations, and General Tests for their conformity to the Japanese Pharmacopoeia. (See the General Notices 5.)

2872   *Official Monographs*   *Supplement I, JP XVIII*

Benzyl Alcohol

ベンジルアルコール

Change the Identification as follows:

Identification   Determine the infrared absorption spectrum of Benzyl Alcohol as directed in the liquid film method under Infrared Spectrophotometry <2.25>, and compare the spectrum with the Reference Spectrum: both spectra exhibit similar intensities of absorption at the same wave numbers.

Add the following:

Bicalutamide Tablets

ビカルタミド錠

Bicalutamide Tablets contain not less than 95.0% and not more than 105.0% of the labeled amount of bicalutamide ($C_{18}H_{14}F_4N_2O_4S$: 430.37).

Method of preparation   Prepare as directed under Tablets, with Bicalutamide.

Identification   To a quantity of powdered Bicalutamide Tablets, equivalent to 5 mg of Bicalutamide, add 250 mL of methanol, shake thoroughly, and filter through a membrane filter with a pore size not exceeding 0.45 μm. To 10 mL of the filtrate add methanol to make 20 mL. Determine the absorption spectrum of the solution as directed under Ultraviolet-visible Spectrophotometry <2.24>: it exhibits a maximum between 269 nm and 273 nm.

Uniformity of dosage units <6.02>   Perform the Mass variation test, or the Content uniformity test according to the following method: it meets the requirement.

To 1 tablet of Bicalutamide Tablets add 10 mL of water, shake until the tablet is disintegrated. Then, add 80 mL of tetrahydrofuran, sonicate, add tetrahydrofuran to make exactly 100 mL, and filter through a membrane filter with a pore size 0.45 μm. Discard 1 mL of the first filtrate, pipet V mL of the subsequent filtrate, add a solution of sodium lauryl sulfate (3 in 200) to make exactly V' mL so that each mL contains about 8 μg of bicalutamide ($C_{18}H_{14}F_4N_2O_4S$), and use this solution as the sample solution. Separately, weigh accurately about 16 mg of Bicalutamide RS (separately determine the loss on drying <2.41> in the same conditions as Bicalutamide), dissolve in 2 mL of tetrahydrofuran, and add a solution of sodium lauryl sulfate (3 in 200) to make exactly 200 mL. Pipet 5 mL of this solution, add a solution of sodium lauryl sulfate (3 in 200) to make exactly 50 mL, and use this solution as the standard solution. Determine the absorbances, A_T and A_S, of the sample solution and standard solution at 270 nm as directed under Ultraviolet-visible Spectrophotometry <2.24>.

Amount (mg) of bicalutamide ($C_{18}H_{14}F_4N_2O_4S$)
$$= M_S \times A_T/A_S \times V'/V \times 1/20$$

M_S: Amount (mg) of Bicalutamide RS taken, calculated on the dried basis

Dissolution <6.10>   When the test is performed at 50 revolutions per minute according to the Paddle method, using 1000 mL of a solution of sodium lauryl sulfate (3 in 200) as the dissolution medium, the dissolution rate in 45 minutes of Bicalutamide Tablets is not less than 80%.

Start the test with 1 tablet of Bicalutamide Tablets, withdraw not less than 10 mL of the medium at the specified minute after starting the test, and filter through a membrane filter with a pore size not exceeding 0.45 μm. Discard not less than 1 mL of the first filtrate, pipet V mL of the subsequent filtrate, add the dissolution medium to make exactly V' mL so that each mL contains about 8 μg of bicalutamide ($C_{18}H_{14}F_4N_2O_4S$), and use this solution as the sample solution. Separately, weigh accurately about 16 mg of Bicalutamide RS (separately determine the loss on drying <2.41> in the same conditions as Bicalutamide), dissolve in 2 mL of tetrahydrofuran, and add the dissolution medium to make exactly 200 mL. Pipet 5 mL of this solution, add the dissolution medium to make exactly 50 mL, and use this solution as the standard solution. Determine the absorbances, A_T and A_S, of the sample solution and standard solution at 270 nm as directed under Ultraviolet-visible Spectrophotometry <2.24>.

Dissolution rate (%) with respect to the labeled amount of bicalutamide ($C_{18}H_{14}F_4N_2O_4S$)
$$= M_S \times A_T/A_S \times V'/V \times 1/C \times 50$$

M_S: Amount (mg) of Bicalutamide RS taken, calculated on the dried basis
C: Labeled   amount   (mg)   of   bicalutamide ($C_{18}H_{14}F_4N_2O_4S$) in 1 tablet

Assay   Weigh accurately the mass of not less than 20 tablets of Bicalutamide Tablets, and powder. Weigh accurately a portion of the powder, equivalent to about 50 mg of bicalutamide ($C_{18}H_{14}F_4N_2O_4S$), add 50 mL of tetrahydrofuran, sonicate, and add tetrahydrofuran to make exactly 100 mL. Filter this solution through a membrane filter with a pore size not exceeding 0.45 μm. Discard 1 mL of the first filtrate, pipet 4 mL of the subsequent filtrate, add exactly 5 mL of the internal standard solution, then add the mobile phase to make 50 mL, and use this solution as the sample solution. Separately, weigh accurately about 25 mg of Bicalutamide RS (separately determine the loss on drying <2.41> in the same conditions as Bicalutamide), dissolve in tetrahydrofuran to make exactly 50 mL. Pipet 4 mL of this solution, add exactly 5 mL of the internal standard solution, then add the mobile phase to make 50 mL, and use this solution as the standard solution. Perform the test with 10 μL each of the sample solution and standard solution as directed under Liquid Chromatography <2.01> according to the following conditions, and calculate the ratios, Q_T and Q_S, of the peak area of bicalutamide to that of the internal

The JP Drugs are to be tested according to the provisions given in the pertinent monographs, General Notices, General Rules for Crude Drugs, General Rules for Preparations, and General Tests for their conformity to the Japanese Pharmacopoeia. (See the General Notices 5.)

Supplement I, JP XVIII   *Official Monographs*   2873

standard.

     Amount (mg) of bicalutamide ($C_{18}H_{14}F_4N_2O_4S$)
       $= M_S \times Q_T/Q_S \times 2$

M_S: Amount (mg) of Bicalutamide RS taken, calculated
   on the dried basis

Internal standard solution—A solution of propyl parahydroxybenzoate in the mobile phase.

Operating conditions—

  Detector: An ultraviolet absorption photometer (wavelength: 270 nm).

  Column: A stainless steel column 4.6 mm in inside diameter and 12.5 cm in length, packed with octadecylsilanized silica gel for liquid chromatography (3 μm in particle diameter).

  Column temperature: A constant temperature of about 50°C.

  Mobile phase: A mixture of water, tetrahydrofuran and acetonitrile (13:4:3).

  Flow rate: Adjust so that the retention time of bicalutamide is about 7 minutes.

System suitability—

  System performance: When the procedure is run with 10 μL of the standard solution under the above operating conditions, the internal standard and bicalutamide are eluted in this order with the resolution between these peaks being not less than 7.

  System repeatability: When the test is repeated 6 times with 10 μL of the standard solution under the above operating conditions, the relative standard deviation of the ratio of the peak area of bicalutamide to that of the internal standard is not more than 1.0%.

Containers and storage Containers—Well-closed containers.

Bromhexine Hydrochloride

ブロムヘキシン塩酸塩

Change the Purity as follows:

Purity Related substances—Conduct this procedure without exposure to light, using light-resistant vessels. Dissolve 50 mg of Bromhexine Hydrochloride in 10 mL of methanol, and use this solution as the sample solution. Pipet 1 mL of the sample solution, and add the mobile phase to make exactly 20 mL. Pipet 1 mL of this solution, add the mobile phase to make exactly 25 mL, and use this solution as the standard solution. Perform the test with exactly 5 μL each of the sample solution and standard solution as directed under Liquid Chromatography <2.01> according to the following conditions, and determine each peak area by the automatic integration method: each peak area other than bromhexine obtained from the sample solution is not larger than the peak area of bromhexine from the standard solution.

Operating conditions—

  Detector: An ultraviolet absorption photometer (wavelength: 245 nm).

  Column: A stainless steel column 4.6 mm in inside diameter and 15 cm in length, packed with octadecylsilanized silica gel for liquid chromatography (5 μm in particle diameter).

  Column temperature: A constant temperature of about 40°C.

  Mobile phase: Dissolve 1.0 g of potassium dihydrogen phosphate in 900 mL of water, adjust to pH 7.0 with 0.5 mol/L sodium hydroxide TS, and add water to make 1000 mL. To 200 mL of this solution add 800 mL of acetonitrile.

  Flow rate: Adjust so that the retention time of bromhexine is about 6 minutes.

  Time span of measurement: About 2 times as long as the retention time of bromhexine, beginning after the solvent peak.

System suitability—

  Test for required detectability: Pipet 5 mL of the standard solution, and add the mobile phase to make exactly 20 mL. Confirm that the peak area of bromhexine obtained with 5 μL of this solution is equivalent to 17.5 to 32.5% of that with 5 μL of the standard solution.

  System performance: When the procedure is run with 5 μL of the standard solution under the above operating conditions, the number of theoretical plates and the symmetry factor of the peak of bromhexine are not less than 2800 and not more than 1.5, respectively.

  System repeatability: When the test is repeated 6 times with 5 μL of the standard solution under the above operating conditions, the relative standard deviation of the peak area of bromhexine is not more than 2.0%.

Add the following:

Budesonide

ブデソニド

and epimer at C*

$C_{25}H_{34}O_6$: 430.53
16α,17-[(1*RS*)-Butylidenebis(oxy)]-11β,21-dihydroxypregna-1,4-diene-3,20-dione
[*51333-22-3*]

  Budesonide contains not less than 98.0% and not more than 102.0% of budesonide ($C_{25}H_{34}O_6$), calculated on the dried basis.

Description Budesonide occurs as white to pale yellow-white, crystals or crystalline powder.

The JP Drugs are to be tested according to the provisions given in the pertinent monographs, General Notices, General Rules for Crude Drugs, General Rules for Preparations, and General Tests for their conformity to the Japanese Pharmacopoeia. (See the General Notices 5.)

2874　*Official Monographs*

It is soluble in methanol, sparingly soluble in acetonitrile and in ethanol (99.5), and practically insoluble in water.

Optical rotation: $[\alpha]_D^{25}$: $+102 - +109°$ (0.25 g, methanol, 25 mL, 100 mm).

Melting point: about 240°C (with decomposition).

Identification　**(1)**　Determine the absorption spectrum of a solution of Budesonide (1 in 40,000) as directed under Ultraviolet-visible Spectrophotometry <2.24>, and compare the spectrum with the Reference Spectrum or the spectrum of a solution of Budesonide RS prepared in the same manner as the sample solution: both spectra exhibit similar intensities of absorption at the same wavelengths.

(2)　Determine the infrared absorption spectrum of Budesonide as directed in the potassium bromide disk method under Infrared Spectrophotometry <2.25>, and compare the spectrum with the Reference Spectrum or the spectrum of Budesonide RS: both spectra exhibit similar intensities of absorption at the same wave numbers.

Purity　Related substances—Conduct this procedure without exposure to light, using light-resistant vessels. Dissolve 50 mg of Budesonide in 15 mL of acetonitrile, add phosphate buffer solution (pH 3.2) to make 50 mL, and use this solution as the sample solution. Perform the test with 20 μL of the sample solution as directed under Liquid Chromatography <2.01> according to the following conditions. Determine each peak area by the automatic integration method, and calculate the amount of them by the area percentage method: the amounts of the peaks of related substances A and L, having the relative retention times of about 0.1 and about 0.95 to the first eluted peak (epimer B) of the two peaks of budesonide, are not more than 0.2%, respectively, the sum of the amounts of the peaks of related substance D, having the relative retention times of about 0.63 and about 0.67, and the sum of the amounts of the peaks of the related substance K, having the relative retention times of about 2.9 and about 3.0, are not more than 0.2%, respectively, and the amount of the peak other than budesonide and mentioned above is not more than 0.1%. Furthermore, the total amount of the peaks other than budesonide is not more than 0.5%. For the peak areas of the related substances D and K, multiply their correction factors, 1.8 and 1.3, respectively.

Operating conditions—

Detector, column, column temperature and flow rate: Proceed as directed in the operating conditions in the Assay.

Mobile phase A: A mixture of phosphate buffer solution (pH 3.2), acetonitrile for liquid chromatography and ethanol (99.5) (34:16:1).

Mobile phase B: A mixture of phosphate buffer solution (pH 3.2) and acetonitrile for liquid chromatography (1:1).

Flowing of mobile phase: Control the gradient by mixing the mobile phases A and B as directed in the following table.

Time after injection of sample (min)	Mobile phase A (vol%)	Mobile phase B (vol%)
0 – 38	100	0
38 – 50	100 → 0	0 → 100
50 – 60	0	100

Time span of measurement: For 60 minutes after injection, beginning after the solvent peak.

System suitability—

Test for required detectability: Pipet 1 mL of the sample solution add a mixture of phosphate buffer solution (pH 3.2) and acetonitrile (17:8) to make exactly 10 mL. Pipet 1 mL of this solution, add a mixture of phosphate buffer solution (pH 3.2) and acetonitrile (17:8) to make exactly 100 mL, and use this solution as the solution for system suitability test. When the procedure is run with 20 μL of the solution for system suitability test under the above operating conditions, the SN ratio of the second eluted peak (epimer A) of the two peaks of budesonide is not less than 10.

System performance: When the procedure is run with 20 μL of the solution for system suitability test under the above operating conditions, the resolution between the two peaks of budesonide is not less than 1.5.

Loss on drying <2.41>　Not more than 0.5% (1 g, 105°C, 3 hours).

Isomer ratio　Conduct this procedure without exposure to light, using light-resistant vessels. Perform the test with 20 μL of the sample solution obtained in the Assay as directed under Liquid Chromatography <2.01> according to the following conditions. Determine the peak areas, A_b and A_a, where A_b is the area of the early eluted peak and A_a is the area of the lately eluted peak of the two peaks of budesonide: $A_a/(A_a + A_b)$ is between 0.40 and 0.51.

Operating conditions—

Proceed as directed in the operating conditions in the Assay.

System suitability—

System performance: Proceed as directed in the system suitability in the Assay.

Assay　Conduct this procedure without exposure to light, using light-resistant vessels. Weigh accurately about 25 mg each of Budesonide and Budesonide RS (separately determine the loss on drying <2.41> under the same conditions as Budesonide), dissolve each in 15 mL of acetonitrile, add phosphate buffer solution (pH 3.2) to make exactly 50 mL, and use these solutions as the sample solution and the standard solution, respectively. Perform the test with exactly 20 μL each of the sample solution and standard solution as directed under Liquid Chromatography <2.01> according to the following conditions, and determine the peak areas, A_T and A_S, of the sum of the two peak areas of budesonide in each solution.

The JP Drugs are to be tested according to the provisions given in the pertinent monographs, General Notices, General Rules for Crude Drugs, General Rules for Preparations, and General Tests for their conformity to the Japanese Pharmacopoeia. (See the General Notices 5.)

Supplement I, JP XVIII *Official Monographs* 2875

Amount (mg) of budesonide ($C_{25}H_{34}O_6$) = $M_S \times A_T/A_S$

M_S: Amount (mg) of Budesonide RS taken, calculated on the dried basis

Operating conditions—

Detector: An ultraviolet absorption photometer (wavelength: 240 nm).

Column: A stainless steel column 4.6 mm in inside diameter and 15 cm in length, packed with octadecylsilanized silica gel for liquid chromatography (3 μm in particle diameter).

Column temperature: A constant temperature of about 50°C.

Mobile phase: A mixture of phosphate buffer solution (pH 3.2), acetonitrile for liquid chromatography and ethanol (99.5) (34:16:1).

Flow rate: 1.0 mL per minute (the retention times of two peaks of budesonide are about 17 and about19 minutes).

System suitability—

System performance: When the procedure is run with 20 μL of the standard solution under the above operating conditions, the resolution between the two peaks of budesonide is not less than 1.5.

System repeatability: When the test is repeated 6 times with 20 μL of the standard solution under the above operating conditions, the relative standard deviation of the sum of the two peak areas of budesonide is not more than 1.0%.

Containers and storage Containers—Tight containers.
Storage—Light-resistant.

Others

Related substance A:
11β,16α,17,21-Tetrahydroxypregna-1,4-diene-3,20-dione

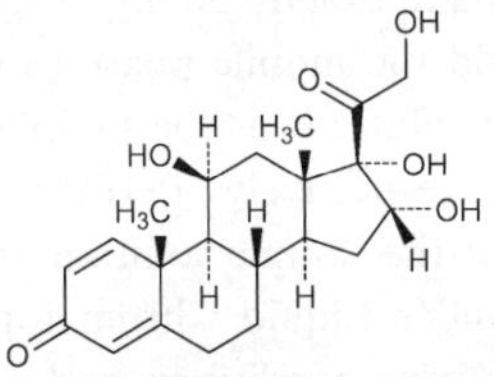

Related substance D:
16α,17-[(1RS)-Butylidenebis(oxy)]-11β-hydroxy-3,20-dioxopregna-1,4-dien-21-al

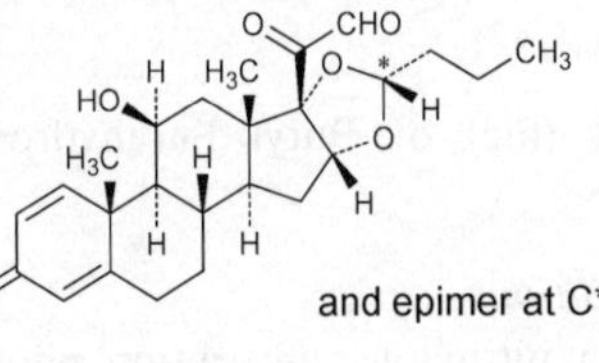

and epimer at C*

Related substance K:
16α,17-[(1RS)-Butylidenebis(oxy)]-11β,21-dihydroxypregna-1,4-diene-3,20-dione 21-acetate

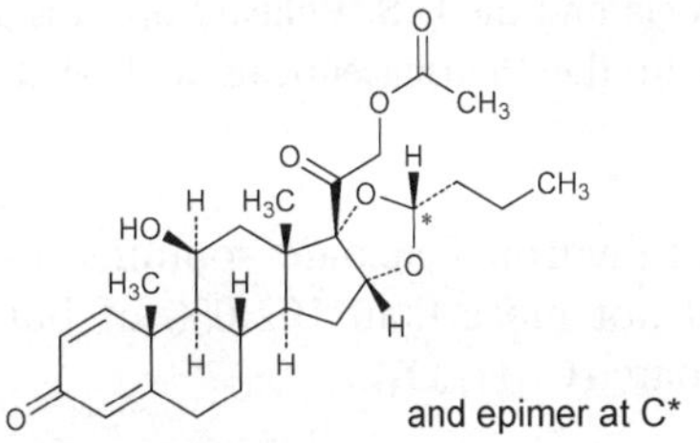

and epimer at C*

Related substance L:
16α,17-[(1RS)-Butylidenebis(oxy)]-21-hydroxypregna-1,4-diene-3,11,20-trione

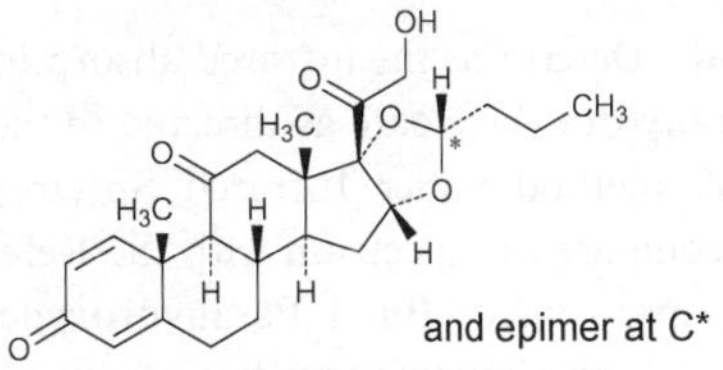

and epimer at C*

Butropium Bromide

ブトロピウム臭化物

Change the Assay as follows:

Assay Weigh accurately about 0.8 g of Butropium Bromide, previously dried, dissolve in 5 mL of formic acid, add 100 mL of acetic anhydride, and titrate <2.50> with 0.1 mol/L perchloric acid VS (potentiometric titration). Perform a blank determination in the same manner, and make any necessary correction.

Each mL of 0.1 mol/L perchloric acid VS
= 53.25 mg of $C_{28}H_{38}BrNO_4$

Change the following as follows:

Butyl Parahydroxybenzoate

パラオキシ安息香酸ブチル

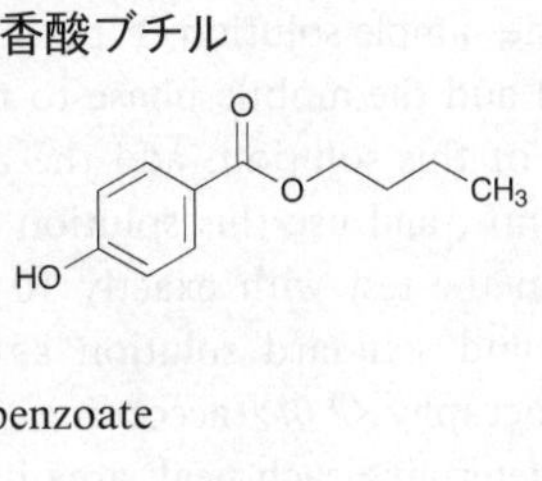

$C_{11}H_{14}O_3$: 194.23
Butyl 4-hydroxybenzoate
[94-26-8]

This monograph is harmonized with the European Pharmacopoeia and the U.S. Pharmacopeia.

The corresponding part of the attributes/provisions which are agreed as non-harmonized within the scope of the harmonization is marked with symbols (♦ ♦), and the corresponding parts which are agreed as the JP local require-

The JP Drugs are to be tested according to the provisions given in the pertinent monographs, General Notices, General Rules for Crude Drugs, General Rules for Preparations, and General Tests for their conformity to the Japanese Pharmacopoeia. (See the General Notices 5.)

2876   *Official Monographs*   *Supplement I, JP XVIII*

ment other than the scope of the harmonization are marked with symbols (◇ ◇).

Information on the harmonization with the European Pharmacopoeia and the U.S. Pharmacopeia is available on the website of the Pharmaceuticals and Medical Devices Agency.

Butyl Parahydroxybenzoate contains not less than 98.0% and not more than 102.0% of butyl parahydroxybenzoate ($C_{11}H_{14}O_3$).

◆**Description**   Butyl Parahydroxybenzoate occurs as colorless crystals or white crystalline powder.

It is very soluble in methanol, freely soluble in ethanol (95) and in acetone, and practically insoluble in water.◆

Identification   Determine the infrared absorption spectrum of Butyl Parahydroxybenzoate as directed in the potassium bromide disk method under Infrared Spectrophotometry <2.25>, and compare the spectrum with the Reference Spectrum or the spectrum of Butyl Parahydroxybenzoate RS: both spectra exhibit similar intensities of absorption at the same wave numbers.

Melting point <2.60>   68 – 71°C

Purity   (1)   Clarity and color of solution—Dissolve 1.0 g of Butyl Parahydroxybenzoate in ethanol (95) to make 10 mL: the solution is clear and not more intensely colored than ethanol (95) or the following control solution.

Control solution: To 5.0 mL of Cobalt (II) Chloride CS, 12.0 mL of Iron (III) Chloride CS and 2.0 mL of Copper (II) Sulfate CS add diluted dilute hydrochloric acid (1 in 10) to make 1000 mL.

(2)   Acidity—To 2 mL of the solution of Butyl Parahydroxybenzoate obtained in (1) add 3 mL of ethanol (95), add 5 mL of freshly boiled and cooled water and 0.1 mL of bromocresol green-sodium hydroxide-ethanol TS, then add 0.1 mol/L sodium hydroxide VS until the solution shows a blue color: the volume of 0.1 mol/L sodium hydroxide VS used does not exceed 0.1 mL.

(3)   Related substances—Dissolve 50.0 mg of Butyl Parahydroxybenzoate in 2.5 mL of methanol, and add the mobile phase to make exactly 50 mL. Pipet 10 mL of this solution, add the mobile phase to make exactly 100 mL, and use this solution as the sample solution. Pipet 1 mL of the sample solution, and add the mobile phase to make exactly 20 mL. Pipet 1 mL of this solution, add the mobile phase to make exactly 10 mL, and use this solution as the standard solution. Perform the test with exactly 10 μL each of the sample solution and standard solution as directed under Liquid Chromatography <2.01> according to the following conditions, and determine each peak area by the automatic integration method: the peak area of parahydroxybenzoic acid having the relative retention time of about 0.1 to butyl parahydroxybenzoate obtained from the sample solution is not larger than the peak area of butyl parahydroxybenzoate from the standard solution (0.5%). For the area of the peak of parahydroxybenzoic acid multiply the correction factor, 1.4. Furthermore, the area of the peak other than butyl par-

ahydroxybenzoate and parahydroxybenzoic acid from the sample solution is not larger than the peak area of butyl parahydroxybenzoate from the standard solution (0.5%), and the total area of the peaks other than butyl parahydroxybenzoate is not larger than 2 times the peak area of butyl parahydroxybenzoate from the standard solution (1.0%). For this calculation the peak area not larger than 1/5 times the peak area of butyl parahydroxybenzoate from the standard solution is excluded (0.1%).

Operating conditions—

Detector, column, column temperature, mobile phase, and flow rate: Proceed as directed in the operating conditions in the Assay.

Time span of measurement: 1.5 times as long as the retention time of butyl parahydroxybenzoate.

System suitability—

System performance: Proceed as directed in the system suitability in the Assay.

◇Test for required detectability: To exactly 2 mL of the standard solution add the mobile phase to make exactly 10 mL. Confirm that the peak area of butyl parahydroxybenzoate obtained with 10 μL of this solution is equivalent to 14 to 26% of that with 10 μL of the standard solution.◇

◇System repeatability: When the test is repeated 6 times with 10 μL of the standard solution under the above operating conditions, the relative standard deviation of the peak area of butyl parahydroxybenzoate is not more than 2.0%.◇

Residue on ignition <2.44>   Not more than 0.1% (1 g).

Assay   Weigh accurately about 50 mg each of Butyl Parahydroxybenzoate and Butyl Parahydroxybenzoate RS, dissolve separately in 2.5 mL each of methanol, and add the mobile phase to make exactly 50 mL. Pipet 10 mL each of these solutions, add the mobile phase to make exactly 100 mL, and use these solutions as the sample solution and the standard solution, respectively. Perform the test with exactly 10 μL each of the sample solution and standard solution as directed under Liquid Chromatography <2.01> according to the following conditions, and determine the peak areas, A_T and A_S, of butyl parahydroxybenzoate in each solution.

Amount (mg) of butyl parahydroxybenzoate ($C_{11}H_{14}O_3$)
$$= M_S \times A_T/A_S$$

M_S: Amount (mg) of Butyl Parahydroxybenzoate RS taken

Operating conditions—

Detector: An ultraviolet absorption photometer (wavelength: 272 nm).

Column: A stainless steel column 4.6 mm in inside diameter and 15 cm in length, packed with octadecylsilanized silica gel for liquid chromatography (5 μm in particle diameter).

Column temperature: A constant temperature of about 35°C.

Mobile phase: A mixture of potassium dihydrogen phos-

The JP Drugs are to be tested according to the provisions given in the pertinent monographs, General Notices, General Rules for Crude Drugs, General Rules for Preparations, and General Tests for their conformity to the Japanese Pharmacopoeia. (See the General Notices 5.)

Supplement I, JP XVIII

phate solution (17 in 2500) and methanol (1:1).

Flow rate: 1.3 mL per minute.

System suitability—

System performance: Dissolve 5 mg each of Butyl Parahydroxybenzoate, propyl parahydroxybenzoate and parahydroxybenzoic acid in the mobile phase to make exactly 100 mL. Pipet 1 mL of this solution, add the mobile phase to make exactly 10 mL, and use this solution as the solution for system suitability test (1). Separately, dissolve 5 mg of isobutyl parahydroxybenzoate in the mobile phase to make exactly 100 mL. Pipet 0.5 mL of this solution, add the standard solution to make exactly 50 mL, and use this solution as the solution for system suitability test (2). When the procedure is run with 10 μL each of the solutions for system suitability test (1) and (2) under the above operating conditions, parahydroxybenzoic acid, propyl parahydroxybenzoate, isobutyl parahydroxybenzoate and butyl parahydroxybenzoate are eluted in this order, the relative retention times of parahydroxybenzoic acid, propyl parahydroxybenzoate and isobutyl parahydoxybenzoate to butyl parahydroxybenzoate are about 0.1, about 0.5 and about 0.9, respectively, the resolution between the peaks of propyl parahydroxybenzoate and butyl parahydroxybenzoate is not less than 5.0, and the resolution between the peaks of isobutyl parahydroxybenzoate and butyl parahydroxybenzoate is not less than 1.5.

System repeatability: When the test is repeated 6 times with 10 μL of the standard solution under the above operating conditions, the relative standard deviation of the peak area of butyl parahydroxybenzoate is not more than 0.85%.

◆**Containers** **and** **storage** Containers—Well-closed containers.◆

Croscarmellose Sodium

クロスカルメロースナトリウム

Change the Identification as follows:

Identification (1) Determine the infrared absorption spectrum of Croscarmellose Sodium as directed in the potassium bromide disk method under Infrared Spectrophotometry <2.25>, and compare the spectrum with the Reference Spectrum: both spectra exhibit similar intensities of absorption at the same wave numbers. If there is an absorption at about 1750 cm^{-1}, disregard the absorption.

(2) To 1 g of Croscarmellose Sodium add 100 mL of a solution of methylene blue (1 in 250,000), stir thoroughly, and allow to stand: blue cotton-like precipitates appear.

(3) Dissolve 0.1 g of the residue obtained in the Residue on ignition in 2 mL of water, add 2 mL of potassium carbonate solution (3 in 20), and heat to boiling: no precipitate is formed. To this solution add 4 mL of potassium hexahydroxoantimonate (V) TS, heat to boiling, and cool immediately in ice water, if necessary, rubbing the inside wall of the test tube with a glass rod: a white crystalline precipitate is formed.

Delete the Purity (1) and move up the section number sequentially, and change as follows:

Purity ◆(1) Sodium chloride and sodium glycolate—The total amount of sodium chloride and sodium glycolate is not more than 0.5%, calculated on the dried basis.

(i) Sodium chloride: Weigh accurately about 5 g of Croscarmellose Sodium, add 50 mL of water and 5 mL of hydrogen peroxide (30), and heat on a water bath for 20 minutes with occasional stirring. After cooling, add 100 mL of water and 10 mL of nitric acid, and titrate <2.50> with 0.1 mol/L silver nitrate VS (potentiometric titration). Perform a blank determination in the same manner, and make any necessary correction.

Each mL of 0.1 mol/L silver nitrate VS
= 5.844 mg of NaCl

(ii) Sodium glycolate: Weigh accurately about 0.5 g of Croscarmellose Sodium, add 2 mL of acetic acid (100) and 5 mL of water, and stir for 15 minutes. Add gradually 50 mL of acetone with stirring, then add 1 g of sodium chloride, stir for 3 minutes, and filter through a filter paper moistened with acetone. Wash the residue thoroughly with 30 mL of acetone, combine the filtrate and washings, add acetone to make exactly 100 mL, and use this solution as the sample stock solution. Separately, dissolve 0.100 g of glycolic acid in water to make exactly 200 mL. Pipet 0.5 mL, 1 mL, 2 mL, 3 mL and 4 mL of this solution, add water to make them exactly 5 mL, then add 5 mL of acetic acid (100) and acetone to make exactly 100 mL, and designate them standard stock solution (1), standard stock solution (2), standard stock solution (3), standard stock solution (4) and standard stock solution (5), respectively. Pipet 2 mL each of the sample stock solution and the standard stock solutions (1), (2), (3), (4) and (5), and heat them in a water bath for 20 minutes to evaporate acetone. After cooling, add exactly 5 mL of 2,7-dihydroxynaphthalene TS, mix, then add 15 mL of 2,7-dihydroxynaphthalene TS, mix, cover the mouth of the vessels with aluminum foil, and heat in a water bath for 20 minutes. After cooling, add sulfuric acid to make exactly 25 mL, mix, and use them as the sample solution, standard solution (1), standard solution (2), standard solution (3), standard solution (4) and standard solution (5), respectively. Separately, to 10 mL of a mixture of water and acetic acid (100) (1:1) add acetone to make exactly 100 mL, and proceed with exactly 2 mL of this solution in the same manner for preparation of the sample solution, and use the solution so obtained as the blank solution. Determine the absorbances, A_T, A_{S1}, A_{S2}, A_{S3}, A_{S4} and A_{S5}, of the sample solution and the standard solutions (1), (2), (3), (4) and (5), respectively, at 540 nm as directed under Ultraviolet-visible Spectrophotometry <2.24>, using the blank solution as the control. Determine the amount (g) of glycolic acid, X, in 100 mL of the sample stock solution from the calibration curve obtained with the standard solutions, and calculate the amount of sodium glycolate by the following formula.

The JP Drugs are to be tested according to the provisions given in the pertinent monographs, General Notices, General Rules for Crude Drugs, General Rules for Preparations, and General Tests for their conformity to the Japanese Pharmacopoeia. (See the General Notices 5.)

2878 *Official Monographs*

Amount (%) of sodium glycolate
= $X/M \times 100 \times 1.289$

M: Amount (g) of sample taken, calculated on the dried basis.

◆(2)　Water-soluble substance—Weigh accurately about 10 g of Croscarmellose Sodium, disperse in 800 mL of water by stirring for 1 minute every 10 minutes during 30 minutes. If precipitation is slow, allow to stand another 1 hour. Filter by suction or centrifuge. Weigh accurately the mass of about 150 mL of the filtrate or supernatant liquid. Heat to concentrate this liquid avoiding to dryness, then dry at 105° C for 4 hours, and weigh the mass of the residue accurately. Calculate the amount of the water-soluble substance by the following formula: not less than 1.0% and not more than 10.0%.

Amount (%) of water-soluble substance
= $100 \times M_3 \times (800 + M_1)/(M_1 \times M_2)$

M_1: Amount (g) of sample taken, calculated on the dried basis

M_2: Amount (g) of the filtrate or supernatant liquid of about 150 mL

M_3: Amount (g) of the residue.

Change the Residue on ignition, Containers and storage as follows:

Residue on ignition ⟨2.44⟩　14.0 – 28.0% (1 g calculated on the dried basis).

◆**Containers and storage**　Containers—Tight containers.◆

Cefoperazone Sodium and Sulbactam Sodium for Injection

注射用セフォペラゾンナトリウム・スルバクタムナトリウム

Change the description of Uniformity of dosage units as follows:

Uniformity of dosage units ⟨6.02⟩　It meets the requirement of the Mass variation test (*T*: Being specified separately when the drug is granted approval based on the Law.).

Change the following as follows:

Powdered Cellulose

粉末セルロース

[*9004-34-6*, Cellulose]

This monograph is harmonized with the European Pharmacopoeia and the U.S. Pharmacopeia.

The corresponding part of the attributes/provisions which are agreed as non-harmonized within the scope of the harmonization is marked with symbols (◆ ◆), and the corresponding parts which are agreed as the JP local requirement other than the scope of the harmonization are marked with symbols (◇ ◇).

Information on the harmonization with the European Pharmacopoeia and the U.S. Pharmacopeia is available on the website of the Pharmaceuticals and Medical Devices Agency.

Powdered Cellulose is a purified, mechanically disintegrated alpha cellulose obtained as a pulp, ◇after partial hydrolysis as occasion demands◇, from fibrous plant materials.

◆The label indicates the mean degree of polymerization value with a range.◆

◆**Description**　Powdered Cellulose occurs as a white powder.

It is practically insoluble in water, in ethanol (95) and in diethyl ether.◆

Identification　(1)　Dissolve 20 g of zinc chloride and 6.5 g of potassium iodide in 10.5 mL of water, add 0.5 g of iodine, and shake for 15 minutes. Place about 10 mg of Powdered Cellulose on a watch glass, and disperse in 2 mL of this solution: the substance develops a blue-violet color.

◇(2)　Mix 30 g of Powdered Cellulose with 270 mL of water in a high-speed (18,000 revolutions per minute or more) blender for 5 minutes, transfer 100 mL of the dispersion to a 100-mL graduated cylinder, and allow to stand for 1 hour: a supernatant liquid appears above the layer of the cellulose.◇

(3)　Transfer 0.25 g of Powdered Cellulose, accurately weighed, to a 125-mL conical flask, add exactly 25 mL each of water and 1 mol/L cupriethylenediamine TS, and proceed as directed in the Identification (3) under Microcrystalline Cellulose. The mean degree of polymerization, *P*, is not less than 440 ◆and is within the labeled specification.◆

pH ⟨2.54⟩　Mix 10 g of Powdered Cellulose with 90 mL of water, and allow to stand for 1 hour with occasional stirring: the pH of the supernatant liquid is between 5.0 and 7.5.

Purity　(1)　Water-soluble substances—Shake 6.0 g of Powdered Cellulose with 90 mL of recently boiled and cooled water, and allow to stand for 10 minutes with occasional shaking. Filter, with the aid of vacuum through a filter paper, discard the first 10 mL of the filtrate, and pass the subsequent filtrate through the same filter, if necessary, to obtain a clear filtrate. Evaporate a 15.0-mL portion of the filtrate in a tared evaporating dish to dryness without charring, dry at 105°C for 1 hour, and weigh after allowing to cool in a desiccator: the difference between the mass of the residue and the mass obtained from a blank determination does not exceed 15.0 mg (1.5%).

(2)　Diethyl ether-soluble substances—Place 10.0 g of

The JP Drugs are to be tested according to the provisions given in the pertinent monographs, General Notices, General Rules for Crude Drugs, General Rules for Preparations, and General Tests for their conformity to the Japanese Pharmacopoeia. (See the General Notices 5.)

Supplement I, JP XVIII   *Official Monographs*   2879

Powdered Cellulose in a column having an internal diameter of about 20 mm, and pass 50 mL of peroxide-free diethyl ether through the column. Evaporate the eluate to dryness in a previously dried and tared evaporation dish. Dry the residue at 105°C for 30 minutes, and weigh after allowing to cool in a desiccator: the difference between the mass of the residue and the mass obtained from a blank determination does not exceed 15.0 mg (0.15%).

Loss on drying <2.41> Not more than 6.5% (1 g, 105°C, 3 hours).

Residue on ignition <2.44> Not more than 0.3% (1 g calculated on the dried basis).

◆**Microbial limit** <4.05> The acceptance criteria of TAMC and TYMC are 10^3 CFU/g and 10^2 CFU/g, respectively. *Escherichia coli, Salmonella, Pseudomonas aeruginosa* and *Staphylococcus aureus* are not observed.◆

◆**Containers and storage** Containers—Tight containers.◆

Enviomycin Sulfate

エンビオマイシン硫酸塩

Change the Content ratio of the active principle as follows:

Content ratio of the active principle Dissolve about 50 mg of Enviomycin Sulfate in water to make 100 mL, and use this solution as the sample solution. Perform the test with 5 μL of the sample solution as directed under Liquid Chromatography <2.01> according to the following conditions, and determine the peak areas, A_{T1} and A_{T2}, of tuberactinomycin N and tuberactinomycin O, having the relative retention time, about 1.2, to tuberactinomycin N, by the automatic integration method: $A_{T2}/(A_{T1} + A_{T2})$ is between 0.090 and 0.150.
Operating conditions—
  Detector: An ultraviolet absorption photometer (wavelength: 254 nm).
  Column: A stainless steel column 4.6 mm in inside diameter and 25 cm in length, packed with octadecylsilanized silica gel for liquid chromatography (3 μm in particle diameter).
  Column temperature: A constant temperature of about 40°C.
  Mobile phase: A mixture of water and trifluoroacetic acid (1000:1).
  Flow rate: Adjust so that the retention time of tuberactinomycin N is about 15 minutes.
System suitability—
  System performance: When the procedure is run with 5 μL of the sample solution under the above operating conditions, tuberactinomycin N and tuberactinomycin O are eluted in this order with the resolution between these peaks being not less than 3.
  System repeatability: When the test is repeated 6 times

with 5 μL of the sample solution under the above operating conditions, the relative standard deviation of the peak area of tuberactinomycin N is not more than 2.0%.

Epoetin Beta (Genetical Recombination)

エポエチン ベータ（遺伝子組換え）

Change the Identification (1) as follows:

Identification (1) Desalt an appropriate volume each of Epoetin Beta (Genetical Recombination) and Epoetin Beta RS by a suitable method, add water if necessary, to make solutions so that each mL contains about 1 mg of each protein, and use these solutions as the sample solution and the standard solution, respectively. When perform a capillary electrophoresis with the sample solution and standard solution according to the following conditions, the relative migration time of each peak to the peak of the electroosmotic flow obtained from both solutions is the same and their electropherograms are similar to each other.
Operating conditions—
  Detector: An ultraviolet absorption photometer (wavelength: 214 nm).
  Column: A silica capillary tube 50 μm in inside diameter and about 110 cm in length (about 100 cm in effective length, washed with a suitable alkaline solution and pretreated with the electrolyte solution).
  Electrolyte solution: Dissolve 0.58 g of sodium chloride, 1.79 g of tricine and 0.82 g of anhydrous sodium acetate in water to make 100 mL, and use this solution as the electrolyte stock solution. Separately, dissolve 42 g of urea in 50 mL of water, add 10 mL of the electrolyte stock solution and 250 μL of 1 mol/L 1,4-diaminobutane solution, add water to make 100 mL, adjust to pH 5.6 with diluted acetic anhydride (1 in 20), and filter through a membrane filter with a pore size of 0.45 μm.
  Running temperature: A constant temperature of about 35°C.
  Running conditions: Migration voltage (applied voltage of about 17 kV), migration time (100 minutes).
  Injection of sample and standard solutions: 15 seconds (pressurization: 10.3 kPa).
  Time span of measurement: For 100 minutes after injection.
System suitability—
  System performance: When the procedure is run with the standard solution under the above operating conditions, more than 4 major peaks of epoetin beta are detected, and the resolution between the first and second eluted major peaks is not less than 0.8.
  System repeatability: When the test is repeated 3 times with the standard solution under the above operating conditions, the relative standard deviation of the relative migration time of the first eluted major peak to the peak of the electroosmotic flow detected before the peak of epoetin beta

The JP Drugs are to be tested according to the provisions given in the pertinent monographs, General Notices, General Rules for Crude Drugs, General Rules for Preparations, and General Tests for their conformity to the Japanese Pharmacopoeia. (See the General Notices 5.)

2880 *Official Monographs* *Supplement I, JP XVIII*

is not more than 2%.

Ethanol

エタノール

Change the description of the international harmonization at the beginning of the text, containers and storage, and shelf life as follows:

This monograph is harmonized with the European Pharmacopoeia and the U.S. Pharmacopeia.

The corresponding part of the attributes/provisions which are agreed as non-harmonized within the scope of the harmonization is marked with symbols (♦ ♦), and the corresponding parts which are agreed as the JP local requirement other than the scope of the harmonization are marked with symbols (◇ ◇).

Information on the harmonization with the European Pharmacopoeia and the U.S. Pharmacopeia is available on the website of the Pharmaceuticals and Medical Devices Agency.

Containers and storage ◇Containers—Tight containers.◇ Storage—Without exposure to light.

◇**Shelf life** In not glass containers: Unless otherwise specified, 24 months after preparation.◇

Anhydrous Ethanol

無水エタノール

Change the description of the international harmonization at the beginning of the text, containers and storage, and shelf life as follows:

This monograph is harmonized with the European Pharmacopoeia and the U.S. Pharmacopeia.

The corresponding part of the attributes/provisions which are agreed as non-harmonized within the scope of the harmonization is marked with symbols (♦ ♦), and the corresponding parts which are agreed as the JP local requirement other than the scope of the harmonization are marked with symbols (◇ ◇).

Information on the harmonization with the European Pharmacopoeia and the U.S. Pharmacopeia is available on the website of the Pharmaceuticals and Medical Devices Agency.

Containers and storage ◇Containers—Tight containers.◇ Storage—Without exposure to light.

◇**Shelf life** In not glass containers: Unless otherwise specified, 24 months after preparation.◇

Change the following as follows:

Ethyl Parahydroxybenzoate

パラオキシ安息香酸エチル

$C_9H_{10}O_3$: 166.17
Ethyl 4-hydroxybenzoate
[*120-47-8*]

This monograph is harmonized with the European Pharmacopoeia and the U.S. Pharmacopeia.

The corresponding part of the attributes/provisions which are agreed as non-harmonized within the scope of the harmonization is marked with symbols (♦ ♦), and the corresponding parts which are agreed as the JP local requirement other than the scope of the harmonization are marked with symbols (◇ ◇).

Information on the harmonization with the European Pharmacopoeia and the U.S. Pharmacopeia is available on the website of the Pharmaceuticals and Medical Devices Agency.

Ethyl Parahydroxybenzoate contains not less than 98.0% and not more than 102.0% of ethyl parahydroxybenzoate ($C_9H_{10}O_3$).

♦**Description** Ethyl Parahydroxybenzoate occurs as colorless crystals or a white, crystalline powder.

It is freely soluble in methanol, in ethanol (95) and in acetone, and very slightly soluble in water.♦

Identification Determine the infrared absorption spectrum of Ethyl Parahydroxybenzoate as directed in the potassium bromide disk method under Infrared Spectrophotometry ⟨*2.25*⟩, and compare the spectrum with the Reference Spectrum or the spectrum of Ethyl Parahydroxybenzoate RS: both spectra exhibit similar intensities of absorption at the same wave numbers.

Melting point ⟨*2.60*⟩ 115 – 118°C

Purity (1) Clarity and color of solution—Dissolve 1.0 g of Ethyl Parahydroxybenzoate in ethanol (95) to make 10 mL: the solution is clear and not more intensely colored than ethanol (95) or the following control solution.

Control solution: To 5.0 mL of Cobalt (II) Chloride CS, 12.0 mL of Iron (III) Chloride CS and 2.0 mL of Copper (II) Sulfate CS add diluted dilute hydrochloric acid (1 in 10) to make 1000 mL.

(2) Acidity—To 2 mL of the solution of Ethyl Parahydroxybenzoate obtained in (1) add 3 mL of ethanol (95), add 5 mL of freshly boiled and cooled water and 0.1 mL of bromocresol green-sodium hydroxide-ethanol TS, then add 0.1 mol/L sodium hydroxide VS until the solution shows a blue color: the volume of 0.1 mol/L sodium hydroxide VS used does not exceed 0.1 mL.

The JP Drugs are to be tested according to the provisions given in the pertinent monographs, General Notices, General Rules for Crude Drugs, General Rules for Preparations, and General Tests for their conformity to the Japanese Pharmacopoeia. (See the General Notices 5.)

Supplement I, JP XVIII   *Official Monographs* 2881

(3) Related substances—Dissolve 50.0 mg of Ethyl Parahydroxybenzoate in 2.5 mL of methanol, and add the mobile phase to make exactly 50 mL. Pipet 10 mL of this solution, add the mobile phase to make exactly 100 mL, and use this solution as the sample solution. Pipet 1 mL of the sample solution, and add the mobile phase to make exactly 20 mL. Pipet 1 mL of this solution, add the mobile phase to make exactly 10 mL, and use this solution as the standard solution. Perform the test with exactly 10 μL each of the sample solution and standard solution as directed under Liquid Chromatography <2.01> according to the following conditions, and determine each peak area by the automatic integration method: the peak area of parahydroxybenzoic acid having the relative retention time of about 0.5 to ethyl parahydroxybenzoate obtained from the sample solution is not larger than the peak area of ethyl parahydroxybenzoate from the standard solution (0.5%). For the peak area of parahydroxybenzoic acid, multiply the correction factor, 1.4. Furthermore, the area of the peak other than ethyl parahydroxybenzoate and parahydroxybenzoic acid from the sample solution is not larger than the peak area of ethyl parahydroxybenzoate from the standard solution (0.5%), and the total area of the peaks other than ethyl parahydroxybenzoate is not larger than 2 times the peak area of ethyl parahydroxybenzoate from the standard solution (1.0%). For this calculation the peak area not larger than 1/5 times the peak area of ethyl parahydroxybenzoate from the standard solution is excluded (0.1%).

Operating conditions—

Detector, column, column temperature, mobile phase, and flow rate: Proceed as directed in the operating conditions in the Assay.

Time span of measurement: 4 times as long as the retention time of ethyl parahydroxybenzoate.

System suitability—

System performance: Proceed as directed in the system suitability in the Assay.

◇Test for required detectability: To exactly 2 mL of the standard solution add the mobile phase to make exactly 10 mL. Confirm that the peak area of ethyl parahydroxybenzoate obtained with 10 μL of this solution is equivalent to 14 to 26% of that with 10 μL of the standard solution.◇

◇System repeatability: When the test is repeated 6 times with 10 μL of the standard solution under the above operating conditions, the relative standard deviation of the peak area of ethyl parahydroxybenzoate is not more than 2.0%.◇

Residue on ignition <2.44> Not more than 0.1% (1 g).

Assay Weigh accurately about 50 mg each of Ethyl Parahydroxybenzoate and Ethyl Parahydroxybenzoate RS, dissolve separately in 2.5 mL each of methanol, and add the mobile phase to make exactly 50 mL. Pipet 10 mL each of these solutions, add the mobile phase to make exactly 100 mL, and use these solutions as the sample solution and the standard solution, respectively. Perform the test with exactly 10 μL each of the sample solution and standard solution as directed under Liquid Chromatography <2.01> according to the following conditions, and determine the peak

areas, A_T and A_S, of ethyl parahydroxybenzoate in each solution.

Amount (mg) of ethyl parahydroxybenzoate ($C_9H_{10}O_3$)
= $M_S \times A_T/A_S$

M_S: Amount (mg) of Ethyl Parahydroxybenzoate RS taken

Operating conditions—

Detector: An ultraviolet absorption photometer (wavelength: 272 nm).

Column: A stainless steel column 4.6 mm in inside diameter and 15 cm in length, packed with octadecylsilanized silica gel for liquid chromatography (5 μm in particle diameter).

◇Column temperature: A constant temperature of about 35°C.◇

Mobile phase: A mixture of methanol and potassium dihydrogen phosphate solution (17 in 2500) (13:7).

Flow rate: 1.3 mL per minute.

System suitability—

System performance: Dissolve 5 mg each of Ethyl Parahydroxybenzoate, methyl parahydroxybenzoate and parahydroxybenzoic acid in the mobile phase to make exactly 100 mL. Pipet 1 mL of this solution, and add the mobile phase to make exactly 10 mL. When the procedure is run with 10 μL of this solution under the above operating conditions, parahydroxybenzoic acid, methyl parahydroxybenzoate and ethyl parahydroxybenzoate are eluted in this order, the relative retention times of parahydroxybenzoic acid and methyl parahydroxybenzoate to ethyl parahydroxybenzoate are about 0.5 and about 0.8, respectively, and the resolution between the peaks of methyl parahydroxybenzoate and ethyl parahydroxybenzoate is not less than 2.0.

System repeatability: When the test is repeated 6 times with 10 μL of the standard solution under the above operating conditions, the relative standard deviation of the peak area of ethyl parahydroxybenzoate is not more than 0.85%.

◆**Containers and storage** Containers—Well-closed containers.◆

Formoterol Fumarate Hydrate

ホルモテロールフマル酸塩水和物

Change the Chemical name and Purity as follows:

($C_{19}H_{24}N_2O_4$)$_2$.$C_4H_4O_4$.2H_2O: 840.91
N-(2-Hydroxy-5-{(1RS)-1-hydroxy-2-[(2RS)-1-(4-methoxyphenyl)propan-2-ylamino]ethyl}phenyl)formamide hemifumarate monohydrate

Purity (1) Related Substances—Dissolve 20 mg of Formoterol Fumarate Hydrate in the diluting solution to make 100 mL, and use this solution as the sample solution. Perform the test with 20 μL of the sample solution as directed under Liquid Chromatography <2.01> according to the fol-

---

The JP Drugs are to be tested according to the provisions given in the pertinent monographs, General Notices, General Rules for Crude Drugs, General Rules for Preparations, and General Tests for their conformity to the Japanese Pharmacopoeia. (See the General Notices 5.)

lowing conditions. Determine each peak area by the automatic integration method, and calculate their amounts by the area percentage method: the amount of the peak of the related substance A, having the relative retention time of about 0.5 to formoterol, is not more than 0.3%, the amounts of the peaks of the related substances B, C, D and F, having the relative retention times of about 0.7, about 1.2, about 1.3 and about 2.0, are not more than 0.2%, respectively, the amount of the peak of the related substance E, having the relative retention time of about 1.8, is not more than 0.1%, and the amount of the peak other than formoterol and the peaks mentioned above is not more than 0.1%. Furthermore, the total amount of the peaks other than formoterol is not more than 0.5%. For the peak area of the related substance A, multiply the correction factor, 1.75.

Diluting solution: Dissolve 6.9 g of sodium dihydrogen phosphate dihydrate and 0.8 g of anhydrous disodium hydrogen phosphate in water to make 1000 mL, and adjust to pH 6.0 with 0.5 mol/L disodium hydrogen phosphate TS or diluted phosphoric acid (27 in 400). To 21 volumes of this solution add 4 volumes of acetonitrile.

Operating conditions—

Detector: An ultraviolet absorption photometer (wavelength: 214 nm).

Column: A stainless steel column 4.6 mm in inside diameter and 15 cm in length, packed with octylsilanized silica gel for liquid chromatography (5 μm in particle diameter).

Column temperature: A constant temperature of about 22°C.

Mobile phase A: Dissolve 4.2 g of sodium dihydrogen phosphate dihydrate and 0.35 g of phosphoric acid in water to make 1000 mL, and adjust to pH 3.1 with a solution prepared by dissolving 156 g of sodium dihydrogen phosphate dihydrate in water to make 1000 mL or diluted phosphoric acid (27 in 400).

Mobile phase B: Acetonitrile for liquid chromatography.

Flowing of mobile phase: Control the gradient by mixing the mobile phases A and B as directed in the following table.

Time after injection of sample (min)	Mobile phase A (vol%)	Mobile phase B (vol%)
0 – 10	84	16
10 – 37	84 → 30	16 → 70

Flow rate: 1.0 mL per minute (the retention time of formoterol is about 10 minutes).

Time span of measurement: For 37 minutes after injection, beginning after the peak of fumaric acid.

System suitability—

Test for required detectability: Pipet 1 mL of the sample solution, and add the diluting solution to make exactly 100 mL. Pipet 1 mL of this solution, add the diluting solution to make exactly 20 mL. When the procedure is run with 20 μL of this solution under the above operating conditions, the SN ratio of the peak of formoterol is not less than 10.

System performance: When the procedure is run with 20 μL of the sample solution under the above operating conditions, the number of theoretical plates and the symmetry factor of the peak of formoterol are not less than 2000 and not more than 3.0, respectively.

(2) Diastereomer—Dissolve 5 mg of Formoterol Fumarate Hydrate in water to make 50 mL, and use this solution as the sample solution. Perform the test with 20 μL of the sample solution as directed under Liquid Chromatography <2.01> according to the following conditions. Determine the peak areas, A_f and A_d, of formoterol and the related substance I (diastereomer), having the relative retention time of about 1.2 to formoterol, in the sample solution by the automatic integration method, and calculate the amount of the diastereomer by the following equation: not more than 0.3%.

$$\text{Amount (\%) of diastereomer} = A_d/(A_d + A_f) \times 100$$

Operating conditions—

Detector: An ultraviolet absorption photometer (wavelength: 225 nm).

Column: A stainless steel column 4.6 mm in inside diameter and 15 cm in length, packed with octadecylsilanized polyvinyl alcohol gel polymer for liquid chromatography (5 μm in particle diameter).

Column temperature: A constant temperature of about 22°C.

Mobile phase: Dissolve 5.3 g of potassium phosphate trihydrate in water to make 1000 mL, and adjust to pH 12.0 with a solution of potassium hydroxide (281 in 1000) or phosphoric acid. To 22 volumes of this solution add 3 volumes of acetonitrile for liquid chromatography.

Flow rate: 0.5 mL per minute (the retention time of formoterol is about 22 minutes).

System suitability—

Test for required detectability: Pipet 1 mL of the sample solution, and add water to make exactly 20 mL. Pipet 1 mL of this solution, and add water to make exactly 25 mL. When the procedure is run with 20 μL of this solution under the above operating conditions, the SN ratio of the peak of formoterol is not less than 10.

System performance: When the procedure is run with 20 μL of the sample solution under the above operating conditions, the number of theoretical plates and the symmetry factor of the peak of formoterol are not less than 4300 and not more than 1.7, respectively.

The JP Drugs are to be tested according to the provisions given in the pertinent monographs, General Notices, General Rules for Crude Drugs, General Rules for Preparations, and General Tests for their conformity to the Japanese Pharmacopoeia. (See the General Notices 5.)

Supplement I, JP XVIII 　　　　　　　　　　　　　　　　*Official Monographs*　2883

Add the following next to the Containers and storage:

Others

Related substance A:
2-Amino-4-{1-hydroxy-2-[1-(4-methoxyphenyl)propan-2-ylamino]ethyl}phenol

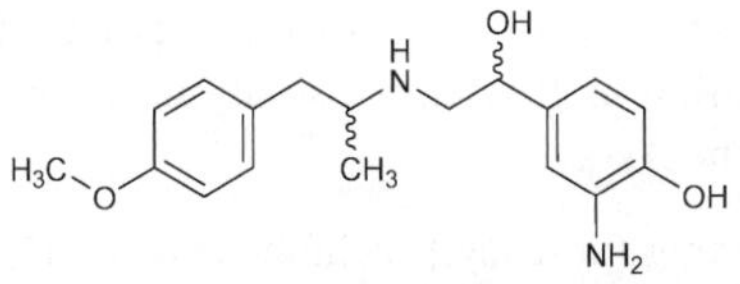

Related substance B:
N-(2-Hydroxy-5-{1-hydroxy-2-[2-(4-methoxyphenyl)ethylamino]ethyl}phenyl)formamide

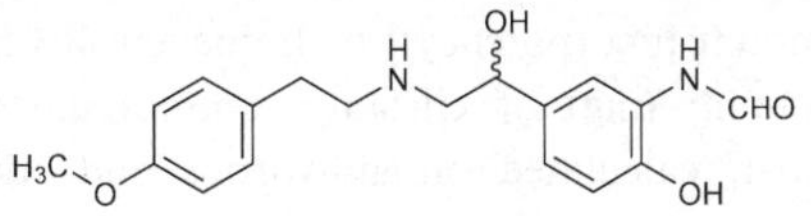

Related substance C:
N-(2-Hydroxy-5-{1-hydroxy-2-[1-(4-methoxyphenyl)propan-2-ylamino]ethyl}phenyl)acetamide

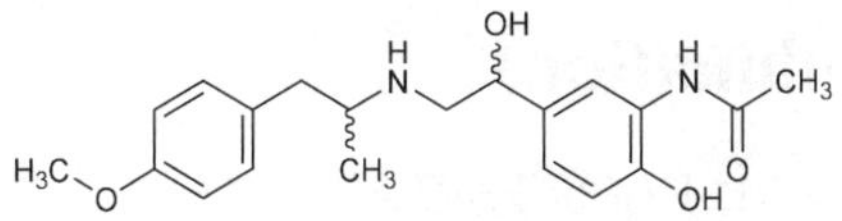

Related substance D:
N-(2-Hydroxy-5-{1-hydroxy-2-[1-(4-methoxyphenyl)propan-2-ylmethylamino]ethyl}phenyl)formamide

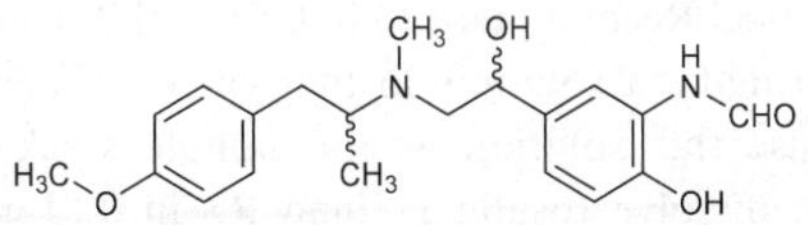

Related substance E:
N-(2-Hydroxy-5-{1-hydroxy-2-[1-(4-methoxy-3-methylphenyl)propan-2-ylamino]ethyl}phenyl)formamide

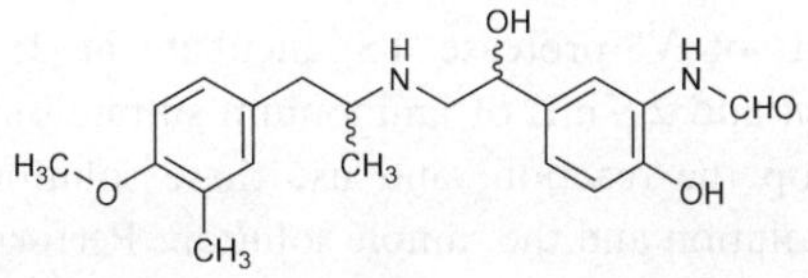

Related substance F:
N-(2-Hydroxy-5-{1-(2-hydroxy-5-{1-hydroxy-2-[1-(4-methoxyphenyl)propan-2-ylamino]ethyl}phenyl)amino-2-[1-(4-methoxyphenyl)propan-2-ylamino]ethyl}phenyl)formamide

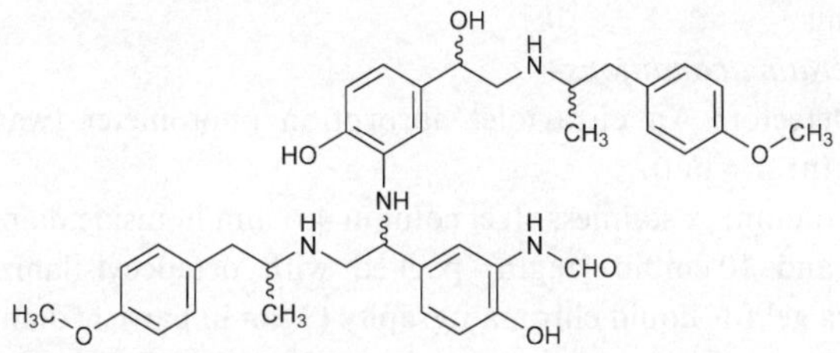

Related substance I (diastereomer):
N-(2-Hydroxy-5-{(1*RS*)-1-hydroxy-2-[(2*SR*)-1-(4-methoxyphenyl)propan-2-ylamino]ethyl}phenyl)formamide

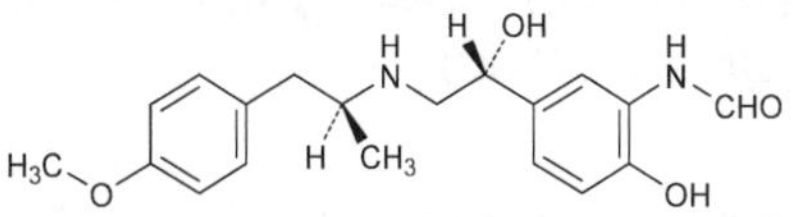

Glyceryl Monostearate

モノステアリン酸グリセリン

Delete the Identification (1), and change as follows:

Identification　Dissolve 0.1 g of Glyceryl Monostearate in 2 mL of ethanol (95) by warming, heat with 5 mL of dilute sulfuric acid in a water bath for 30 minutes, and cool; a white to yellow solid is produced. This separated solid dissolves when shaken with 3 mL of diethyl ether.

Hypromellose Phthalate

ヒプロメロースフタル酸エステル

Change the preamble concerning the harmonization to the beginning of the text, and change the Description and the Viscosity:

This monograph is harmonized with the European Pharmacopoeia and the U.S. Pharmacopeia.

The corresponding part of the attributes/provisions which are agreed as non-harmonized within the scope of the harmonization is marked with symbols (♦　♦), and the corresponding parts which are agreed as the JP local requirement other than the scope of the harmonization are marked with symbols (◇　◇).

Information on the harmonization with the European Pharmacopoeia and the U.S. Pharmacopeia is available on the website of the Pharmaceuticals and Medical Devices Agency.

♦**Description**　Hypromellose Phthalate occurs as white, powder or granules.

It is practically insoluble in water, in acetonitrile and in ethanol (99.5).

It becomes a viscous liquid when a mixture of methanol and dichloromethane (1:1 in mass ratio) or a mixture of ethanol (99.5) and acetone (1:1) is added.

It dissolves in sodium hydroxide TS.♦

Viscosity ⟨2.53⟩　To 10 g of Hypromellose Phthalate, previously dried at 105°C for 1 hour, add 90 g of a mixture of methanol and dichloromethane (1:1 in mass ratio), stir, and shake to dissolve. Determine the viscosity at 20 ± 0.1°C as directed in Method 1 under Viscosity Determination: the viscosity is not less than 80% and not more than 120% of the labeled unit.

The JP Drugs are to be tested according to the provisions given in the pertinent monographs, General Notices, General Rules for Crude Drugs, General Rules for Preparations, and General Tests for their conformity to the Japanese Pharmacopoeia. (See the General Notices 5.)

2884 *Official Monographs*

Supplement I, JP XVIII

Delete the Purity (2) and move up the after section, and change as follows:

Purity

(2) Phthalic acid—Weigh accurately about 0.2 g of Hypromellose Phthalate, add about 50 mL of acetonitrile to dissolve partially by sonicating, add 10 mL of water, and dissolve further by sonicating. After cooling, add acetonitrile to make exactly 100 mL, and use this solution as the sample solution. Separately, weigh accurately about 12.5 mg of phthalic acid, dissolve in about 125 mL of acetonitrile by mixing, add 25 mL of water, then add acetonitrile to make exactly 250 mL, and use this solution as the standard solution. Perform the test with exactly 10 μL each of the sample solution and standard solution as directed under Liquid Chromatography <2.01> according to the following conditions, and determine the peak areas, A_T and A_S, of phthalic acid in each solution: amount of phthalic acid ($C_8H_6O_4$: 166.13) is not more than 1.0%.

Amount (%) of phthalic acid = $M_S/M_T \times A_T/A_S \times 40$

M_S: Amount (mg) of phthalic acid taken

M_T: Amount (mg) of Hypromellose Phthalate taken, calculated on the anhydrous basis

Operating conditions—

Detector: An ultraviolet absorption photometer (wavelength: 235 nm).

Column: A stainless steel column about 4.6 mm in inside diameter and 25 cm in length, packed with octadecylsilanized silica gel for liquid chromatography (3 to 10 μm in particle diameter).

Column temperature: A constant temperature of about 20°C.

Mobile phase: A mixture of 0.1% trifluoroacetic acid and acetonitrile (9:1).

Flow rate: About 2.0 mL per minute.

System suitability—

◇System performance: When the procedure is run with 10 μL of the standard solution under the above operating conditions, the number of theoretical plates and the symmetry factor of the peak of phthalic acid are not less than 2500 and not more than 1.5, respectively.◇

System repeatability: When repeat the test 5 times with 10 μL of the standard solution under the above operating conditions, the relative standard deviation of the peak area of phthalic acid is not more than 1.0%.

Imipenem and Cilastatin Sodium for Injection

注射用イミペネム・シラスタチンナトリウム

Change the description of Uniformity of dosage units as follows:

Uniformity of dosage units <6.02> Perform the test according to the following method: it meets the requirement of the Content uniformity test (*T*: Being specified separately when the drug is granted approval based on the Law.).

Dissolve the total amount of the content of 1 Imipenem and Cilastatin Sodium for Injection in isotonic sodium chloride solution to make exactly 100 mL. Pipet *V* mL of this solution, equivalent to about 25 mg (potency) of Imipenem Hydrate, add 0.1 mol/L 3-(*N*-morpholino) propanesulfonic acid buffer solution (pH 7.0) to make exactly 50 mL, and use this solution as the sample solution. Then, proceed as directed in the Assay.

Amount [mg (potency)] of imipenem ($C_{12}H_{17}N_3O_4S$)
= $M_{SI} \times A_{TI}/A_{SI} \times 100/V$

Amount (mg) of cilastatin ($C_{16}H_{26}N_2O_5S$)
= $M_{SC} \times A_{TC}/A_{SC} \times 100/V \times 0.955$

M_{SI}: Amount [mg (potency)] of Imipenem RS taken

M_{SC}: Amount (mg) of cilastatin ammonium for assay taken, calculated on anhydrous and ethanol-free basis

Insulin Human (Genetical Recombination)

インスリン　ヒト（遺伝子組換え）

Change the Identification and Assay as follows:

Identification Dissolve a suitable amount of Insulin Human (Genetical Recombination) in 0.01 mol/L hydrochloric acid TS to make a solution so that each mL contains 2.0 mg, and use this solution as the sample stock solution. Separately, dissolve Insulin Human RS in 0.01 mol/L hydrochloric acid TS to make a solution so that each mL contains 2.0 mg, and use this solution as the standard stock solution. Transfer 500 μL each of these solutions into a clean test tube, add 2.0 mL of HEPES buffer solution (pH 7.5) and 400 μL of V8-protease TS, incubate at 25°C for 6 hours, then add 2.9 mL of ammonium sulfate buffer solution to stop the reaction, and use these solutions as the standard solution and the sample solution. Perform the test with 50 μL each of the sample solution and standard solution as directed under Liquid Chromatography <2.01> according to the following conditions, and compare the chromatograms obtained from these solutions: a similar peak is observed at the same retention time in the both chromatograms.

Operating conditions—

Detector: An ultraviolet absorption photometer (wavelength: 214 nm).

Column: A stainless steel column 4.6 mm in inside diameter and 10 cm in length, packed with octadecylsilanized silica gel for liquid chromatography (3 μm in particle diameter).

Column temperature: A constant temperature of about 40°C.

Mobile phase A: A mixture of water, ammonium sulfate

The JP Drugs are to be tested according to the provisions given in the pertinent monographs, General Notices, General Rules for Crude Drugs, General Rules for Preparations, and General Tests for their conformity to the Japanese Pharmacopoeia. (See the General Notices 5.)

Supplement I, JP XVIII

buffer solution and acetonitrile (7:2:1).

Mobile phase B: A mixture of water, acetonitrile and ammonium sulfate buffer solution (2:2:1).

Flowing of mobile phase: Change the mixing ratio of the mobile phase A and B linearly from 9:1 to 3:7 in 60 minutes after sample injection, further change to 0:10 linearly in 5 minutes, and then flow the mobile phase B only for 5 minutes.

Flow rate: 1.0 mL per minute.

System suitability—

System performance: When the procedure is run with 50 μL of the standard solution under the above operating conditions, the symmetry factor of the two larger peaks which appear next to the first peak just after the solvent peak are not more than 1.5 respectively, and the resolution between these peaks is not less than 3.4.

Assay Perform this procedure quickly. Weigh accurately about 7.5 mg of Insulin Human (Genetical Recombination), dissolve in 0.01 mol/L hydrochloric acid TS to make exactly 5 mL, and use this solution as the sample solution. Separately, dissolve exactly Insulin Human RS in 0.01 mol/L hydrochloric acid TS to make a solution so that each mL contains about 40 Insulin Units, and use this solution as the standard solution. Perform the test with exactly 20 μL each of the sample solution and standard solution as directed under Liquid Chromatography <2.01> according to the following conditions, and determine the peak areas of human insulin, A_{TI} and A_{SI}, and the peak areas of the desamido substance having the relative retention time of 1.3 to human insulin, A_{TD} and A_{SD}, respectively, of these solutions.

Amount (Insulin Unit/mg) of human insulin ($C_{257}H_{383}N_{65}O_{77}S_6$)
$$= M_S/M_T \times (A_{TI} + A_{TD})/(A_{SI} + A_{SD}) \times 5$$

M_T: Amount (mg) of Insulin Human (Genetical Recombination) taken, calculated on the dried basis

M_S: Amount (Insulin Unit) of insulin human in 1 mL of the standard solution

Operating conditions—

Detector: An ultraviolet absorption photometer (wavelength: 214 nm).

Column: A stainless steel column 4.6 mm in inside diameter and 15 cm in length, packed with octadecylsilanized silica gel for liquid chromatography (5 μm in particle diameter).

Column temperature: A constant temperature of about 40°C.

Mobile phase: A mixture of phosphoric acid-sodium sulfate buffer solution (pH 2.3) and acetonitrile for liquid chromatography (3:1). Adjust the mixing ratio of the component of the mobile phase so that the retention time of human insulin is between 10 minutes and 17 minutes.

Flow rate: 1.0 mL per minute.

System suitability—

System performance: When the procedure is run with 20 μL of human insulin desamido substance-containing TS under the above operating conditions, human insulin and

Official Monographs 2885

human insulin desamido substance are eluted in this order with the resolution between these peaks being not less than 2.0, and the symmetry factor of the peak of human insulin is not more than 1.8.

System repeatability: When the test is repeated 6 times with 20 μL of the standard solution under the above operating conditions, the relative standard deviation of the peak areas of human insulin is not more than 1.6%.

Insulin Human (Genetical Recombination) Injection

インスリン　ヒト（遺伝子組換え）注射液

Change the Assay as follows:

Assay To exactly 10 mL of Insulin Human (Genetical Recombination) Injection add exactly 40 μL of 6 mol/L hydrochloric acid TS. Pipet 2 mL of this solution, add 0.01 mol/L hydrochloric acid TS to make exactly 5 mL, and use this solution as the sample solution. Then, proceed as directed in the Assay under Insulin Human (Genetical Recombination).

Amount (Insulin Unit) of human insulin ($C_{257}H_{383}N_{65}O_{77}S_6$) in 1 mL
$$= M_S \times (A_{TI} + A_{TD})/(A_{SI} + A_{SD}) \times 1.004 \times 5/2$$

M_S: Amount (Insulin Unit) of insulin human in 1 mL of the standard solution

Isophane Insulin Human (Genetical Recombination) Injectable Aqueous Suspension

イソフェンインスリン　ヒト（遺伝子組換え）水性懸濁注射液

Change the Purity (2) and Assay (1) as follows:

Purity

(2) Dissolved insulin human—Centrifuge Isophane Insulin Human (Genetical Recombination) Injectable Aqueous Suspension, and use the supernatant liquid as the sample solution. Separately, dissolve exactly Insulin Human RS in 0.01 mol/L hydrochloric acid TS to make a solution so that each mL contains about 1.0 Insulin Units, and use this solution as the standard solution. Perform the test with exactly 20 μL each of the sample solution and standard solution as directed under Liquid Chromatography <2.01> according to the following conditions. Determine the peak areas, A_T and A_S, of insulin human by the automatic integration method, and calculate the amount of dissolved insulin human by the following equation: not more than 0.5 Insulin Units per mL.

The JP Drugs are to be tested according to the provisions given in the pertinent monographs, General Notices, General Rules for Crude Drugs, General Rules for Preparations, and General Tests for their conformity to the Japanese Pharmacopoeia. (See the General Notices 5.)

2886 *Official Monographs*

Amount (mg) of dissolved insulin human'
(Insulin Unit/mL)

$$= M_S \times A_T/A_S$$

M_S: Amount (Insulin Unit) of insulin human in 1 mL of
the standard solution

Operating conditions—

Proceed as directed in the operating conditions in the
Assay (1).

System suitability—

System performance: When the procedure is run with 20
μL of insulin human desamido substance-containing TS
under the above operating conditions, insulin human and
insulin human desamido substance are eluted in this order
with the resolution between these peaks being not less than
2.0, and the symmetry factor of the peak of insulin human
is not more than 1.6.

System repeatability: When the test is repeated 4 times
with 20 μL of the standard solution under the above operating conditions, the relative standard deviation of the peak
area of insulin human is not more than 6.0%.

Assay (1) Insulin human—Pipet 10 mL of gently shaken
Isophane Insulin Human (Genetical Recombination) Injectable Aqueous Suspension, and add exactly 40 μL of 6
mol/L hydrochloric acid TS. Pipet 2 mL of this solution,
add 0.01 mol/L hydrochloric acid TS to make exactly 5 mL,
and use this solution as the sample solution. Then, proceed
as directed in the Assay under Insulin Human (Genetical
Recombination).

Amount (Insulin Unit) of insulin human ($C_{257}H_{383}N_{65}O_{77}S_6$)
in 1 mL

$$= M_S \times (A_{TI} + A_{TD})/(A_{SI} + A_{SD}) \times 1.004 \times 5/2$$

M_S: Amount (Insulin Unit) of insulin human in 1 mL of
the standard solution

Biphasic Isophane Insulin Human (Genetical Recombination) Injectable Aqueous Suspension

二相性イソフェンインスリン　ヒト（遺伝子組換え）水性
懸濁注射液

Change the Assay (1) as follows:

Assay (1) Insulin human—Pipet 10 mL of gently shaken
Biphasic Isophane Insulin Human (Genetical Recombination) Injectable Aqueous Suspension, and add exactly 40 μL
of 6 mol/L hydrochloric acid TS. Pipet 2 mL of this solution, add 0.01 mol/L hydrochloric acid TS to make exactly
5 mL, and use this solution as the sample solution. Then,
proceed as directed in the Assay under Insulin Human (Genetical Recombination).

Amount (Insulin Unit) of insulin human ($C_{257}H_{383}N_{65}O_{77}S_6$)
in 1 mL

$$= M_S \times (A_{TI} + A_{TD})/(A_{SI} + A_{SD}) \times 1.004 \times 5/2$$

M_S: Amount (Insulin Unit) of insulin human in 1 mL of
the standard solution

Change the following as follows:

Magnesium Stearate

ステアリン酸マグネシウム

This monograph is harmonized with the European Pharmacopoeia and the U.S. Pharmacopeia.

The corresponding part of the attributes/provisions
which are agreed as non-harmonized within the scope of the
harmonization is marked with symbols (◆　◆), and the corresponding parts which are agreed as the JP local requirement other than the scope of the harmonization are marked
with symbols (◇　◇).

Information on the harmonization with the European
Pharmacopoeia and the U. S. Pharmacopeia is available on
the website of the Pharmaceuticals and Medical Devices
Agency.

Magnesium Stearate is a compound of magnesium
with a mixture of solid fatty acids, and consists chie-
fly of variable proportions of magnesium stearate and
magnesium palmitate obtained from sources of veget-
able or animal origin.

It contains not less than 4.0% and not more than
5.0% of magnesium (Mg: 24.31), calculated on the
dried basis.

◆Description Magnesium Stearate occurs as a white, light,
bulky powder.

It is smooth to the touch and sticky to the skin. It has no
odor or a faint, characteristic odor.

It is practically insoluble in water and in ethanol (99.5).◆

Identification Mix 5.0 g of Magnesium Stearate with 50
mL of peroxide-free diethyl ether, 20 mL of dilute nitric
acid, and 20 mL of water in a round-bottom flask, and heat
to dissolve completely under a reflux condenser. After cooling, transfer the contents of the flask to a separator, shake,
allow the layers to separate, and transfer the aqueous layer
to a flask. Extract the diethyl ether layer with two 4-mL
portions of water, and combine these extracts to the main
aqueous extract. After washing the combined aqueous extract with 15 mL of peroxide-free diethyl ether, transfer to a
50-mL volumetric flask, add water to make 50 mL, and use
this solution as the sample solution. To 1 mL of the sample
solution add 1 mL of ammonia TS: A white precipitate is
formed that dissolves on addition of 1 mL of ammonium
chloride TS. By further addition of 1 mL of a solution of
disodium hydrogen phosphate dodecahydrate (3 in 25) a
white crystalline precipitate is formed.

Purity (1) Acidity or alkalinity—Heat 1.0 g of Magnesium Stearate in 20 mL of freshly boiled and cooled water on

*The JP Drugs are to be tested according to the provisions given in the pertinent monographs, General Notices, General Rules for Crude Drugs,
General Rules for Preparations, and General Tests for their conformity to the Japanese Pharmacopoeia. (See the General Notices 5.)*

Supplement I, JP XVIII   *Official Monographs*   **2887**

a water bath for 1 minute while shaking, cool, and filter. Add 0.05 mL of bromothymol blue TS to 10 mL of the filtrate: not more than 0.05 mL of 0.1 mol/L hydrochloric acid VS or 0.1 mol/L sodium hydroxide VS is required to change the color of the solution.

(2) Chloride ⟨*1.03*⟩—To 10.0 mL of the sample solution obtained in Identification add 1 mL of dilute nitric acid and water to make 50 mL. Perform the test using this solution as the test solution. Prepare the control solution with 1.4 mL of 0.02 mol/L hydrochloric acid VS (not more than 0.1%).

(3) Sulfate ⟨*1.14*⟩—Perform the test with 6.0 mL of the sample solution obtained in Identification. Prepare the control solution with 3.0 mL of 0.02 mol/L sulfuric acid VS. To the test and control solutions add 3 mL of barium chloride TS (not more than 1.0%).

Loss on drying ⟨*2.41*⟩   Not more than 6.0% (2 g, 105°C, constant mass).

◆**Microbial limit** ⟨*4.05*⟩   The acceptance criteria of TAMC and TYMC are 10^3 CFU/g and 5×10^2 CFU/g, respectively. *Salmonella* and *Escherichia coli* are not observed.◆

Relative content of stearic acid and palmitic acid   Transfer 0.10 g of Magnesium Stearate to a small conical flask fitted with a reflux condenser. Add 5.0 mL of boron trifluoride-methanol TS, mix, and reflux for 10 minutes to dissolve the solids. Add 4 mL of heptane through the condenser, and reflux for 10 minutes. After cooling, add 20 mL of saturated sodium chloride solution, shake, and allow the layers to separate. Pass the heptane layer through about 0.1 g of anhydrous sodium sulfate, previously washed with heptane, into another flask. Transfer 1.0 mL of this solution to a 10-mL volumetric flask, dilute with heptane to volume, and use this solution as the sample solution. Perform the test with 1 μL of the sample solution as directed under Gas chromatography ⟨*2.02*⟩ according to the following conditions, and determine the area, *A*, of the methyl stearate peak and the sum of the areas, *B*, of all of the fatty acid ester peaks. Calculate the percentage of stearic acid in the fatty acid fraction of Magnesium Stearate by the following formula.

$$\text{Content (\%) of stearic acid} = A/B \times 100$$

Similarly, calculate the percentage of palmitic acid in the portion of Magnesium Stearate taken. The methyl stearate peak, and the sum of the stearate and palmitate peaks are not less than 40% and not less than 90% of the total area of all fatty acid ester peaks, respectively.

Operating conditions—

Detector: A hydrogen flame-ionization detector.

Column: A fused silica capillary column 0.32 mm in inside diameter and 30 m in length, the inside coated with a 0.5-μm layer of polyethylene glycol 15000-diepoxide for gas chromatography.

Column temperature: Maintain at 70°C for 2 minutes after injection, then program to increase the temperature at the rate of 5°C per minute to 240°C and to maintain 240°C

for 5 minutes.

Injection port temperature: A constant temperature of about 220°C.

Detector temperature: A constant temperature of about 260°C.

Carrier gas: Helium.

Flow rate: 2.4 mL per minute.

Splitless.

◇Time span of measurement: For 41 minutes after the solvent peak.◇

System suitability—

◇Test for required detectability:◇ Place about 50 mg each of stearic acid for gas chromatography and palmitic acid for gas chromatography in a small conical flask fitted with a reflux condenser. Add 5.0 mL of boron trifluoride-methanol TS, mix, and proceed in the same manner as directed for the preparation of the sample solution, and use the solution so obtained as the solution for system suitability test. ◇To exactly 1 mL of the solution for system suitability test add heptane to make exactly 10 mL. To exactly 1 mL of this solution add heptane to make exactly 10 mL. Further, to exactly 1 mL of this solution add heptane to make exactly 10 mL. Confirm that the peak area of methyl stearate obtained with 1 μL of this solution is equivalent to 0.05 to 0.15% of that with 1 μL of the solution for system suitability test.◇

System performance: When the procedure is run with 1 μL of the solution for system suitability test under the above operating conditions, the relative retention time of methyl palmitate to methyl stearate is about 0.9, and the resolution between these peaks is not less than 5.0.

System repeatability: When the test is repeated 6 times with the solution for system suitability test under the above operating conditions, the relative standard deviation of the peak areas of methyl palmitate and methyl stearate are not more than 3.0%, respectively, and the relative standard deviation of the ratios of the peak area of methyl palmitate to methyl stearate is not more than 1.0%.

Assay   Transfer about 0.5 g of Magnesium Stearate, accurately weighed, to a 250-mL flask, add 50 mL of a mixture of ethanol (99.5) and 1-butanol (1:1), 5 mL of ammonia solution (28), 3 mL of ammonium chloride buffer solution (pH 10), 30.0 mL of 0.1 mol/L disodium dihydrogen ethylenediamine tetraacetate VS and 1 to 2 drops of eriochrome black T TS, and mix. Heat at 45–50°C to make the solution clear, and after cooling, titrate ⟨*2.50*⟩ the excess disodium dihydrogen ethylenediamine tetraacetate with 0.1 mol/L zinc sulfate VS until the solution changes from blue to violet in color. Perform a blank determination in the same manner.

Each mL of 0.1 mol/L disodium dihydrogen
ethylenediamine tetraacetate VS
= 2.431 mg of Mg

◆**Containers and storage**   Containers—Tight containers.◆

The JP Drugs are to be tested according to the provisions given in the pertinent monographs, General Notices, General Rules for Crude Drugs, General Rules for Preparations, and General Tests for their conformity to the Japanese Pharmacopoeia. (See the General Notices 5.)

2888 *Official Monographs*

Supplement I, JP XVIII

Change the following as follows:

D-**Mannitol**

D-マンニトール

$C_6H_{14}O_6$: 182.17
D-Mannitol
[69-65-8]

This monograph is harmonized with the European Pharmacopoeia and the U.S. Pharmacopeia.

The corresponding part of the attributes/provisions which are agreed as non-harmonized within the scope of the harmonization is marked with symbols (♦ ♠), and the corresponding parts which are agreed as the JP local requirement other than the scope of the harmonization are marked with symbols (◇ ◇).

Information on the harmonization with the European Pharmacopoeia and the U.S. Pharmacopeia is available on the website of Pharmaceuticals and Medical Devices Agency.

D-Mannitol contains not less than 97.0% and not more than 102.0% of D-mannitol ($C_6H_{14}O_6$), calculated on the dried basis.

♦**Description** D-Mannitol occurs as white, crystals, powder or grain. It has a sweet taste with a cold sensation.

It is freely soluble in water, and practically insoluble in ethanol (99.5).

It dissolves in sodium hydroxide TS.

It shows crystal polymorphism.♠

Identification Determine the infrared absorption spectrum of D-Mannitol as directed in the potassium bromide disk method under Infrared Spectrophotometry <2.25>, and compare the spectrum with the Reference Spectrum or the spectrum of D-Mannitol RS: both spectra exhibit similar intensities of absorption at the same wave numbers. If any difference appears between the spectra, put 25 mg each of D-Mannitol and D-Mannitol RS in glass vessels, dissolve in 0.25 mL of water without heating, dry them in a 600 – 700 W microwave oven for 20 minutes or in a drying chamber at 100°C for 1 hour, then further dry by gradual reducing pressure, and perform the same test as above with so obtained non-sticky white to pale yellow powders: both spectra exhibit similar intensities of absorption at the same wave numbers.

Melting point <2.60> 165 – 170°C

Purity (1) Clarity and color of solution—Dissolve 5.0 g of D-Mannitol in water to make 50 mL, and use this solution as the test solution. Perform the test with the test solution as directed under Turbidity Measurement <2.61>: the solution is clear. Perform the test with the test solution ac-

cording to Method 2 under Methods for Color Matching <2.65>: the solution is colorless.

(2) Nickel—Shake 10.0 g of D-Mannitol with 30 mL of 2 mol/L acetic acid TS, and add water to make exactly 100 mL. Add 2.0 mL of a saturated solution of ammonium pyrrolidinedithiocarbamate (about 10 g/L) and 10.0 mL of water-saturated 4-methyl-2-pentanone, and shake for 30 seconds without exposure to light. Allow the layers to separate, and use the 4-methyl-2-pentanone layer as the sample solution. Separately, put 10.0 g each of D-Mannitol in three vessels, add 30 mL of 2 mol/L acetic acid TS to them, shake, add a suitable amount of water and exactly 0.5 mL, 1.0 mL and 1.5 mL respectively of Standard Nickel Solution for Atomic Absorption Spectrophotometry, and add water to make them exactly 100 mL. Then, proceed in the same manner as the sample solution, and use so obtained three 4-methyl-2-pentanone layers as the standard solutions. Additionally, prepare a 4-methyl-2-pentanone layer by proceeding in the same manner as the sample solution without using D-Mannitol, and use this layer as the blank solution. Perform the test with the sample solution and standard solutions as directed in the standard addition method under Atomic Absorption Spectrophotometry <2.23> according to the following conditions. Set the zero of the instrument using the blank solution, and between each measurement, rinse with water and ascertain that the readings return to zero with the blank solution: amount of nickel is not more than 1 ppm.

Gas: Combustible gas—Acetylene.
     Supporting gas—Air.
Lamp: Nickel hollow-cathode lamp.
Wavelength: 232.0 nm.

(3) Related substances—Dissolve 0.50 g of D-Mannitol in water to make 10 mL, and use this solution as the sample solution. Pipet 2 mL of the sample solution, add water to make exactly 100 mL, and use this solution as the standard solution (1). Pipet 0.5 mL of the standard solution (1), add water to make exactly 20 mL, and use this solution as the standard solution (2). Perform the test with exactly 20 μL each of the sample solution and standard solutions (1) and (2) as directed under Liquid Chromatography <2.01> according to the following conditions. Determine each peak area by the automatic integration method: the peak area of D-sorbitol, having the relative retention time of about 1.2 to D-mannitol, obtained from the sample solution is not larger than that of D-mannitol from the standard solution (1) (not more than 2.0%), the total peak area of maltitol, having the relative retention time of about 0.69, and isomalt, having the relative retention times of about 0.6 and about 0.73, is not larger than the peak area of D-mannitol from the standard solution (1) (not more than 2.0%), and the area of the peak other than D-mannitol and the peaks mentioned above is not larger than 2 times the peak area of D-mannitol from the standard solution (2) (not more than 0.1%). Furthermore, the total area of the peak other than D-mannitol from the sample solution is not larger than the peak area of D-mannitol from the standard solution (1) (not more than 2.0%). For these calculations exclude the peak of which

The JP Drugs are to be tested according to the provisions given in the pertinent monographs, General Notices, General Rules for Crude Drugs, General Rules for Preparations, and General Tests for their conformity to the Japanese Pharmacopoeia. (See the General Notices 5.)

Supplement I, JP XVIII   *Official Monographs* 2889

area is not larger than the peak area of D-mannitol from the standard solution (2) (not more than 0.05%).

Operating conditions—

Detector, column, column temperature, mobile phase, and flow rate: Proceed as directed in the operating conditions in the Assay.

Time span of measurement: About 1.5 times as long as the retention time of D-mannitol.

System suitability—

System performance: Proceed as directed in the system suitability in the Assay.

◇Test for required detectability: Confirm that the peak area of D-mannitol obtained with 20 μL of the standard solution (2) is equivalent to 1.75 to 3.25% of that with 20 μL of the standard solution (1).

System repeatability: When the test is repeated 6 times with 20 μL of the standard solution (1) under the above operating conditions, the relative standard deviation of the peak area of D-mannitol is not more than 1.0%.◇

(4) Glucose—To 7.0 g of D-Mannitol add 13 mL of water and 40 mL of Fehling's TS, boil gently for 3 minutes, and allow to stand for 2 minutes to precipitate copper (I) oxide. Separate the supernatant liquid, filter through a sintered glass filter for cupric oxide filtration coated with siliceous earth or a sintered glass filter (G4). Wash the precipitates with 50 – 60°C hot water until the washing no longer alkaline, and filter the washings through the filter described above. Discard all the filtrate at this step. Immediately, dissolve the precipitate with 20 mL of iron (III) sulfate TS, filter through the filter described above in a clean flask, and wash the filter with 15 – 20 mL of water. Combine the filtrate and the washings, heat to 80°C, and titrate <2.50> with 0.02 mol/L potassium permanganate VS until the green color turns to light red and the color persists at least 10 seconds: not more than 3.2 mL is required to change the color of the solution (not more than 0.1% expressed as glucose).

Conductivity <2.51> Dissolve 20.0 g of D-Mannitol in a fleshly boiled and cooled water prepared from distilled water by heating to 40 – 50°C, add the same water to make 100 mL, and use this solution as the sample solution. After cooling, measure the conductivity of the sample solution at 25 ± 0.1°C while gently stirring with a magnetic stirrer: not more than 20 μS·cm^{-1}.

Loss on drying <2.41> Not more than 0.5% (1 g, 105°C, 4 hours).

Assay Weigh accurately about 0.5 g each of D-Mannitol and D-Mannitol RS (separately determine the loss on drying <2.41> under the same conditions as D-Mannitol), dissolve separately in water to make exactly 10 mL, and use these solutions as the sample solution and the standard solution, respectively. Perform the test with exactly 20 μL each of the sample solution and standard solution as directed under Liquid Chromatography <2.01> according to the following conditions, and determine the peak areas, A_T and A_S, of D-mannitol in each solution.

Amount (g) of D-mannitol ($C_6H_{14}O_6$)
= $M_S \times A_T/A_S$

M_S: Amount (g) of D-Mannitol RS taken, calculated on the dried basis

Operating conditions—

Detector: A differential refractometer maintained at a constant temperature (40°C for example).

Column: A stainless steel column 7.8 mm in inside diameter and 30 cm in length, packed with strongly acidic ion-exchange resin for liquid chromatography (calcium type) composed with a sulfonated polystyrene cross-linked with 8% of divinylbenzene (9 μm in particle diameter).

Column temperature: 85 ± 2°C.

Mobile phase: Water.

Flow rate: 0.5 mL per minute (the retention time of D-mannitol is about 20 minutes).

System suitability—

System performance: Dissolve 0.25 g each of D-Mannitol and D-sorbitol in water to make 10 mL, and use this solution as the solution for system suitability test (1). Separately, dissolve 0.5 g each of maltitol and isomalt in water to make 100 mL. To 2 mL of this solution add water to make 10 mL, and use this solution as the solution for system suitability test (2). When proceed with 20 μL each of the solution for system suitability test (1) and the solution for system suitability test (2) as directed under the above operating conditions, isomalt (first peak), maltitol, isomalt (second peak), D-mannitol and D-sorbitol are eluted in this order, the relative retention time of isomalt (first peak), maltitol, isomalt (second peak) and D-sorbitol to D-mannitol is about 0.6, about 0.69, about 0.73 and about 1.2, respectively, and the resolution between the peaks of D-mannitol and D-sorbitol is not less than 2.0. Coelution of maltitol and the second peak of isomalt may be observed.

◇System repeatability: When the test is repeated 6 times with 20 μL of the standard solution under the above operating conditions, the relative standard deviation of the peak area of D-mannitol is not more than 1.0%.◇

♦**Containers   and   storage** Containers—Well-closed containers.♦

dl-Menthol

dl-メントール

Change the Containers and storage as follows:

Containers and storage Containers—Tight containers.

The JP Drugs are to be tested according to the provisions given in the pertinent monographs, General Notices, General Rules for Crude Drugs, General Rules for Preparations, and General Tests for their conformity to the Japanese Pharmacopoeia. (See the General Notices 5.)

2890 *Official Monographs*

Supplement I, JP XVIII

l-Menthol

l-メントール

Change the Containers and storage as follows:

Containers and storage Containers—Tight containers.

Change the following as follows:

Methyl Parahydroxybenzoate

パラオキシ安息香酸メチル

$C_8H_8O_3$: 152.15
Methyl 4-hydroxybenzoate
[*99-76-3*]

This monograph is harmonized with the European Pharmacopoeia and the U.S. Pharmacopeia.

The corresponding part of the attributes/provisions which are agreed as non-harmonized within the scope of the harmonization is marked with symbols (♦　♦), and the corresponding parts which are agreed as the JP local requirement other than the scope of the harmonization are marked with symbols (◇　◇).

Information on the harmonization with the European Pharmacopoeia and the U.S. Pharmacopeia is available on the website of the Pharmaceuticals and Medical Devices Agency.

Methyl Parahydroxybenzoate contains not less than 98.0% and not more than 102.0% of methyl parahydroxybenzoate ($C_8H_8O_3$).

♦**Description** Methyl Parahydroxybenzoate, occurs as colorless crystals or a white crystalline powder.

It is freely soluble in methanol, in ethanol (95) and in acetone, and slightly soluble in water.♦

Identification Determine the infrared absorption spectrum of Methyl Parahydroxybenzoate as directed in the potassium bromide disk method under Infrared Spectrophotometry <2.25>, and compare the spectrum with the Reference Spectrum or the spectrum of Methyl Parahydroxybenzoate RS: both spectra exhibit similar intensities of absorption at the same wave numbers.

Melting point <2.60>　125 – 128°C

Purity (1) Clarity and color of solution—Dissolve 1.0 g of Methyl Parahydroxybenzoate in ethanol (95) to make 10 mL: the solution is clear and not more intensely colored than ethanol (95) or the following control solution.

Control solution: To 5.0 mL of Cobalt (II) Chloride CS, 12.0 mL of Iron (III) Chloride CS and 2.0 mL of Copper

(II) Sulfate CS add diluted dilute hydrochloric acid (1 in 10) to make 1000 mL.

(2) Acidity—To 2 mL of the solution of Methyl Parahydroxybenzoate obtained in (1) add 3 mL of ethanol (95), add 5 mL of freshly boiled and cooled water and 0.1 mL of bromocresol green-sodium hydroxide-ethanol TS, then add 0.1 mol/L sodium hydroxide VS until the solution shows a blue color: the volume of 0.1 mol/L sodium hydroxide VS used does not exceed 0.1 mL.

(3) Related substances—Dissolve 50.0 mg of Methyl Parahydroxybenzoate in 2.5 mL of methanol, and add the mobile phase to make exactly 50 mL. Pipet 10 mL of this solution, add the mobile phase to make exactly 100 mL, and use this solution as the sample solution. Pipet 1 mL of the sample solution, and add the mobile phase to make exactly 20 mL. Pipet 1 mL of this solution, add the mobile phase to make exactly 10 mL, and use this solution as the standard solution. Perform the test with exactly 10 μL each of the sample solution and standard solution as directed under Liquid Chromatography <2.01> according to the following conditions, and determine each peak area by the automatic integration method: the peak area of parahydroxybenzoic acid having the relative retention time of about 0.6 to methyl parahydroxybenzoate obtained from the sample solution is not larger than the peak area of methyl parahydroxybenzoate from the standard solution (0.5%). For the peak area of parahydroxybenzoic acid, multiply the correction factor, 1.4. Furthermore, the area of the peak other than methyl parahydroxybenzoate and parahydroxybenzoic acid from the sample solution is not larger than the peak area of methyl parahydroxybenzoate from the standard solution (0.5%), and the total area of the peaks other than methyl parahydroxybenzoate from the sample solution is not larger than 2 times the peak area of methyl parahydroxybenzoate from the standard solution (1.0%). For this calculation the peak area not larger than 1/5 times the peak area of methyl parahydroxybenzoate from the standard solution is excluded (0.1%).

Operating conditions—

Detector, column, column temperature, mobile phase, and flow rate: Proceed as directed in the operating conditions in the Assay.

Time span of measurement: 5 times as long as the retention time of methyl parahydroxybenzoate.

System suitability—

System performance: Proceed as directed in the system suitability in the Assay.

◇Test for required detectability: To exactly 2 mL of the standard solution add the mobile phase to make exactly 10 mL. Confirm that the peak area of methyl parahydroxybenzoate obtained with 10 μL of this solution is equivalent to 14 to 26% of that with 10 μL of the standard solution.◇

◇System repeatability: When the test is repeated 6 times with 10 μL of the standard solution under the above operating conditions, the relative standard deviation of the peak area of methyl parahydroxybenzoate is not more than 2.0%.◇

The JP Drugs are to be tested according to the provisions given in the pertinent monographs, General Notices, General Rules for Crude Drugs, General Rules for Preparations, and General Tests for their conformity to the Japanese Pharmacopoeia. (See the General Notices 5.)

Supplement I, JP XVIII　　　　　　　　　　　　　　　　　　　　*Official Monographs*　2891

Residue on ignition <2.44>　Not more than 0.1% (1 g).

Assay　Weigh accurately about 50 mg each of Methyl Parahydroxybenzoate and Methyl Parahydroxybenzoate RS, dissolve separately in 2.5 mL each of methanol, and add the mobile phase to make exactly 50 mL. Pipet 10 mL each of these solutions, add the mobile phase to make exactly 100 mL, and use these solutions as the sample solution and the standard solution, respectively. Perform the test with exactly 10 μL each of the sample solution and standard solution as directed under Liquid Chromatography <2.01> according to the following conditions, and determine the peak areas, A_T and A_S, of methyl parahydroxybenzoate in each solution.

Amount (mg) of methyl parahydroxybenzoate ($C_8H_8O_3$)
　= $M_S \times A_T/A_S$

　M_S: Amount (mg) of Methyl Parahydroxybenzoate RS taken

Operating conditions—

Detector: An ultraviolet absorption photometer (wavelength: 272 nm).

Column: A stainless steel column 4.6 mm in inside diameter and 15 cm in length, packed with octadecylsilanized silica gel for liquid chromatography (5 μm in particle diameter).

◇Column temperature: A constant temperature of about 35°C.◇

Mobile phase: A mixture of methanol and potassium dihydrogen phosphate solution (17 in 2500) (13:7).

Flow rate: 1.3 mL per minute.

System suitability—

System performance: Dissolve 5 mg each of Methyl Parahydroxybenzoate and parahydroxybenzoic acid in the mobile phase to make exactly 100 mL. Pipet 1 mL of this solution, and add the mobile phase to make exactly 10 mL. When the procedure is run with 10 μL of this solution under the above operating conditions, parahydroxybenzoic acid and methyl parahydroxybenzoate are eluted in this order, the relative retention time of parahydroxybenzoic acid to methyl parahydroxybenzoate is about 0.6, and the resolution between these peaks is not less than 2.0.

System repeatability: When the test is repeated 6 times with 10 μL of the standard solution under the above operating conditions, the relative standard deviation of the peak area of methyl parahydroxybenzoate is not more than 0.85%.

◆**Containers and storage**　Containers—Well-closed containers.◆

Delete the following Monographs:

Nartograstim (Genetical Recombination)

ナルトグラスチム（遺伝子組換え）

Nartograstim for Injection (Genetical Recombination)

注射用ナルトグラスチム（遺伝子組換え）

Add the following:

Oxybutynin Hydrochloride

オキシブチニン塩酸塩

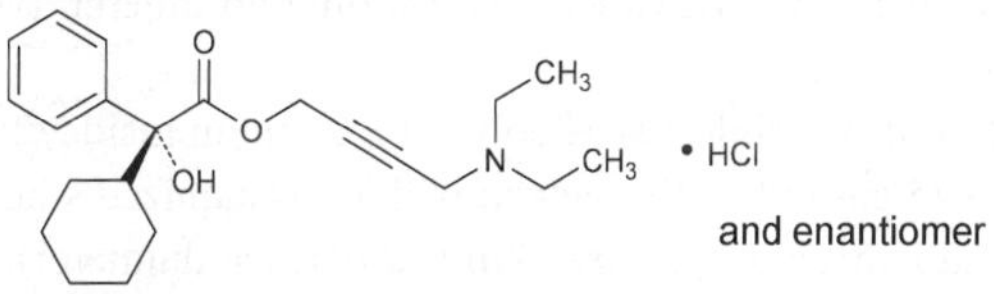

C$_{22}$H$_{31}$NO$_3$.HCl: 393.95
4-(Diethylamino)but-2-yn-1-yl (2*RS*)-2-cyclohexyl-2-hydroxy-2-phenylacetate monohydrochloride
[*1508-65-2*]

Oxybutynin Hydrochloride, when dried, contains not less than 98.0% and not more than 101.0% of oxybutynin hydrochloride (C$_{22}$H$_{31}$NO$_3$.HCl).

Description　Oxybutynin Hydrochloride occurs as a white crystalline powder.

It is freely soluble in water and in ethanol (99.5).

A solution of Oxybutynin Hydrochloride (1 in 50) shows no optical rotation.

Identification　(1)　Determine the absorption spectrum of a solution of Oxybutynin Hydrochloride (3 in 100,000) as directed under Ultraviolet-visible Spectrophotometry <2.24>, and compare the spectrum with the Reference Spectrum: both spectra exhibit similar intensities of absorption at the same wavelengths.

(2)　Determine the infrared absorption spectrum of Oxybutynin Hydrochloride, previously dried, as directed in the potassium chloride disk method under Infrared Spectrophotometry <2.25>, and compare the spectrum with the Reference Spectrum: both spectra exhibit similar intensities of absorption at the same wave numbers.

(3)　A solution of Oxybutynin Hydrochloride (1 in 50) responds to Qualitative Tests <1.09> for chloride.

Melting point <2.60>　124 – 129°C

Purity　Related substances—Dissolve 50 mg of Oxybutynin Hydrochloride in 10 mL of the mobile phase, and use this

The JP Drugs are to be tested according to the provisions given in the pertinent monographs, General Notices, General Rules for Crude Drugs, General Rules for Preparations, and General Tests for their conformity to the Japanese Pharmacopoeia. (See the General Notices 5.)

2892　*Official Monographs*

solution as the sample solution. Pipet 1 mL of the sample solution, add the mobile phase to make exactly 200 mL, and use this solution as the standard solution. Perform the test with exactly 10 μL each of the sample solution and standard solution as directed under Liquid Chromatography <2.01> according to the following conditions, and determine each peak area by the automatic integration method: the peak area of the related substance A, having the relative retention time of about 1.6 to oxybutynin, obtained from the sample solution is not larger than 3 times the peak area of oxybutynin from the standard solution, and the area of the peak other than oxybutynin and the peak mentioned above from the sample solution is not larger than 1/5 times the peak area of oxybutynin from the standard solution. Furthermore, the total area of the peaks other than oxybutynin and the related substance A from the sample solution is not larger than the peak area of oxybutynin from the standard solution. For the peak area of the related substance A, multiply the correction factor, 2.3.

Operating conditions—

Detector: An ultraviolet absorption photometer (wavelength: 210 nm).

Column: A stainless steel column 3.9 mm in inside diameter and 15 cm in length, packed with octylsilanized silica gel for liquid chromatography (5 μm in particle diameter).

Column temperature: A constant temperature of about 25°C.

Mobile phase: Dissolve 3.4 g of potassium dihydrogen phosphate and 4.36 g of dipotassium hydrogen phosphate in water to make 1000 mL. To 490 mL of this solution add 510 mL of acetonitrile for liquid chromatography.

Flow rate: Adjust so that the retention time of oxybutynin is about 15 minutes.

Time span of measurement: About 2 times as long as the retention time of oxybutynin.

System suitability—

Test for required detectability: Pipet 2 mL of the standard solution, and add the mobile phase to make exactly 20 mL. Confirm that the peak area of oxybutynin obtained with 10 μL of this solution is equivalent to 7 to 13% of that with 10 μL of the standard solution.

System performance: When the procedure is run with 10 μL of the standard solution under the above operating conditions, the number of theoretical plates and the symmetry factor of the peak of oxybutynin are not less than 5000 and not more than 1.5, respectively.

System repeatability: When the test is repeated 6 times with 10 μL of the standard solution under the above operating conditions, the relative standard deviation of the peak area of oxybutynin is not more than 2.0%.

Loss on drying <2.41>　Not more than 3.0% (0.5 g, 105°C, 4 hours).

Residue on ignition <2.44>　Not more than 0.1% (1 g).

Assay　Weigh accurately about 0.5 g of Oxybutynin Hydrochloride, previously dried, dissolve in 70 mL of a mixture of acetic anhydride and acetic acid (100) (7:3), and

Supplement I, JP XVIII

titrate <2.50> with 0.1 mol/L perchloric acid VS (potentiometric titration). Perform a blank determination in the same manner, and make any necessary correction.

Each mL of 0.1 mol/L perchloric acid VS
= 39.40 mg of $C_{22}H_{31}NO_3 \cdot HCl$

Containers and storage　Containers—Tight containers.
Storage—Light-resistant.

Others
Related substance A:
4-(Diethylamino)but-2-yn-1-yl (2*R*)-2-(cyclohex-3-en-1-yl)-2-cyclohexyl-2-hydroxyacetate

4-(Diethylamino)but-2-yn-1-yl (2*S*)-2-(cyclohex-3-en-1-yl)-2-cyclohexyl-2-hydroxyacetate

Change the following as follows:

White Petrolatum

白色ワセリン

This monograph is harmonized with the European Pharmacopoeia and the U.S. Pharmacopeia.

The corresponding part of the attributes/provisions which are agreed as non-harmonized within the scope of the harmonization is marked with symbol (◆　◆), and the corresponding parts which are agreed as the JP local requirement other than the scope of the harmonization are marked with symbols (◇　◇).

Information on the harmonization with the European Pharmacopoeia and the U.S. Pharmacopeia is available on the website of the Pharmaceuticals and Medical Devices Agency.

White Petrolatum is a purified and wholly or nearly decolorized semi-solid mixture of hydrocarbons obtained from petroleum.

It may contain a suitable antioxidant ◇such as dibutylhydroxytoluene or an appropriate type of tocopherol.◇ ◆If an antioxidant is added, the label states the name and amount of the antioxidant.◆

◆**Description**　White Petrolatum occurs as a white to pale yellow, homogeneous, unctuous mass. It is odorless and tasteless.

It is practically insoluble in water and in ethanol (95).

The JP Drugs are to be tested according to the provisions given in the pertinent monographs, General Notices, General Rules for Crude Drugs, General Rules for Preparations, and General Tests for their conformity to the Japanese Pharmacopoeia. (See the General Notices 5.)

Supplement I, JP XVIII   *Official Monographs*   2893

It becomes a clear liquid when warmed.◆

Identification Place about 2 mg of White Petrolatum on an optical plate, place the plate upon another optical plate to spread the sample, and determine the infrared absorption spectrum as directed in the liquid film method under Infrared Spectrophotometry <2.25>, and compare the spectrum with the Reference Spectrum: both spectra exhibit similar intensities of absorption at the same wave numbers.

◇**Melting point** <2.60> 38 – 60°C (Method 3).◇

Purity **(1)** Color—Melt about 10 g of White Petrolatum on a water bath, and pour 5 mL of it into a clear glass 15 × 150 mm test tube, and keep the content in melted condition: the liquid has no more color than the following control solution, when observed transversely in reflected light against a white background.

Control solution: Pipet 0.5 mL of Iron (III) Chloride CS and 4.5 mL of diluted dilute hydrochloric acid (1 in 10), respectively, and mix in a clear glass 15 × 150 mm test tube.

(2) Acidity or alkalinity—To 10 g of White Petrolatum add 20 mL of hot water, shake vigorously for 1 minute, and cool. To the 10 mL of aqueous layer add 0.1 mL of phenolphthalein TS: the solution is colorless. Add 0.01 mol/L sodium hydroxide VS until a light red or red color develops: the necessary volume of the VS is not more than 0.5 mL.

(3) Polycyclic aromatic hydrocarbons—Dissolve 1.0 g of White Petrolatum in the solution prepared by adding 50 mL of hexane for ultraviolet-visible spectrophotometry to 10 mL of dimethylsulfoxide for ultraviolet-visible spectrophotometry and shaking twice. Transfer this solution to a separator with unlubricated ground-glass parts (stopper, stopcock). To this separator add 20 mL of dimethylsulfoxide for ultraviolet-visible spectrophotometry, shake vigorously for 1 minute, and allow to stand until two clear layers are formed. Transfer the lower layer to a second separator, repeat the extraction with a further 20 mL of dimethylsulfoxide for ultraviolet-visible spectrophotometry. Combine the lower layers obtained by the extraction procedures, shake vigorously with 20 mL of hexane for ultraviolet-visible spectrophotometry for 1 minute. Allow to stand until two clear layers are formed, separate the lower layer, add dimethylsulfoxide for ultraviolet-visible spectrophotometry to make exactly 50 mL, and use this solution as the sample solution. Determine the absorbance between 265 nm and 420 nm in a layer of 1 cm. Shake vigorously 25 mL of hexane for ultraviolet-visible spectrophotometry and 10 mL of dimethylsulfoxide for ultraviolet-visible spectrophotometry for 1 minute, allow to stand until two clear layers are formed, and use the lower layer thus obtained as the control solution. Separately, weigh accurately about 6 mg of naphthalene, dissolve in dimethylsulfoxide for ultraviolet-visible spectrophotometry to make exactly 100 mL. Pipet 10 mL of this solution, add dimethylsulfoxide for ultraviolet-visible spectrophotometry to make exactly 100 mL, and use this solution as the standard solution. Determine the absorbance of the standard solution at 278 nm in a layer of 1 cm in length and the absorption spectrum between 265 nm and

420 nm of the sample solution as directed under Ultraviolet-visible Spectrophotometry <2.24>: the maximum absorbance of the sample solution is not more than 1/4 the absorbance at 278 nm of the standard solution.

Residue on ignition <2.44> Not more than 0.05% (2 g).

◆**Containers and storage** Containers—Tight containers.◆

Change the following as follows:

Yellow Petrolatum

Petrolatum

黄色ワセリン

This monograph is harmonized with the European Pharmacopoeia and the U.S. Pharmacopeia.

The corresponding part of the attributes/provisions which are agreed as non-harmonized within the scope of the harmonization is marked with symbol (◆ ◆), and the corresponding parts which are agreed as the JP local requirement other than the scope of the harmonization are marked with symbols (◇ ◇).

Information on the harmonization with the European Pharmacopoeia and the U.S. Pharmacopeia is available on the website of the Pharmaceuticals and Medical Devices Agency.

Yellow Petrolatum is a purified semi-solid mixture of hydrocarbons obtained from petroleum.

It may contain a suitable antioxidant ◇such as dibutylhydroxytoluene or an appropriate type of tocopherol.◇ ◆If an antioxidant is added, the label states the name and amount of the antioxidant.◆

◆**Description** Yellow Petrolatum occurs as a yellow, homogeneous, unctuous mass. It is odorless and tasteless.

It is slightly soluble in ethanol (95), and practically insoluble in water.

It becomes a yellow, clear liquid with slight fluorescence when warmed.◆

Identification Place about 2 mg of Yellow Petrolatum on an optical plate, place the plate upon another optical plate to spread the sample, and determine the infrared absorption spectrum as directed in the liquid film method under Infrared Spectrophotometry <2.25>, and compare the spectrum with the Reference Spectrum: both spectra exhibit similar intensities of absorption at the same wave numbers.

◇**Melting point** <2.60> 38 – 60°C (Method 3).◇

Purity **(1)** Color—Melt about 10 g of Yellow Petrolatum on a water bath, and pour 5 mL of it into a clear glass 15 × 150 mm test tube, and keep the content in melted condition: the liquid has no more color than the following control solution (1) and has equal color to or more color than the following control solution (2), when observed transversely in

---

The JP Drugs are to be tested according to the provisions given in the pertinent monographs, General Notices, General Rules for Crude Drugs, General Rules for Preparations, and General Tests for their conformity to the Japanese Pharmacopoeia. (See the General Notices 5.)

2894　*Official Monographs*　　　　　　　　　　　　　　*Supplement I, JP XVIII*

reflected light against a white background.

Control solution (1): Pipet 3.8 mL of Iron (III) Chloride CS and 1.2 mL of Cobalt (II) Chloride CS, and mix in a clear glass 15 × 150 mm test tube.

Control solution (2): Pipet 0.5 mL of Iron (III) Chloride CS and 4.5 mL of diluted dilute hydrochloric acid (1 in 10), and mix in a clear glass 15 × 150 mm test tube.

(2) Acidity or alkalinity—To 10 g of Yellow Petrolatum add 20 mL of hot water, shake vigorously for 1 minute, and cool. To the 10 mL of aqueous layer add 0.1 mL of phenolphthalein TS: the solution is colorless. Add 0.01 mol/L sodium hydroxide VS until a light red or red color develops: the necessary volume of the VS is not more than 0.5 mL.

(3) Polycyclic aromatic hydrocarbons—Dissolve 1.0 g of Yellow Petrolatum in the solution prepared by adding 50 mL of hexane for ultraviolet-visible spectrophotometry to 10 mL of dimethylsulfoxide for ultraviolet-visible spectrophotometry and shaking twice. Transfer this solution to a separator with unlubricated ground-glass parts (stopper, stopcock). To this separator add 20 mL of dimethylsulfoxide for ultraviolet-visible spectrophotometry, shake vigorously for 1 minute, and allow to stand until two clear layers are formed. Transfer the lower layer to a second separator, repeat the extraction with a further 20 mL of dimethylsulfoxide for ultraviolet-visible spectrophotometry. Combine the lower layers obtained by the extraction procedures, shake vigorously with 20 mL of hexane for ultraviolet-visible spectrophotometry for 1 minute. Allow to stand until two clear layers are formed, separate the lower layer, add dimethylsulfoxide for ultraviolet-visible spectrophotometry to make exactly 50 mL, and use this solution as the sample solution. Determine the absorbance between 265 nm and 420 nm in a layer of 1 cm. Shake vigorously 25 mL of hexane for ultraviolet-visible spectrophotometry and 10 mL of dimethylsulfoxide for ultraviolet-visible spectrophotometry for 1 minute, allow to stand until two clear layers are formed, and use the lower layer thus obtained as the control solution. Separately, weigh accurately about 6 mg of naphthalene, dissolve in dimethylsulfoxide for ultraviolet-visible spectrophotometry to make exactly 100 mL. Pipet 10 mL of this solution, add dimethylsulfoxide for ultraviolet-visible spectrophotometry to make exactly 100 mL, and use this solution as the standard solution. Determine the absorbance of the standard solution at 278 nm in a layer of 1 cm in length and the absorption spectrum between 265 nm and 420 nm of the sample solution as directed under Ultraviolet-visible Spectrophotometry <2.24>: the maximum absorbance of the sample solution is not more than 1/4 the absorbance at 278 nm of the standard solution.

Residue on ignition <2.44>　Not more than 0.05% (2 g).

◆**Containers and storage**　Containers—Tight containers.◆

Change the following as follows:

Polysorbate 80

ポリソルベート 80

This monograph is harmonized with the European Pharmacopoeia and the U.S. Pharmacopeia.

The corresponding part of the attributes/provisions which are agreed as non-harmonized within the scope of the harmonization is marked with symbols (◆ ◆), and the corresponding parts which are agreed as the JP local requirement other than the scope of the harmonization are marked with symbols (◇ ◇).

Information on the harmonization with the European Pharmacopoeia and the U.S. Pharmacopeia is available on the website of the Pharmaceuticals and Medical Devices Agency.

Polysorbate 80 is a mixture of partial esters of fatty acids, mainly oleic acid, with sorbitol and its anhydrides ethoxylated with approximately 20 moles of ethylene oxide for each mole of sorbitol and sorbitol anhydrides.

◆**Description**　Polysorbate 80 is a colorless or brownish yellow, clear or slightly opalescent, oily liquid.

It is miscible with water, with methanol, with ethanol (99.5) and with ethyl acetate.

It is practically insoluble in fatty oils and in liquid paraffin.

Viscosity: about 400 mPa·s (25°C).

Specific gravity d_{20}^{20} : about 1.10◆

Identification　It meets the requirements of the Composition of fatty acids.

Composition of fatty acids　Dissolve 0.10 g of Polysorbate 80 in 2 mL of a solution of sodium hydroxide in methanol (1 in 50) in a 25-mL conical flask, and boil under a reflux condenser for 30 minutes. Add 2.0 mL of boron trifluoride-methanol TS through the condenser, and boil for 30 minutes. Add 4 mL of heptane through the condenser, and boil for 5 minutes. After cooling, add 10.0 mL of saturated sodium chloride solution, shake for about 15 seconds, and add a quantity of saturated sodium chloride solution such that the upper layer is brought into the neck of the flask. Collect 2 mL of the upper layer, wash with three 2-mL portions of water, dry with anhydrous sodium sulfate, and use this solution as the sample solution. Perform the test with 1 μL each of the sample solution and fatty acid methyl esters mixture TS as directed under Gas Chromatography <2.02> according to the following conditions. Identify each peak obtained with the sample solution using the chromatogram with fatty acid methyl esters mixture TS. Determine each peak area with the sample solution by the automatic integration method, and calculate the composition of fatty acids by the area percentage method: myristic acid is not more than 5.0%, palmitic acid is not more than 16.0%, palmitoleic acid is not more than 8.0%, stearic acid is not

The JP Drugs are to be tested according to the provisions given in the pertinent monographs, General Notices, General Rules for Crude Drugs, General Rules for Preparations, and General Tests for their conformity to the Japanese Pharmacopoeia. (See the General Notices 5.)

Supplement I, JP XVIII · *Official Monographs* 2895

more than 6.0%, oleic acid is not less than 58.0%, linoleic acid is not more than 18.0% and linolenic acid is not more than 4.0%.

Operating conditions—

Detector: A hydrogen flame-ionization detector.

Column: A fused silica column 0.32 mm in inside diameter and 30 m in length, coated with polyethylene glycol 20 M for gas chromatography 0.5 μm in thickness.

Column temperature: Inject at a constant temperature of about 80°C, raise the temperature to 220°C at a rate of 10°C per minute, and maintain at 220°C for 40 minutes.

Injection port temperature: A constant temperature of about 250°C.

Detector temperature: A constant temperature of about 250°C.

Carrier gas: Helium.

Flow rate: 50 cm per second.

Split ratio: 1: 50.

System suitability—

Test for required detectability: Dissolve 0.50 g of the mixture of fatty acid methyl esters described in the following table in heptane to make exactly 50 mL, and use this solution as the solution for system suitability test. Pipet 1 mL of the solution for system suitability test add heptane to make exactly 10 mL. When the procedure is run with 1 μL of this solution under the above operating conditions, the SN ratio of methyl myristate is not less than 5.

Mixture of fatty acid methyl esters	Composition (%)
Methyl myristate for gas chromatography	5
Methyl palmitate for gas chromatography	10
Methyl stearate for gas chromatography	15
Methyl arachidate for gas chromatography	20
Methyl oleate for gas chromatography	20
Methyl eicosenoate for gas chromatography	10
Methyl behenate	10
Methyl lignocerate for gas chromatography	10

System performance: When the procedure is run with 1 μL of the solution for system suitability test under the above operating conditions, $^\diamond$methyl stearate and methyl oleate are eluted in this order,$_\diamond$ the resolution between these peaks is not less than 1.8, and the number of theoretical plates of the peak of methyl stearate is not less than 30,000.

Acid value ⟨1.13⟩ Not more than 2.0 (using ◆ethanol (95)◆ instead).

Saponification value Introduce about 4 g of Polysorbate 80, accurately weighed, into a 250-mL borosilicate glass flask. Add exactly 30 mL of 0.5 mol/L potassium hydroxide-ethanol VS and a few glass beads. Attach a reflux condenser, and heat for 60 minutes. Add 1 mL of phenolphthalein TS and 50 mL of ethanol (99.5), and titrate ⟨2.50⟩ immediately with 0.5 mol/L hydrochloric acid VS. Perform a blank determination in the same manner. Calculate the saponification value by the following equation: 45 – 55.

Saponification value = $(a - b) \times 28.05/M$

M: Amount (g) of Polysorbate 80 taken

a: Volume (mL) of 0.5 mol/L hydrochloric acid VS required for blank determination

b: Volume (mL) of 0.5 mol/L hydrochloric acid VS required for sample determination

Hydroxyl value Introduce about 2 g of Polysorbate 80, accurately weighed, into a 150-mL round bottom flask, add exactly 5 mL of acetic anhydride-pyridine TS, and attach an air condenser. Heat the flask in a water bath for 1 hour keeping the level of the water about 2.5 cm above the level of the liquid in the flask. Withdraw the flask and allow to cool. Add 5 mL of water through the condenser. If a cloudiness appears add sufficient pyridine to clear it, noting the volume added. Shake the flask, and heat in the water bath for 10 minutes. Withdraw the flask and allow to cool. Rinse the condenser and the walls of the flask with 5 mL of neutralized ethanol, and titrate ⟨2.50⟩ with 0.5 mol/L potassium hydroxide-ethanol VS (indicator: 0.2 mL of phenolphthalein TS). Perform a blank determination in the same manner. Calculate the hydroxyl value by the following equation: 65 – 80.

Hydroxyl value = $(a - b) \times 28.05/M$ + acid value

M: Amount (g) of Polysorbate 80 taken

a: Volume (mL) of 0.5 mol/L potassium hydroxide-ethanol VS required for blank determination

b: Volume (mL) of 0.5 mol/L potassium hydroxide-ethanol VS required for sample determination

Purity (1) Ethylene oxide and 1,4-dioxane—Transfer exactly 1.00 g of Polysorbate 80 into a 10-mL headspace vial, add exactly 2 mL of water, seal the vial immediately with a septum of silicon rubber coated with fluororesin and an aluminum cap. Mix carefully, and use the content as the sample solution. Separately, pipet 0.5 mL of a solution, prepared by dissolving ethylene oxide in dichloromethane so that each mL contains 50 mg, and add water to make exactly 50 mL. Allow to stand to reach room temperature. Pipet 1 mL of this solution, add water to make exactly 250 mL, and use this solution as ethylene oxide stock solution. Separately, pipet 1 mL of 1,4-dioxane, add water to make exactly 200 mL. Pipet 1 mL of this solution, add water to make exactly 100 mL, and use this solution as 1,4-dioxane stock solution. To exact 6 mL of ethylene oxide stock solution and exact 2.5 mL of 1,4-dioxane stock solution add water to make exactly 25 mL, and use this solution as ethylene oxide-1,4-dioxane standard stock solution. Separately, transfer exactly 1.00 g of Polysorbate 80 into a 10-mL headspace vial, add exactly 2 mL of ethylene oxide-1,4-dioxane standard stock solution, seal the vial immediately with a septum of silicon rubber coated the surface with fluororesin and an aluminum cap. Mix carefully, and use the content as the standard solution. Perform the test with the sample solution and standard solution as directed in the head-space method under Gas Chromatography ⟨2.02⟩ according to the following conditions. The amounts of ethylene oxide and

The JP Drugs are to be tested according to the provisions given in the pertinent monographs, General Notices, General Rules for Crude Drugs, General Rules for Preparations, and General Tests for their conformity to the Japanese Pharmacopoeia. (See the General Notices 5.)

2896　*Official Monographs*　　　　　　　　　　*Supplement I, JP XVIII*

1,4-dioxane, calculated by the following equations, are not more than 1 ppm and not more than 10 ppm, respectively.

$$\text{Amount (ppm) of ethylene oxide} = 2 \times C_{\text{EO}} \times A_a/(A_b - A_a)$$

C_{EO}: Concentration (μg/mL) of added ethylene oxide in the standard solution

A_a: Peak area of ethylene oxide obtained with the sample solution

A_b: Peak area of ethylene oxide obtained with the standard solution

$$\text{Amount (ppm) of 1,4-dioxane} = 2 \times 1.03 \times C_D \times A'_a \times 1000/(A'_b - A'_a)$$

C_D: Concentration (μL/mL) of added 1,4-dioxane in the standard solution

1.03: Density (g/mL) of 1,4-dioxane

A'_a: Peak area of 1,4-dioxane obtained with the sample solution

A'_b: Peak area of 1,4-dioxane obtained with the standard solution

Head-space injection conditions—

Equilibration temperature in vial: A constant temperature of about 80°C.

Equilibration time in vial: 30 minutes.

Carrier gas: Helium.

Injection volume of sample: 1.0 mL.

Operating conditions—

Detector: A hydrogen flame-ionization detector.

Column: A fused silica column 0.53 mm in inside diameter and 50 m in length, coated the inside surface with 5% diphenyl-95% dimethylpolysiloxane for gas chromatography 5 μm in thickness.

Column temperature: Inject at a constant temperature of about 70°C, raise the temperature to 250°C at a rate of 10°C per minute, and maintain at 250°C for 5 minutes.

Injection port temperature: A constant temperature of about 85°C.

Detector temperature: A constant temperature of about 250°C.

Carrier gas: Helium.

Flow rate: 4.0 mL per minute.

Split ratio: 1:3.5.

System suitability—

System performance: Introduce 0.100 g of acetaldehyde in a 100-mL volumetric flask, and add water to make 100 mL. To exact 1 mL of this solution add water to make exactly 100 mL. Transfer exactly 2 mL of this solution and exactly 2 mL of ethylene oxide stock solution into a 10-mL headspace vial, seal the vial immediately with a fluororesin coated silicon septum and an aluminum cap. Mix carefully, and use the content as the solution for system suitability test. When perform the test with the standard solution and the solution for system suitability test under the above conditions, acetaldehyde, ethylene oxide and 1,4-dioxane are eluted in this order, and the resolution between the peaks of acetaldehyde and ethylene oxide is not less than 2.0.

(2)　Peroxide value—Introduce about 10 g of Polysorbate 80, accurately weighed, into a 100-mL beaker, dissolve in 20 mL of acetic acid (100). Add 1 mL of saturated potassium iodide solution and allow to stand for 1 minute. Add 50 mL of fleshly boiled and cooled water, and titrate <2.50> with 0.01 mol/L sodium thiosulfate VS, while stirring with a magnetic stirrer (potentiometric titration). Perform a blank determination in the same manner, and make any necessary correction. Calculate peroxide value by the following equation: not more than 10.0.

$$\text{Peroxide value} = (a - b) \times 10/M$$

M: Amount (g) of Polysorbate 80 taken

a: Volume (mL) of 0.01 mol/L sodium thiosulfate VS required for sample determination

b: Volume (mL) of 0.01 mol/L sodium thiosulfate VS required for blank determination

Water <2.48>　Not more than 3.0% (1 g, volumetric titration, direct titration).

Residue on ignition　Heat a quartz or platinum crucible to redness for 30 minutes, allow to cool in a desiccator (silica gel or other appropriate desiccants), and weigh accurately. Evenly distribute 2.00 g of Polysorbate 80 in the crucible, dry at 100 – 105°C for 1 hour, ◇and gradually heat with as lower temperature as possible to carbonize completely.◇ Then after igniting to constant mass in an electric furnace at 600 ± 25°C, allow the crucible to cool in a desiccator, and weigh the mass accurately. Flames should not be produced at any time during the procedure. If after prolonged ignition the ash still contains black particles, take up the ash with hot water, filter through a filter paper for quantitative analysis, and ignite the residue and the filter paper. Combine the filtrate with the ash, carefully evaporate to dryness, and ignite to constant mass: not more than 0.25%.

Containers and storage　Containers—Tight containers.

Storage—Light-resistant.

Change the following as follows:

Propyl Parahydroxybenzoate

パラオキシ安息香酸プロピル

$C_{10}H_{12}O_3$: 180.20
Propyl 4-hydroxybenzoate
[*94-13-3*]

This monograph is harmonized with the European Pharmacopoeia and the U.S. Pharmacopeia.

The corresponding part of the attributes/provisions which are agreed as non-harmonized within the scope of the harmonization is marked with symbols (♦　♦), and the cor-

The JP Drugs are to be tested according to the provisions given in the pertinent monographs, General Notices, General Rules for Crude Drugs, General Rules for Preparations, and General Tests for their conformity to the Japanese Pharmacopoeia. (See the General Notices 5.)

Supplement I, JP XVIII   *Official Monographs* 2897

responding parts which are agreed as the JP local requirement other than the scope of the harmonization are marked with symbols ($^\diamond$ $_\diamond$).

Information on the harmonization with the European Pharmacopoeia and the U.S. Pharmacopeia is available on the website of the Pharmaceuticals and Medical Devices Agency.

Propyl Parahydroxybenzoate contains not less than 98.0% and not more than 102.0% of propyl parahydroxybenzoate ($C_{10}H_{12}O_3$).

◆**Description** Propyl Parahydroxybenzoate occurs as colorless crystals or a white crystalline powder.

It is freely soluble in methanol, in ethanol (95) and in acetone, and very slightly soluble in water.◆

Identification Determine the infrared absorption spectrum of Propyl Parahydroxybenzoate as directed in the potassium bromide disk method under Infrared Spectrophotometry ⟨2.25⟩, and compare the spectrum with the Reference Spectrum or the spectrum of Propyl Parahydroxybenzoate RS: both spectra exhibit similar intensities of absorption at the same wave numbers.

Melting point ⟨2.60⟩ 96 – 99°C

Purity (1) Clarity and color of solution—Dissolve 1.0 g of Propyl Parahydroxybenzoate in ethanol (95) to make 10 mL: the solution is clear and not more intensely colored than ethanol (95) or the following control solution.

Control solution: To 5.0 mL of Cobalt (II) Chloride CS, 12.0 mL of Iron (III) Chloride CS and 2.0 mL of Copper (II) Sulfate CS add diluted dilute hydrochloric acid (1 in 10) to make 1000 mL.

(2) Acidity—To 2 mL of the solution of Propyl Parahydroxybenzoate obtained in (1) add 3 mL of ethanol (95), add 5 mL of freshly boiled and cooled water and 0.1 mL of bromocresol green-sodium hydroxide-ethanol TS, then add 0.1 mol/L sodium hydroxide VS until the solution shows a blue color: the volume of 0.1 mol/L sodium hydroxide VS used does not exceed 0.1 mL.

(3) Related substances—Dissolve 50.0 mg of Propyl Parahydroxybenzoate in 2.5 mL of methanol, and add the mobile phase to make exactly 50 mL. Pipet 10 mL of this solution, add the mobile phase to make exactly 100 mL, and use this solution as the sample solution. Pipet 1 mL of the sample solution, and add the mobile phase to make exactly 20 mL. Pipet 1 mL of this solution, add the mobile phase to make exactly 10 mL, and use this solution as the standard solution. Perform the test with exactly 10 μL each of the sample solution and standard solution as directed under Liquid Chromatography ⟨2.01⟩ according to the following conditions, and determine each peak area by the automatic integration method: the peak area of parahydroxybenzoic acid having the relative retention time of about 0.3 to propyl parahydroxybenzoate obtained from the sample solution is not larger than the peak area of propyl parahydroxybenzoate from the standard solution (0.5%). For the peak area of parahydroxybenzoic acid, multiply the correc-

tion factor, 1.4. Furthermore, the area of the peak other than propyl parahydroxybenzoate and parahydroxybenzoic acid from the sample solution is not larger than the peak area of propyl parahydroxybenzoate from the standard solution (0.5%), and the total area of the peaks other than propyl parahydroxybenzoate from the sample solution is not larger than 2 times the peak area of propyl parahydroxybenzoate from the standard solution (1.0%). For this calculation the peak area not larger than 1/5 times the peak area of propyl parahydroxybenzoate from the standard solution is excluded (0.1%).

Operating conditions—

Detector, column, column temperature, mobile phase, and flow rate: Proceed as directed in the operating conditions in the Assay.

Time span of measurement: 2.5 times as long as the retention time of propyl parahydroxybenzoate.

System suitability—

System performance: Proceed as directed in the system suitability in the Assay.

$^\diamond$Test for required detectability: To exactly 2 mL of the standard solution add the mobile phase to make exactly 10 mL. Confirm that the peak area of propyl parahydroxybenzoate obtained with 10 μL of this solution is equivalent to 14 to 26% of that with 10 μL of the standard solution.$_\diamond$

$^\diamond$System repeatability: When the test is repeated 6 times with 10 μL of the standard solution under the above operating conditions, the relative standard deviation of the peak area of propyl parahydroxybenzoate is not more than 2.0%.$_\diamond$

Residue on ignition ⟨2.44⟩ Not more than 0.1% (1 g).

Assay Weigh accurately about 50 mg each of Propyl Parahydroxybenzoate and Propyl Parahydroxybenzoate RS, dissolve separately in 2.5 mL each of methanol, and add the mobile phase to make exactly 50 mL. Pipet 10 mL each of these solutions, add the mobile phase to make exactly 100 mL, and use these solutions as the sample solution and the standard solution, respectively. Perform the test with exactly 10 μL each of the sample solution and standard solution as directed under Liquid Chromatography ⟨2.01⟩ according to the following conditions, and determine the peak areas, A_T and A_S, of propyl parahydroxybenzoate in each solution.

Amount (mg) of propyl parahydroxybenzoate ($C_{10}H_{12}O_3$)
$$= M_S \times A_T/A_S$$

M_S: Amount (mg) of Propyl Parahydroxybenzoate RS taken

Operating conditions—

Detector: An ultraviolet absorption photometer (wavelength: 272 nm).

Column: A stainless steel column 4.6 mm in inside diameter and 15 cm in length, packed with octadecylsilanized silica gel for liquid chromatography (5 μm in particle diameter).

$^\diamond$Column temperature: A constant temperature of about

The JP Drugs are to be tested according to the provisions given in the pertinent monographs, General Notices, General Rules for Crude Drugs, General Rules for Preparations, and General Tests for their conformity to the Japanese Pharmacopoeia. (See the General Notices 5.)

2898 *Official Monographs*

35°C.◇

Mobile phase: A mixture of methanol and potassium dihydrogen phosphate solution (17 in 2500) (13:7).

Flow rate: 1.3 mL per minute.

System suitability—

System performance: Dissolve 5 mg each of Propyl Parahydroxybenzoate, ethyl parahydroxybenzoate and parahydroxybenzoic acid in the mobile phase to make exactly 100 mL. Pipet 1 mL of this solution, and add the mobile phase to make exactly 10 mL. When the procedure is run with 10 μL of this solution under the above operating conditions, parahydroxybenzoic acid, ethyl parahydroxybenzoate and propyl parahydroxybenzoate are eluted in this order, the relative retention times of parahydroxybenzoic acid and ethyl parahydroxybenzoate to propyl parahydroxybenzoate are about 0.3 and about 0.7, respectively, and the resolution between the peaks of ethyl parahydroxybenzoate and propyl parahydroxybenzoate is not less than 3.0.

System repeatability: When the test is repeated 6 times with 10 μL of the standard solution under the above operating conditions, the relative standard deviation of the peak area of propyl parahydroxybenzoate is not more than 0.85%.

◆**Containers and storage** Containers—Well-closed containers.◆

Sarpogrelate Hydrochloride Fine Granules

サルポグレラート塩酸塩細粒

Change the Uniformity of dosage units and Assay as follows:

Uniformity of dosage units ⟨*6.02*⟩ Perform the test according to the following method: Sarpogrelate Hydrochloride Fine Granules in single-dose packages meet the requirement of the Content uniformity test.

To the total amount of the content of 1 package of Sarpogrelate Hydrochloride Fine Granules add $4V/5$ mL of the mobile phase, disperse the particles by sonicating, then add the mobile phase to make exactly V mL so that each mL contains about 1 mg of sarpogrelate hydrochloride ($C_{24}H_{31}NO_6.HCl$), and centrifuge. Pipet 5 mL of the supernatant liquid, add the mobile phase to make exactly 50 mL, and use this solution as the sample solution. Then, proceed as directed in the Assay.

Amount (mg) of sarpogrelate hydrochloride
($C_{24}H_{31}NO_6.HCl$)
$= M_S \times A_T/A_S \times V/50$

M_S: Amount (mg) of Sarpogrelate Hydrochloride RS taken, calculated on the anhydrous basis

Assay Powder Sarpogrelate Hydrochloride Fine Granules. Weigh accurately a portion of the powder, equivalent to about 0.25 g of sarpogrelate hydrochloride ($C_{24}H_{31}NO_6.HCl$), add 200 mL of the mobile phase, and disperse the particles by sonicating. To this solution add the mobile phase to make exactly 250 mL, and centrifuge. Pipet 5 mL of the supernatant liquid, add the mobile phase to make exactly 50 mL, and use this solution as the sample solution. Separately, weigh accurately about 50 mg of Sarpogrelate Hydrochloride RS (separately determine the water ⟨*2.48*⟩ in the same manner as Sarpogrelate Hydroxide), and add the mobile phase to make exactly 50 mL. Pipet 5 mL of this solution, add the mobile phase to make exactly 50 mL, and use this solution as the standard solution. Perform the test with exactly 10 μL each of the sample solution and standard solution as directed under Liquid Chromatography ⟨*2.01*⟩ according to the following conditions, and determine the peak areas, A_T and A_S, of sarpogrelate in each solution.

Amount (mg) of sarpogrelate hydrochloride
($C_{24}H_{31}NO_6.HCl$)
$= M_S \times A_T/A_S \times 5$

M_S: Amount (mg) of Sarpogrelate Hydrochloride RS taken, calculated on the anhydrous basis

Operating conditions—

Proceed as directed in the operating conditions in the Assay under Sarpogrelate Hydrochloride.

System suitability—

System performance: When the procedure is run with 10 μL of the standard solution under the above operating conditions, the number of theoretical plates and the symmetry factor of the peak of sarpogrelate are not less than 5000 and not more than 1.8, respectively.

System repeatability: When the test is repeated 6 times with 10 μL of the standard solution under the above operating conditions, the relative standard deviation of the peak area of sarpogrelate is not more than 1.0%.

Sodium Chloride

塩化ナトリウム

Change the Identification as follows:

Identification (1) A solution of Sodium Chloride (1 in 20) responds to Qualitative Tests (2) ⟨*1.09*⟩ for sodium salt.

(2) A solution of Sodium Chloride (1 in 20) responds to Qualitative Tests (2) ⟨*1.09*⟩ for chloride.

The JP Drugs are to be tested according to the provisions given in the pertinent monographs, General Notices, General Rules for Crude Drugs, General Rules for Preparations, and General Tests for their conformity to the Japanese Pharmacopoeia. (See the General Notices 5.)

Supplement I, JP XVIII   *Official Monographs* 2899

Spectinomycin Hydrochloride for Injection

注射用スペクチノマイシン塩酸塩

Change the description of Uniformity of dosage units as follows:

Uniformity of dosage units *⟨6.02⟩* It meets the requirement of the Mass variation test (*T*: Being specified separately when the drug is granted approval based on the Law.).

Wheat Starch

コムギデンプン

Change the Purity (5) as follows:

Purity

(5) Total protein—Weigh accurately about 3 g of Wheat Starch, place it in a Kjeldahl flask, add 4 g of a decomposition accelerator (a powdered mixture of 100 g of potassium sulfate, 3 g of copper (II) sulfate pentahydrate and 3 g of titanium (IV) oxide), wash down any adhering substances from the neck of the flask with a fine jet of water. Add 25 mL of sulfuric acid allowing to flow down the inside wall of the flask, and mix the contents. Close the mouth of the flask loosely, for example by means of a glass bulb with a short stem, to avoid excessive loss of the sulfuric acid. Heat the flask gradually at first, then increase the temperature until there is vigorous boiling with condensation of sulfuric acid in the neck of the flask, preventing the upper part of the flask from becoming overheated. Continue the heating until the solution becomes clear, and the inside wall of the flask is free from a carbonaceous material. After cooling, dissolve the solid material by adding cautiously 25 mL of water, cool again, and place in a steam-distillation apparatus previously washed by passing steam. Add exactly 25 mL of 0.01 mol/L hydrochloric acid VS and a suitable amount of water into the receiver, and immerse the tip of the condenser in this acid solution. Add the same quantity of a solution of sodium hydroxide (21 in 50) as used for a blank determination through the funnel, and distill immediately by passing steam through the mixture. Collect about 40 mL of distillate, lower the receiver so that the tip of the condenser is above the surface of the acid solution, then continue the distillation for a while, and rinse the end part of the condenser with a small amount of water. Titrate *⟨2.50⟩* the excessive hydrochloric acid with 0.025 mol/L sodium hydroxide VS until the color of the solution changes from red-purple through grayish blue to green (indicator: 3 drops of methyl red-methylene blue TS). Perform a blank determination in the same manner. The amount of a solution of sodium hydroxide (21 in 50) to be added from the funnel is sufficient to change the color of the solution in the flask from bluish green to dark brown or black.

$$\text{Amount (\%) of nitrogen} = (a - b) \times 0.035/M$$

M: Amount (g) of Wheat Starch taken
a: Volume (mL) of 0.025 mol/L sodium hydroxide VS consumed in a blank determination
b: Volume (mL) of 0.025 mol/L sodium hydroxide VS consumed in the sample determination

The amount of total protein is not more than 0.3% [0.048% as nitrogen (N: 14.01) (using conversion factor of nitrogen to protein, 6.25)].

Stearic Acid

ステアリン酸

Change the Congealing point as follows:

Congealing point The apparatus consists of a test tube about 25 mm in diameter and 150 mm long placed inside a test tube about 40 mm in diameter and 160 mm long. The inner tube is closed by a stopper which carries a thermometer about 175 mm long and graduated in 0.2°C fixed so that ◆the upper end of◆ the bulb is about 15 mm above the bottom of the tube. The stopper has a hole allowing the passage of the stem of a stirrer made from a glass rod or other suitable material formed at one end into a loop of about 18 mm overall diameter at right angles to the rod. The inner tube with its jacket is supported centrally in a 1-L beaker containing a suitable cooling liquid to within 20 mm of the top. A thermometer is supported in the cooling bath. Place in the inner tube sufficient quantity of the liquid or previously melted substance to be examined, to cover the thermometer bulb and determine the approximate congealing point by cooling rapidly. Place the inner tube in a bath about 5°C above the approximate congealing point until all but the last traces of crystals are melted. Fill the beaker with water or a saturated solution of sodium chloride, at a temperature about 5°C lower than the expected congealing point, insert the inner tube into the outer tube, ensuring that some seed crystals are present, and stir thoroughly until solidification takes place. Note the highest temperature observed during solidification.

The apparatus directed under Congealing Point Determination *⟨2.42⟩* can also be used. Transfer the melted sample into sample container B up to the marked line C. Adjust the immersion line H of thermometer F to the same level of the meniscus of the sample, and then determine the approximate congealing point by cooling rapidly. Place the sample container B in a bath at a temperature about 5°C above the approximate congealing point until all but the last traces of crystals are melted. Fill bath D with water or a saturated solution of sodium chloride, at a temperature about 5°C lower than the expected congealing point, and set the sample container B in A. Ensuring that some seed crystals are present, stir thoroughly until solidification takes place. Note the highest temperature observed during solidification.

The JP Drugs are to be tested according to the provisions given in the pertinent monographs, General Notices, General Rules for Crude Drugs, General Rules for Preparations, and General Tests for their conformity to the Japanese Pharmacopoeia. (See the General Notices 5.)

2900 *Official Monographs* *Supplement I, JP XVIII*

The congealing point of stearic acid 50 is 53 – 59°C, of stearic acid 70 is 57 – 64°C, and of stearic acid 95 is 64 – 69°C.

Add the following:

Temozolomide

テモゾロミド

H_3C ... O, N, N, N, N, NH$_2$, O

C$_6$H$_6$N$_6$O$_2$: 194.15
3-Methyl-4-oxo-3,4-dihydroimidazo[5,1-*d*][1,2,3,5]tetrazine-8-carboxamide
[*85622-93-1*]

Temozolomide contains not less than 98.0% and not more than 102.0% of temozolomide (C$_6$H$_6$N$_6$O$_2$).

Description Temozolomide occurs as a white to pale red or light yellow-brown, crystalline powder or powder.

It is sparingly soluble in dimethyl sulfoxide, slightly soluble in water and in acetonitrile, and very slightly soluble in ethanol (99.5).

Melting point: 180°C (with decomposition).

It shows crystal polymorphism.

Identification (1) Determine the absorption spectrum of a solution of Temozolomide (1 in 100,000) as directed under Ultraviolet-visible Spectrophotometry <2.24>, and compare the spectrum with the Reference Spectrum or the spectrum of a solution of Temozolomide RS prepared in the same manner as the sample solution: both spectra exhibit similar intensities of absorption at the same wavelengths.

(2) Determine the infrared absorption spectrum of Temozolomide as directed in the potassium bromide disk method under Infrared Spectrophotometry <2.25>, and compare the spectrum with the Reference Spectrum or the spectrum of Temozolomide RS: both spectra exhibit similar intensities of absorption at the same wave numbers. If any difference appears between the spectra, dissolve Temozolomide in acetonitrile, evaporate the acetonitrile, dry the residue, and perform the test with the residue.

Purity (1) Related substances—Use the sample solution obtained in the Assay as the sample solution. Pipet 1 mL of the sample solution, add dimethyl sulfoxide to make exactly 100 mL, and use this solution as the standard solution. Perform the test with exactly 10 μL each of the sample solution and standard solution as directed under Liquid Chromatography <2.01> according to the following conditions, and determine each peak area by the automatic integration method: the peak area of the related substance E, having the relative retention time of about 0.4 to temozolomide, obtained from the sample solution is not larger than 1/5

times the peak area of temozolomide from the standard solution, the peak area of the related substance D, having the relative retention time of about 0.5, from the sample solution is not larger than 1/2 times the peak area of temozolomide from the standard solution, and the area of the peak other than temozolomide and the peaks mentioned above from the sample solution is not larger than 1/10 times the peak area of temozolomide from the standard solution. Furthermore, the total area of the peaks other than temozolomide from the sample solution is not larger than 4/5 times the peak area of temozolomide from the standard solution. For the peak area of the related substance E, multiply the correction factor 0.63.

Operating conditions—

Detector, column, column temperature, mobile phase and flow rate: Proceed as directed in the operating conditions in the Assay.

Time span of measurement: About 3 times as long as the retention time of temozolomide, beginning after the solvent peak.

System suitability—

System performance: Proceed as directed in the system suitability in the Assay.

Test for required detectability: Pipet 1 mL of the standard solution, and add dimethyl sulfoxide to make exactly 20 mL. Confirm that the peak area of temozolomide obtained with 10 μL of this solution is equivalent to 3.5 to 6.5% of that with 10 μL of the standard solution.

System repeatability: When the test is repeated 6 times with 10 μL of the standard solution under the above operating conditions, the relative standard deviation of the peak area of temozolomide is not more than 2.0%.

(2) Residual solvent—Being specified separately when the drug is granted approval based on the Law.

Water <2.48> Not more than 0.4% (0.5 g, coulometric titration).

Residue on ignition <2.44> Not more than 0.1% (1 g).

Assay Weigh accurately about 25 mg each of Temozolomide and Temozolomide RS, to each add 20 mL of dimethyl sulfoxide, shake to dissolve, add dimethyl sulfoxide to make exactly 25 mL, and use these solutions as the sample solution and the standard solution, respectively. Perform the test with exactly 10 μL each of the sample solution and standard solution as directed under Liquid Chromatography <2.01> according to the following conditions, and determine the peak areas, A_T and A_S, of temozolomide in each solution.

Amount (mg) of temozolomide (C$_6$H$_6$N$_6$O$_2$)
= $M_S \times A_T/A_S$

M_S: Amount (mg) of Temozolomide RS taken

Operating conditions—

Detector: An ultraviolet absorption photometer (wavelength: 270 nm).

Column: A stainless steel column 4.6 mm in inside diameter and 15 cm in length, packed with octadecylsilanized

The JP Drugs are to be tested according to the provisions given in the pertinent monographs, General Notices, General Rules for Crude Drugs, General Rules for Preparations, and General Tests for their conformity to the Japanese Pharmacopoeia. (See the General Notices 5.)

Supplement I, JP XVIII   *Official Monographs*   2901

silica gel for liquid chromatography (5 μm in particle diameter).

Column temperature: A constant temperature of about 25°C.

Mobile phase: To 5 mL of acetic acid (100) add 1000 mL of water. To 24 volumes of this solution add 1 volume of methanol. Dissolve 0.94 g of sodium 1-hexanesulfonate in 1000 mL of this solution.

Flow rate: Adjust so that the retention time of temozolomide is about 9.5 minutes.

System suitability—

System performance: To 5 mL of the sample solution add 5 mL of 0.1 mol/L hydrochloric acid TS, heat on a water bath for 1 hour, and cool to 4°C. When the procedure is run with 10 μL of this solution under the above operating conditions, the resolution between the peak of temozolomide and the peak having the relative retention time of about 1.4 to temozolomide is not less than 2.5, and the symmetry factor of the peak of temozolomide is not more than 1.9.

System repeatability: When the test is repeated 6 times with 10 μL of the standard solution under the above operating conditions, the relative standard deviation of the peak area of temozolomide is not more than 1.0%.

Containers and storage   Containers—Well-closed containers (moisture-proof packaging).

Others
Related substance E:
3,7-Dihydro-4*H*-imidazo[4,5-*d*][1,2,3]triazin-4-one

Related substance D:
4-Diazo-4*H*-imidazole-5-carboxamide

Add the following:

Temozolomide Capsules

テモゾロミドカプセル

Temozolomide Capsules contain not less than 95.0% and not more than 105.0% of the labeled amount of temozolomide ($C_6H_6N_6O_2$: 194.15).

Method of preparation   Prepare as directed under Capsules, with Temozolomide.

Identification   Perform the test with 20 μL each of the sample solution and standard solution obtained in the Assay as directed under Liquid Chromatography <2.01> according to the following conditions: the retention times of the principal peaks in the chromatograms obtained from these solutions are the same, and the absorption spectra of these peaks exhibit similar intensities of absorption at the same wavelengths.

Operating conditions—

Column, column temperature, mobile phase and flow rate: Proceed as directed in the operating conditions in the Assay.

Detector: A photodiode array detector (wavelength: 270 nm, spectrum range of measurement: 210 – 400 nm).

System suitability—

System performance: Proceed as directed in the system suitability in the Assay.

Purity   Related substances—Use the sample solution obtained in the Assay as the sample solution. Pipet 1 mL of the sample solution, add dimethyl sulfoxide to make exactly 100 mL, and use this solution as the standard solution. Perform the test with exactly 20 μL each of the sample solution and standard solution as directed under Liquid Chromatography <2.01> according to the following conditions, and determine each peak area by the automatic integration method: the peak area of the related substance E, having the relative retention time of about 0.4 to temozolomide, obtained from the sample solution is not larger than 3/5 times the peak area of temozolomide from the standard solution, the peak area of the related substance CA, having the relative retention time of about 1.4, from the sample solution is not larger than the peak area of temozolomide from the standard solution, and the area of the peak other than temozolomide and the peaks mentioned above from the sample solution is not larger than 1/5 times the peak area of temozolomide from the standard solution. Furthermore, the total area of the peaks other than temozolomide from the sample solution is not larger than 1.2 times the peak area of temozolomide from the standard solution. For the peak areas of the related substances E and CA, multiply the correction factors, 0.63 and 0.30, respectively.

Operating conditions—

Detector, Column, column temperature, mobile phase and flow rate: Proceed as directed in the operating conditions in the Assay under Temozolomide.

Time span of measurement: About 3 times as long as the retention time of temozolomide, beginning after the solvent peak.

System suitability—

System performance: Proceed as directed in the system suitability in the Assay.

Test for required detectability: Pipet 2 mL of the standard solution, and add the mobile phase to make exactly 20 mL. Confirm that the peak area of temozolomide obtained with 20 μL of this solution is equivalent to 7 to 13% of that with 20 μL of the standard solution.

System repeatability: When the test is repeated 6 times with 20 μL of the standard solution under the above operat-

The JP Drugs are to be tested according to the provisions given in the pertinent monographs, General Notices, General Rules for Crude Drugs, General Rules for Preparations, and General Tests for their conformity to the Japanese Pharmacopoeia. (See the General Notices 5.)

2902 *Official Monographs*

ing conditions, the relative standard deviation of the peak area of temozolomide is not more than 2.0%.

Uniformity of dosage units $\langle 6.02 \rangle$ Perform the Mass variation test, or the Content uniformity test according to the following method: it meets the requirement.

To 1 capsule of Temozolomide Capsules add exactly V mL of the mobile phase so that each mL contains about 1 mg of temozolomide ($C_6H_6N_6O_2$), and shake until the capsule is completely disintegrated. Shake until the content is dispersed, centrifuge for 10 minutes, and filter the supernatant liquid through a membrane filter with a pore size of 0.45 μm. Discard the first 3 mL of the filtrate, pipet 10 mL of the subsequent filtrate, add the mobile phase to make exactly 100 mL, and use this solution as the sample solution. Then, proceed as directed in the Assay.

Amount (mg) of temozolomide ($C_6H_6N_6O_2$)
= $M_S \times A_T/A_S \times V/25$

M_S: Amount (mg) of Temozolomide RS taken

Dissolution $\langle 6.10 \rangle$ When the test is performed at 100 revolutions per minute according to the Basket method, using 900 mL of water as the dissolution medium, the Q value in 30 minutes of Temozolomide Capsules is 80%.

Start the test with 1 capsule of Temozolomide Capsules, withdraw not less than 10 mL of the medium at the specified minute after starting the test, and filter through a membrane filter with a pore size not exceeding 0.8 μm. Discard not less than 3 mL of the first filtrate, pipet V mL of the subsequent filtrate, add water to make V' mL so that each mL contains about 22 μg of temozolomide ($C_6H_6N_6O_2$), and use this solution as the sample solution. Separately, weigh accurately about 22 mg of Temozolomide RS, and dissolve in water to make exactly 100 mL. Pipet 10 mL of this solution, add water to make exactly 100 mL, and use this solution as the standard solution. Determine the absorbances, A_T and A_S, of the sample solution and standard solution at 328 nm as directed under Ultraviolet-visible Spectrophotometry $\langle 2.24 \rangle$.

Dissolution rate (%) with respect to the labeled amount of temozolomide ($C_6H_6N_6O_2$)
= $M_S \times A_T/A_S \times V'/V \times 1/C \times 90$

M_S: Amount (mg) of Temozolomide RS taken
C: Labeled amount (mg) of temozolomide ($C_6H_6N_6O_2$) in 1 capsule

Assay   To 10 Temozolomide Capsules add the mobile phase, and shake until the capsules are completely disintegrated. Shake until the content is dispersed, and add the mobile phase to make exactly V mL so that each mL contains about 1 mg of temozolomide ($C_6H_6N_6O_2$). Centrifuge this solution for 10 minutes, and filter the supernatant liquid through a membrane filter with a pore size of 0.45 μm. Discard the first 3 mL of the filtrate, pipet 10 mL of the subsequent filtrate, add the mobile phase to make exactly 100 mL, and use this solution as the sample solution. Separately, weigh accurately about 25 mg of Temozolomide RS,

Supplement I, JP XVIII

add 200 mL of the mobile phase, sonicate to dissolve, add the mobile phase to make exactly 250 mL, and use this solution as the standard solution. Perform the test with exactly 20 μL each of the sample solution and standard solution as directed under Liquid Chromatography $\langle 2.01 \rangle$ according to the following conditions, and determine the peak areas, A_T and A_S, of temozolomide in each solution.

Amount (mg) of temozolomide ($C_6H_6N_6O_2$) in 1 capsule
= $M_S \times A_T/A_S \times V/250$

M_S: Amount (mg) of Temozolomide RS taken

Operating conditions—
Proceed as directed in the operating conditions in the Assay under Temozolomide.
System suitability—
System performance: Dissolve 10 mg of temozolomide in 25 mL of the mobile phase. To this solution add 25 mL of 0.1 mol/L hydrochloric acid TS, allow to stand at 80°C for 4 hours, cool to 4°C, and preserve. When the procedure is run with 20 μL of this solution under the above operating conditions, the resolution between the peaks of temozolomide and the related substance CA is not less than 2.5, and the symmetry factor of the peak of temozolomide is not more than 1.9.
System repeatability: When the test is repeated 6 times with 20 μL of the standard solution under the above operating conditions, the relative standard deviation of the peak area of temozolomide is not more than 1.0%.

Containers and storage   Containers—Tight containers.

Others
Related substance E:
Refer to it described in Temozolomide.
Related substance CA:
5-Amino-1H-imidazole-4-carboxamide

Add the following:

Temozolomide for Injection

注射用テモゾロミド

Temozolomide for Injection is a preparation for injection which is dissolved before use.

It contains not less than 95.0% and not more than 105.0% of the labeled amount of temozolomide ($C_6H_6N_6O_2$: 194.15).

Method of preparation   Prepare as directed under Injections, with Temozolomide.

Description   Temozolomide for Injection occurs as a white

The JP Drugs are to be tested according to the provisions given in the pertinent monographs, General Notices, General Rules for Crude Drugs, General Rules for Preparations, and General Tests for their conformity to the Japanese Pharmacopoeia. (See the General Notices 5.)

Supplement I, JP XVIII *Official Monographs* 2903

to pale red or light yellow-brown powder.

Identification Perform the test with 75 μL each of the sample solution and standard solution obtained in the Assay as directed under Liquid Chromatography ⟨2.01⟩ according to the following conditions: the retention times of the principal peaks in the chromatograms obtained from these solutions are the same, and the absorption spectra of these peaks exhibit similar intensities of absorption at the same wavelengths.

Operating conditions—

Column, column temperature, mobile phase and flow rate: Proceed as directed in the operating conditions in the Assay under Temozolomide.

Detector: A photodiode array detector (wavelength: 270 nm, spectrum range of measurement: 210 – 400 nm).

System suitability—

System performance: Proceed as directed in the system suitability in the Assay.

pH Being specified separately when the drug is granted approval based on the Law.

Purity Related substances—Use the sample solution obtained in the Assay as the sample solution. Pipet 1 mL of the sample solution, add the mobile phase to make exactly 100 mL, and use this solution as the standard solution. Perform the test with exactly 75 μL each of the sample solution and standard solution as directed under Liquid Chromatography ⟨2.01⟩ according to the following conditions, and determine each peak area by the automatic integration method: the peak area of the related substance E, having the relative retention time of about 0.4 to temozolomide, obtained from the sample solution is not larger than 2/5 times the peak area of temozolomide from the standard solution, the peak area of the related substance IA, having the relative retention time of about 1.4, from the sample solution is not larger than the peak area of temozolomide from the standard solution, and the area of the peak other than temozolomide and the peaks mentioned above from the sample solution is not larger than 1/5 times the peak area of temozolomide from the standard solution. Furthermore, the total area of the peaks other than temozolomide from the sample solution is not larger than the peak area of temozolomide from the standard solution. For the peak areas of the related substances E and IA, multiply the correction factors, 0.63 and 0.29, respectively.

Operating conditions—

Detector, Column, column temperature, mobile phase and flow rate: Proceed as directed in the operating conditions in the Assay under Temozolomide.

Time span of measurement: About 3 times as long as the retention time of temozolomide, beginning after the solvent peak.

System suitability—

System performance: Proceed as directed in the system suitability in the Assay.

Test for required detectability: Pipet 5 mL of the standard solution obtained in the Assay, and add the mobile

phase to make exactly 200 mL. Pipet 2 mL of this solution, and add the mobile phase to make exactly 100 mL. When the procedure is run with 75 μL of this solution under the above operating conditions, the SN ratio of the peak of temozolomide is not less than 10.

System repeatability: When the test is repeated 6 times with 75 μL of the standard solution under the above operating conditions, the relative standard deviation of the peak area of temozolomide is not more than 2.0%.

Water ⟨2.48⟩ To an amount of Temozolomide for Injection, equivalent to 100 mg of Temozolomide, add exactly 40 mL of methanol to dissolve the content, pipet 2 mL of the solution, and perform the test by coulometric titration: not more than 1.0%. Perform a blank determination in the same manner, and make any necessary correction.

Bacterial endotoxins ⟨4.01⟩ Less than 0.75 EU/mg.

Uniformity of dosage units ⟨6.02⟩ It meets the requirement of the Mass variation test (*T*: being specified separately when the drug is granted approval based on the Law.).

Foreign insoluble matter ⟨6.06⟩ Perform the test according to Method 2: it meets the requirement.

Insoluble particulate matter ⟨6.07⟩ It meets the requirement.

Sterility ⟨4.06⟩ Perform the test according to the Membrane filtration method: it meets the requirement.

Assay Take a number of Temozolomide for Injection, equivalent to 500 mg of temozolomide ($C_6H_6N_6O_2$), dissolve each content in water, wash each container with water, combine the washings with the former solution, and add water to the combined solution to make exactly 200 mL. Pipet 5 mL of this solution, add the mobile phase to make exactly 100 mL, and use this solution as the sample solution. Separately, weigh accurately about 31 mg of Temozolomide RS, and add the mobile phase to make exactly 50 mL. Pipet 10 mL of this solution, add the mobile phase to make exactly 50 mL, and use this solution as the standard solution. Perform the test with exactly 75 μL each of the sample solution and standard solution as directed under Liquid Chromatography ⟨2.01⟩ according to the following conditions, and determine the peak areas, A_T and A_S, of temozolomide in each solution.

$$\text{Amount (mg) of temozolomide } (C_6H_6N_6O_2)$$
$$= M_S \times A_T/A_S \times 16$$

M_S: Amount (mg) of Temozolomide RS taken

Operating conditions—

Proceed as directed in the operating conditions in the Assay under Temozolomide.

System suitability—

System performance: To 1 mg of temozolomide add a mixture of the mobile phase and 0.1 mol/L hydrochloric acid TS (1:1) to make 10 mL, heat at 80°C for about 4 hours, and cool to about 4°C. To this solution add the mo-

The JP Drugs are to be tested according to the provisions given in the pertinent monographs, General Notices, General Rules for Crude Drugs, General Rules for Preparations, and General Tests for their conformity to the Japanese Pharmacopoeia. (See the General Notices 5.)

2904 *Official Monographs*

bile phase to make 25 mL. When the procedure is run with 75 μL of this solution under the above operating conditions, the resolution between the peaks of temozolomide and the related substance IA is not less than 2.5, and the symmetry factor of the peak of temozolomide is not more than 1.9.

System repeatability: When the test is repeated 6 times with 75 μL of the standard solution under the above operating conditions, the relative standard deviation of the peak area of temozolomide is not more than 1.0%.

Containers and storage Containers—Hermetic containers.
Storage—At a temperature between 2°C and 8°C.

Others
Related substance E:
  Refer to it described in Temozolomide.
Related substance IA:
5-Amino-1*H*-imidazole-4-carboxamide

Add the following:

Voglibose Orally Disintegrating Tablets

ボグリボース口腔内崩壊錠

Voglibose Orally Disintegrating Tablets contain not less than 95.0% and not more than 105.0% of the labeled amount of voglibose ($C_{10}H_{21}NO_7$: 267.28).

Method of preparation Prepare as directed under Tablets, with Voglibose.

Identification To 10 tablets of Voglibose Orally Disintegrating Tablets, crushed if necessary, add methanol so that each mL contains about 0.2 mg of voglibose ($C_{10}H_{21}NO_7$), sonicate while shaking to disintegrate the tablets. Filter this solution through a membrane filter with a pore size not exceeding 0.45 μm, discard the first 3 mL of the filtrate, and use the subsequent filtrate as the sample solution. Separately, dissolve 10 mg of voglibose for assay in 2 mL of water, add methanol to make 50 mL, and use this solution as the standard solution. Perform the test with these solutions as directed under Thin-layer Chromatography <2.03>. Spot 10 μL each of the sample solution and standard solution on a plate of silica gel for thin-layer chromatography. Develop the plate with a mixture of methanol, acetone, water and ammonia solution (28) (10:10:4:1) to a distance of about 12 cm, and air-dry the plate. Then, immerse the plate in lead tetraacetate-fluorescein sodium TS, and lift gently to allow the excessive solution to flow out. After air-drying, examine under ultraviolet light (main wavelength: 366 nm): the spots obtained from the sample solution and

Supplement I, JP XVIII

standard solution exhibit a yellow fluorescence and show the same Rf value.

Uniformity of dosage units <6.02> Perform the test according to the following method: it meets the requirement of the Content uniformity test.

To 1 tablet of Voglibose Orally Disintegrating Tablets add exactly V mL of the mobile phase so that each mL contains about 20 μg of voglibose ($C_{10}H_{21}NO_7$), and sonicate to disintegrate the tablet. Centrifuge this solution, and filter the supernatant liquid through a membrane filter with a pore size not exceeding 0.45 μm. Discard the first 5 mL of the filtrate, and use the subsequent filtrate as the sample solution. Then, proceed as directed in the Assay.

$$\text{Amount (mg) of voglibose } (C_{10}H_{21}NO_7)$$
$$= M_S \times A_T/A_S \times V/2500$$

M_S: Amount (mg) of voglibose for assay taken, calculated on the anhydrous basis

Disintegration Being specified separately when the drug is granted approval based on the Law.

Dissolution <6.10> When the test is performed at 50 revolutions per minute according to the Paddle method, using 900 mL of water as the dissolution medium, the dissolution rate in 15 minutes of Voglibose Orally Disintegrating Tablets is not less than 85%.

Start the test with 1 tablet of Voglibose Orally Disintegrating Tablets, withdraw not less than 10 mL of the medium at the specified minute after starting the test, and filter through a membrane filter with a pore size not exceeding 0.45 μm. Discard not less than 5 mL of the first filtrate, pipet V mL of the subsequent filtrate, add the mobile phase to make exactly V' mL so that each mL contains about 0.11 μg of voglibose ($C_{10}H_{21}NO_7$), and use this solution as the sample solution. Separately, weigh accurately about 50 mg of voglibose for assay (separately determine the water <2.48> in the same manner as Voglibose), and dissolve in water to make exactly 50 mL. Pipet 1 mL of this solution, and add water to make exactly 100 mL. Pipet 2 mL of this solution, and add water to make exactly 100 mL. Pipet 10 mL of this solution, add the mobile phase to make exactly 20 mL, and use this solution as the standard solution. Perform the test with 100 μL each of the sample solution and standard solution as directed under Liquid Chromatography <2.01> according to the following conditions, and determine the peak areas, A_T and A_S, of voglibose in each solution.

Dissolution rate (%) with respect to the labeled amount of voglibose ($C_{10}H_{21}NO_7$)
$$= M_S \times A_T/A_S \times V'/V \times 1/C \times 9/50$$

M_S: Amount (mg) of voglibose for assay taken, calculated on the anhydrous basis
C: Labeled amount (mg) of voglibose ($C_{10}H_{21}NO_7$) in 1 tablet

Operating conditions—
  Apparatus, detector, column temperature, reaction coil,

The JP Drugs are to be tested according to the provisions given in the pertinent monographs, General Notices, General Rules for Crude Drugs, General Rules for Preparations, and General Tests for their conformity to the Japanese Pharmacopoeia. (See the General Notices 5.)

Supplement I, JP XVIII   *Official Monographs*   2905

cooling coil, mobile phase, reaction reagent, reaction temperature, cooling temperature and flow rate of reaction reagent: Proceed as directed in the operating conditions in the Assay.

Column: A stainless steel column 4.6 mm in inside diameter and 7.5 cm in length, packed with polyamine silica gel for liquid chromatography (5 μm in particle diameter).

Flow rate of mobile phase: Adjust so that the retention time of voglibose is about 5 minutes.

System suitability—

System performance: When the procedure is run with 100 μL of the standard solution under the above operating conditions, the number of theoretical plates and the symmetry factor of the peak of voglibose are not less than 900 and not more than 1.5, respectively.

System repeatability: When the test is repeated 6 times with 100 μL of the standard solution under the above operating conditions, the relative standard deviation of the peak area of voglibose is not more than 3.0%.

Assay To 20 tablets of Voglibose Orally Disintegrating Tablets add $4V/5$ mL of the mobile phase, and sonicate to disintegrate the tablets. Add the mobile phase to make exactly V mL so that each mL contains about 20 μg of voglibose ($C_{10}H_{21}NO_7$). Centrifuge this solution, and filter the supernatant liquid through a membrane filter with a pore size not exceeding 0.45 μm. Discard the first 5 mL of the filtrate, and use the subsequent filtrate as the sample solution. Separately, weigh accurately about 50 mg of voglibose for assay (separately determine the water <2.48> in the same manner as Voglibose), and dissolve in the mobile phase to make exactly 100 mL. Pipet 2 mL of this solution, add the mobile phase to make exactly 50 mL, and use this solution as the standard solution. Perform the test with 50 μL each of the sample solution and standard solution as directed under Liquid Chromatography <2.01> according to the following conditions, and determine the peak areas, A_T and A_S, of voglibose in each solution.

Amount (mg) of voglibose ($C_{10}H_{21}NO_7$) in 1 tablet
$$= M_S \times A_T/A_S \times V/50000$$

M_S: Amount (mg) of voglibose for assay taken, calculated on the anhydrous basis

Operating conditions—

Apparatus: Use an apparatus consisting of 2 pumps for the mobile phase and reaction reagent transportation, sample injection port, column, reaction coil, cooling coil, detector and recording device, and the reaction coil and cooling coil maintained at a constant temperature.

Detector: A fluorophotometer (excitation wavelength: 350 nm, fluorescence wavelength: 430 nm).

Column: A stainless steel column 4.6 mm in inside diameter and 25 cm in length, packed with polyamine silica gel for liquid chromatography (5 μm in particle diameter).

Column temperature: A constant temperature of about 25°C.

Reaction coil: A polytetrafluoroethylene tube 0.5 mm in inside diameter and 20 m in length.

Cooling coil: A polytetrafluoroethylene tube 0.3 mm in inside diameter and 2 m in length.

Mobile phase: Dissolve 1.56 g of sodium dihydrogen phosphate dihydrate in 500 mL of water, and adjust to pH 6.5 with a solution prepared by dissolving 3.58 g of disodium hydrogen phosphate dodecahydrate in 500 mL of water. To 500 mL of this solution add 500 mL of acetonitrile.

Reaction reagent: Dissolve 6.25 g of taurine and 2.56 g of sodium periodate in water to make 1000 mL.

Reaction temperature: A constant temperature of about 100°C.

Cooling temperature: A constant temperature of about 25°C.

Flow rate of mobile phase: Adjust so that the retention time of voglibose is about 15 minutes.

Flow rate of reaction reagent: Same as the flow rate of the mobile phase.

System suitability—

System performance: When the procedure is run with 50 μL of the standard solution under the above operating conditions, the number of theoretical plates and the symmetry factor of the peak of voglibose are not less than 3000 and not more than 1.5, respectively.

System repeatability: When the test is repeated 6 times with 50 μL of the standard solution under the above operating conditions, the relative standard deviation of the peak area of voglibose is not more than 1.0%.

Containers and storage Containers—Tight containers.

Voglibose Tablets

ボグリボース錠

Change the Identification as follows:

Identification Shake vigorously an amount of powdered Voglibose Tablets, equivalent to 5 mg of Voglibose, with 40 mL of water, and centrifuge. Transfer the supernatant liquid to a chromatographic column [prepared by pouring 1.0 mL of strongly acidic ion-exchange resin (H type) for column chromatography (70 to 200 μm in particle diameter) into a chromatographic column 8 mm in inside diameter and 130 mm in height], and allow to flow at a rate of about 5 mL per minute. Then wash the column with 200 mL of water, and allow to flow with 10 mL of diluted ammonia TS (1 in 4) at a rate of about 5 mL per minute. Filter the effluent solution 2 times through a membrane filter with a pore size not exceeding 0.22 μm. Evaporate the filtrate to dryness at 50°C under reduced pressure, dissolve the residue with 0.5 mL of a mixture of water and methanol (1:1), and use this solution as the sample solution. Separately, dissolve 20 mg of voglibose for assay in 2 mL of the mixture of water and methanol (1:1), and use this solution as the standard solution. Perform the test with these solutions as directed under Thin-layer Chromatography <2.03>. Spot 20 μL each of the sample solution and standard solution on a plate of silica gel for thin-layer chromatography. Develop

The JP Drugs are to be tested according to the provisions given in the pertinent monographs, General Notices, General Rules for Crude Drugs, General Rules for Preparations, and General Tests for their conformity to the Japanese Pharmacopoeia. (See the General Notices 5.)

2906   *Official Monographs*   *Supplement I, JP XVIII*

the plate with a mixture of acetone, ammonia water (28) and water (5:3:1) to a distance of about 12 cm, air-dry the plate, and allow to stand in iodine vapors: the principal spot obtained from the sample solution and the spot from the standard solution show a yellow-brown color, and the same Rf value.

The JP Drugs are to be tested according to the provisions given in the pertinent monographs, General Notices, General Rules for Crude Drugs, General Rules for Preparations, and General Tests for their conformity to the Japanese Pharmacopoeia. (See the General Notices 5.)

Crude Drugs and Related Drugs

Achyranthes Root

ゴシツ

Change the Identification as follows:

Identification **(1)** Shake vigorously 0.5 g of pulverized Achyranthes Root with 10 mL of water: a lasting fine foam is produced.

(2) To 1.0 g of pulverized Achyranthes Root add 10 mL of methanol, shake for 10 minutes, centrifuge, and use the supernatant liquid as the sample solution. Perform the test with the sample solution as directed under Thin-layer Chromatography <2.03>. Spot 10 μL of the sample solution on a plate of silica gel for thin-layer chromatography. Develop the plate with a mixture of ethyl acetate, methanol, water and acetic acid (100) (14:4:1:1) to a distance of about 7 cm, and air-dry the plate. Spray evenly 4-dimethylaminobenzaldehyde TS for spraying on the plate, heat the plate at 105°C for 5 minutes, allow to cool, and spray water: a light red to red-orange spot appears at an *R*f value of about 0.5.

Akebia Stem

モクツウ

Change the origin/limits of content as follows:

Akebia Stem is the climbing stem of *Akebia quinata* Decaisne, *Akebia trifoliata* Koidzumi, or their interspecific hybrids (*Lardizabalaceae*), usually cut transversely.

Apricot Kernel

キョウニン

Change the Assay as follows:

Assay Weigh accurately 0.5 g of ground Apricot Kernel, add 40 mL of diluted methanol (9 in 10), heat immediately under a reflux condenser for 30 minutes, and cool. Filter the mixture, add diluted methanol (9 in 10) to make exactly 50 mL. Pipet 5 mL of this solution, add water to make exactly 10 mL, and use this solution as the sample solution. Separately, weigh accurately about 10 mg of amygdalin for assay, dissolve in diluted methanol (1 in 2) to make exactly 50 mL, and use this solution as the standard solution. Perform the test with exactly 10 μL each of the sample solution and standard solution as directed under Liquid Chromatography <2.01> according to the following conditions, and determine the peak areas, A_T and A_S, of amygdalin in each solution.

$$\text{Amount (mg) of amygdalin} = M_S \times A_T/A_S \times 2$$

M_S: Amount (mg) of amygdalin for assay taken

Operating conditions—

Detector: An ultraviolet absorption photometer (wavelength: 210 nm).

Column: A stainless steel column 4.6 mm in inside diameter and 15 cm in length, packed with octadecylsilanized silica gel for liquid chromatography (5 μm in particle diameter).

Column temperature: A constant temperature of about 45°C.

Mobile phase: A mixture of 0.05 mol/L sodium dihydrogen phosphate TS and methanol (5:1).

Flow rate: 0.8 mL per minute (the retention time of amygdalin is about 12 minutes).

System suitability—

System performance: When the procedure is run with 10 μL of the standard solution under the above operating conditions, the number of theoretical plates and the symmetry factor of the peak of amygdalin are not less than 5000 and not more than 1.5, respectively.

System repeatability: When the test is repeated 6 times with 10 μL of the standard solution under the above operating conditions, the relative standard deviation of the peak area of amygdalin is not more than 1.5%.

Artemisia Capillaris Flower

インチンコウ

Change the Description as follows (No effect to English text):

Artemisia Leaf

ガイヨウ

Change the Description as follows (No effect to English text):

The JP Drugs are to be tested according to the provisions given in the pertinent monographs, General Notices, General Rules for Crude Drugs, General Rules for Preparations, and General Tests for their conformity to the Japanese Pharmacopoeia. (See the General Notices 5.)

2908 *Crude Drugs and Related Drugs* *Supplement I, JP XVIII*

Bearberry Leaf

ウワウルシ

Change the Description and Assay as follows (No effect to English text for Description):

Assay Weigh accurately about 0.5 g of pulverized Bearberry Leaf in a glass-stoppered centrifuge tube, add 40 mL of water, shake for 30 minutes, centrifuge, and separate the supernatant liquid. To the residue add 40 mL of water, and proceed in the same manner. To the combined extracts add water to make exactly 100 mL, and use this solution as the sample solution. Separately, weigh accurately about 40 mg of arbutin for assay, dissolve in water to make exactly 100 mL, and use this solution as the standard solution. Perform the test with exactly 10 μL each of the sample solution and standard solution as directed under Liquid Chromatography $\langle 2.01 \rangle$ according to the following conditions. Determine the peak areas, A_T and A_S, of arbutin in each solution.

$$\text{Amount (mg) of arbutin} = M_S \times A_T/A_S$$

M_S: Amount (mg) of arbutin for assay taken

Operating conditions—

Detector: An ultraviolet spectrophotometer (wavelength: 280 nm).

Column: A stainless steel column 4 – 6 mm in inside diameter and 15 – 25 cm in length, packed with octadecylsilanized silica gel (5 – 10 μm in particle diameter).

Column temperature: A constant temperature of about 20°C.

Mobile phase: A mixture of water, methanol and 0.1 mol/L hydrochloric acid TS (94:5:1).

Flow rate: Adjust so that the retention time of arbutin is about 6 minutes.

System suitability—

System performance: Dissolve 50 mg each of arbutin for assay, hydroquinone and gallic acid in water to make 100 mL. When the procedure is run with 10 μL of this solution under the above operating conditions, arbutin, hydroquinone and gallic acid are eluted in this order with the resolutions among these peaks being not less than 1.5.

System repeatability: When the test is repeated 5 times with 10 μL of the standard solution under the above operating conditions, the relative standard deviation of the peak area of arbutin is not more than 1.5%.

Bitter Cardamon

ヤクチ

Add the following next to the Description:

Identification To 1.0 g of pulverized Bitter Cardamon add 6 mL of a mixture of water and methanol (1:1) and 3 mL of hexane, shake for 5 minutes, centrifuge, and use the upper layer of the supernatant liquid as the sample solution. Separately, dissolve 1 mg of nootkatone for thin-layer chromatography in 1 mL of hexane, and use this solution as the standard solution. Perform the test with these solutions as directed under Thin-layer Chromatography $\langle 2.03 \rangle$. Spot 20 μL of the sample solution and 10 μL of the standard solution on a plate of silica gel for thin-layer chromatography. Develop the plate with a mixture of hexane and ethyl acetate (3:1) to a distance of about 7 cm, and air-dry the plate. Spray evenly 2,4-dinitrophenylhydrazine TS on the plate: one of the several spots obtained from the sample solution has the same color tone and Rf value with the spot from the standard solution.

Burdock Fruit

ゴボウシ

Change the Description as follows:

Description Burdock Fruit is slightly curved, long obovate achene, 5 – 7 mm in length, 2.0 – 3.2 mm in width, 0.8 to 1.5 mm in thickness; externally grayish brown to brown, with black spots; hollow about 1 mm in diameter at one broad end; flat, indistinct, longitudinal ridge at the other narrow end. 100 fruits weigh 1.0 – 1.5 g.

Practically odorless; taste, bitter and oily.

Under a microscope $\langle 5.01 \rangle$, transverse section reveals an exocarp composed of an epidermis, mesocarp of slightly sclerified parenchyma, and endocarp of a single layer of stone cells; seed coat composed of radially elongated, sclerified epidermis, and parenchyma of several cellular layers; parenchymatous cells of the mesocarp contain a brown substance; stone cells of endocarp contain solitary, discrete crystals of calcium oxalate; cotyledons with oil drops, aleurone grains, and minute crystals of calcium oxalate.

Cardamon

ショウズク

Change the Japanese commonly used name as follows (No effect to English text):

Cimicifuga Rhizome

ショウマ

Change the Purity (3) as follows:

Purity

(3) Rhizome of *Astilbe* and other species—Under a microscope $\langle 5.01 \rangle$, pulverized Cimicifuga Rhizome does not contain rosette aggregates of calcium oxalate.

The JP Drugs are to be tested according to the provisions given in the pertinent monographs, General Notices, General Rules for Crude Drugs, General Rules for Preparations, and General Tests for their conformity to the Japanese Pharmacopoeia. (See the General Notices 5.)

Supplement I, JP XVIII   *Crude Drugs and Related Drugs*   2909

Clove

チョウジ

Change the origin/limits of content as follows:

Clove is the flowering bud of *Syzygium aromaticum* Merrill et L. M. Perry (*Eugenia caryophyllata* Thunberg) (*Myrtaceae*).

Clove Oil

チョウジ油

Change the origin/limits of content as follows:

Clove Oil is the volatile oil distilled with steam from the flower buds or leaves of *Syzygium aromaticum* Merrill et L. M. Perry (*Eugenia caryophyllata* Thunberg) (*Myrtaceae*).
It contains not less than 80.0 vol% of total eugenol.

Cnidium Monnieri Fruit

ジャショウシ

Change the latin name as follows:

Cnidii Monnieri Fructus

Cornus Fruit

サンシュユ

Change the Assay as follows:

Assay Weigh accurately about 1 g of fine cuttings of Cornus Fruit (separately determine the loss on drying <5.01>), put in a glass-stoppered centrifuge tube, add 30 mL of diluted methanol (1 in 2), shake for 20 minutes, centrifuge, and take the supernatant liquid. To the residue add 30 mL of diluted methanol (1 in 2), and repeat the above process twice more. Combine all the extacts, add diluted methanol (1 in 2) to make exactly 100 mL, and use this solution as the sample solution. Separately, weigh accurately about 10 mg of loganin for assay, dissolve in diluted methanol (1 in 2) to make exactly 100 mL, and use this solution as the standard solution. Perform the test with exactly 10 μL each of the sample solution and standard solution as directed under Liquid Chromatography <2.01> according to the following conditions, and determine the peak areas, A_T and A_S, of loganin in each solution.

$$\text{Amount (mg) of loganin} = M_S \times A_T/A_S$$

M_S: Amount (mg) of loganin for assay taken, calculated

on the basis of the content obtained by qNMR

Operating conditions—
Detector: An ultraviolet absorption photometer (wavelength: 238 nm).
Column: A stainless steel column 4.6 mm in inside diameter and 15 cm in length, packed with octadecylsilanized silica gel for liquid chromatography (5 μm in particle diameter).
Column temperature: A constant temperature of about 50°C.
Mobile phase: A mixture of water, acetonitrile and methanol (55:4:1).
Flow rate: Adjust so that the retention time of loganin is about 25 minutes.
System suitability—
System performance: When the procedure is run with 10 μL of the standard solution under the above operating conditions, the number of theoretical plates and the symmetry factor of the peak of loganin are not less than 5000 and not more than 1.5, respectively.
System repeatability: When the test is repeated 6 times with 10 μL of the standard solution under the above operating conditions, the relative standard deviation of the peak area of loganin is not more than 1.5%.

Corydalis Tuber

エンゴサク

Change the Assay as follows:

Assay Weigh accurately about 1 g of pulverized Corydalis Tuber, add 30 mL of a mixture of methanol and dilute hydrochloric acid (3:1), heat under a reflux condenser for 30 minutes, and filter after cooling. To the residue add 15 mL of a mixture of methanol and dilute hydrochloric acid (3:1), and repeat the above procedure. Combine all the filtrates, add a mixture of methanol and dilute hydrochloric acid (3:1) to make exactly 50 mL, and use this solution as the sample solution. Separately, weigh accurately about 10 mg of dehydrocorydaline nitrate for assay, dissolve in a mixture of methanol and dilute hydrochloric acid (3:1) to make exactly 200 mL, and use this solution as the standard solution. Perform the test with exactly 5 μL each of the sample solution and standard solution as directed under Liquid Chromatography <2.01> according to the following conditions, and determine the peak areas, A_T and A_S, of dehydrocorydaline in each solution.

Amount (mg) of dehydrocorydaline [as dehydrocorydaline nitrate ($C_{22}H_{24}N_2O_7$)]
$$= M_S \times A_T/A_S \times 1/4$$

M_S: Amount (mg) of dehydrocorydaline nitrate for assay taken

Operating conditions—
Detector: An ultraviolet absorption photometer (wave-

The JP Drugs are to be tested according to the provisions given in the pertinent monographs, General Notices, General Rules for Crude Drugs, General Rules for Preparations, and General Tests for their conformity to the Japanese Pharmacopoeia. (See the General Notices 5.)

2910　*Crude Drugs and Related Drugs*

length: 340 nm).

Column: A stainless steel column 4.6 mm in inside diameter and 15 cm in length, packed with octadecylsilanized silica gel for liquid chromatography (5 μm in particle diameter).

Column temperature: A constant temperature of about 40°C.

Mobile phase: Dissolve 17.91 g of disodium hydrogen phosphate dodecahydrate in 970 mL of water, and adjust to pH 2.2 with phosphoric acid. To this solution add 14.05 g of sodium perchlorate, dissolve, and add water to make exactly 1000 mL. To this solution add 450 mL of acetonitrile, then dissolve 0.20 g of sodium lauryl sulfate.

Flow rate: Adjust so that the retention time of dehydrocorydaline is about 24 minutes.

System suitability—

System performance: Dissolve 1 mg each of dehydrocorydaline nitrate for assay and berberine chloride hydrate in 20 mL of a mixture of water and acetonitrile (20:9). When the procedure is run with 5 μL of this solution under the above operating conditions, berberine and dehydrocorydaline are eluted in this order with the resolution between these peaks being not less than 1.5.

System repeatability: When the test is repeated 6 times with 5 μL of the standard solution under the above operating conditions, the relative standard deviation of the peak areas of dehydrocorydaline is not more than 1.5%.

Powdered Corydalis Tuber

エンゴサク末

Change the Assay as follows:

Assay Weigh accurately about 1 g of Powdered Corydalis Tuber, add 30 mL of a mixture of methanol and dilute hydrochloric acid (3:1), heat under a reflux condenser for 30 minutes, and filter after cooling. To the residue add 15 mL of the mixture of methanol and dilute hydrochloric acid (3:1), and proceed in the same way as above. Combine all the filtrates, add the mixture of methanol and dilute hydrochloric acid (3:1) to make exactly 50 mL, and use this solution as the sample solution. Separately, weigh accurately about 10 mg of dehydrocorydaline nitrate for assay, dissolve in the mixture of methanol and dilute hydrochloric acid (3:1) to make exactly 200 mL, and use this solution as the standard solution. Perform the test with exactly 5 μL each of the sample solution and standard solution as directed under Liquid Chromatography <2.01> according to the following conditions, and determine the peak areas, A_T and A_S, of dehydrocorydaline in each solution.

Amount (mg) of dehydrocorydaline [as dehydrocorydaline nitrate ($C_{22}H_{24}N_2O_7$)]
$$= M_S \times A_T/A_S \times 1/4$$

M_S: Amount (mg) of dehydrocorydaline nitrate for assay taken

Supplement I, JP XVIII

Operating conditions—

Detector: An ultraviolet absorption photometer (wavelength: 340 nm).

Column: A stainless steel column 4.6 mm in inside diameter and 15 cm in length, packed with octadecylsilanized silica gel for liquid chromatography (5 μm in particle diameter).

Column temperature: A constant temperature of about 40°C.

Mobile phase: Dissolve 17.91 g of disodium hydrogen phosphate dodecahydrate in 970 mL of water, and adjust to pH 2.2 with phosphoric acid. To this solution add 14.05 g of sodium perchlorate, dissolve, and add water to make exactly 1000 mL. Add 450 mL of acetonitrile, and dissolve 0.20 g of sodium lauryl sulfate in this solution.

Flow rate: Adjust so that the retention time of dehydrocorydaline is about 24 minutes.

System suitability—

System performance: Dissolve 1 mg of dehydrocorydaline nitrate for assay and 1 mg of berberine chloride hydrate in 20 mL of a mixture of water and acetonitrile (20:9). When the procedure is run with 5 μL of this solution under the above operating conditions, berberine and dehydrocorydaline are eluted in this order with the resolution between these peaks being not less than 1.5.

System repeatability: When the test is repeated 6 times with 5 μL of the standard solution under the above operating conditions, the relative standard deviation of the peak area of dehydrocorydaline is not more than 1.5%.

Gardenia Fruit

サンシシ

Change the origin/limits of content as follows:

Gardenia Fruit is the fruit of *Gardenia jasminoides* J. Ellis (*Rubiaceae*), sometimes after being passed through hot water or steamed.

It contains not less than 2.7% of geniposide, calculated on the basis of dried material.

Ginger

ショウキョウ

Change the Assay as follows:

Assay Weigh accurately about 1 g of pulverized Ginger (separately determine the loss on drying <5.01>, at 105°C for 5 hours), place in a centrifuge tube, add 30 mL of a mixture of methanol and water (3:1), shake for 20 minutes, centrifuge, and separate the supernatant liquid. To the residue add 30 mL of a mixture of methanol and water (3:1), and repeat the extraction twice more. To the combined all extracts add a mixture of methanol and water (3:1) to make

The JP Drugs are to be tested according to the provisions given in the pertinent monographs, General Notices, General Rules for Crude Drugs, General Rules for Preparations, and General Tests for their conformity to the Japanese Pharmacopoeia. (See the General Notices 5.)

Supplement I, JP XVIII   *Crude Drugs and Related Drugs*   2911

exactly 100 mL, use this solution as the sample solution. Separately, weigh accurately about 5 mg of [6]-gingerol for assay, dissolve in a mixture of methanol and water (3:1) to make exactly 100 mL, and use this solution as the standard solution. Perform the test with exactly 10 μL each of the sample solution and standard solution as directed under Liquid Chromatography <2.01> according to the following conditions, and determine the peak areas, A_T and A_S, of [6]-gingerol in each solution.

$$\text{Amount (mg) of [6]-gingerol} = M_S \times A_T/A_S$$

M_S: Amount (mg) of [6]-gingerol for assay taken, calculated on the basis of the content obtained by qNMR

Operating conditions—

Detector: An ultraviolet absorption photometer (wavelength: 205 nm).

Column: A stainless steel column 4.6 mm in inside diameter and 15 cm in length, packed with octadecylsilanized silicagel for liquid chromatography (5 μm in particle diameter).

Column temperature: A constant temperature of about 40°C.

Mobile phase: A mixture of water and acetonitrile and phosphoric acid (3800:2200:1).

Flow rate: Adjust so that the retention time of [6]-gingerol is about 19 minutes.

System suitability—

System performance: When the procedure is run with 10 μL of the standard solution under the above operating conditions, the number of theoretical plates and the symmetry factor of the peak of [6]-gingerol are not less than 5000 and not more than 1.5, respectively.

System repeatability: When the test is repeated 6 times with 10 μL of the standard solution under the above operating conditions, the relative standard deviation of the peak area of [6]-gingerol is not more than 1.5%.

Powdered Ginger

ショウキョウ末

Change the Assay as follows:

Assay Weigh accurately about 1 g of Powdered Ginger (separately determine the loss on drying <5.01>, at 105°C for 5 hours), place in a centrifuge tube, add 30 mL of a mixture of methanol and water (3:1), shake for 20 minutes, centrifuge, and separate the supernatant liquid. To the residue add 30 mL of a mixture of methanol and water (3:1), and repeat the extraction twice more. To the combined all extracts add a mixture of methanol and water (3:1) to make exactly 100 mL, use this solution as the sample solution. Separately, weigh accurately about 5 mg of [6]-gingerol for assay, dissolve in a mixture of methanol and water (3:1) to make exactly 100 mL, and use this solution as the standard solution. Perform the test with exactly 10 μL each of the sample solution and standard solution as directed under

Liquid Chromatography <2.01> according to the following conditions, and determine the peak areas, A_T and A_S, of [6]-gingerol in each solution.

$$\text{Amount (mg) of [6]-gingerol} = M_S \times A_T/A_S$$

M_S: Amount (mg) of [6]-gingerol for assay taken, calculated on the basis of the content obtained by qNMR

Operating conditions—

Detector: An ultraviolet absorption photometer (wavelength: 205 nm).

Column: A stainless steel column 4.6 mm in inside diameter and 15 cm in length, packed with octadecylsilanized silica gel for liquid chromatography (5 μm in particle diameter).

Column temperature: A constant temperature of about 40°C.

Mobile phase: A mixture of water and acetonitrile and phosphoric acid (3800:2200:1).

Flow rate: Adjust so that the retention time of [6]-gingerol is about 19 minutes.

System suitability—

System performance: When the procedure is run with 10 μL of the standard solution under the above operating conditions, the number of theoretical plates and the symmetry factor of the peak of [6]-gingerol are not less than 5000 and not more than 1.5, respectively.

System repeatability: When the test is repeated 6 times with 10 μL of the standard solution under the above operating conditions, the relative standard deviation of the peak area of [6]-gingerol is not more than 1.5%.

Glehnia Root and Rhizome

ハマボウフウ

Change the origin/limits of content as follows:

Glehnia Root and Rhizome is the root and rhizome of *Glehnia littoralis* F. Schmidt ex Miquel (*Umbelliferae*).

Goshajinkigan Extract

牛車腎気丸エキス

Change the Assay (1) as follows:

Assay (1) Loganin—Weigh accurately about 0.5 g of the dry extract (or an amount of the viscous extract, equivalent to about 0.5 g of the dried substance), add exactly 50 mL of diluted methanol (1 in 2), shake for 15 minutes, filter, and use the filtrate as the sample solution. Separately, weigh accurately about 10 mg of loganin for assay, dissolve in diluted methanol (1 in 2) to make exactly 100 mL, and use this solution as the standard solution. Perform the test with exactly 10 μL each of the sample solution and standard so-

The JP Drugs are to be tested according to the provisions given in the pertinent monographs, General Notices, General Rules for Crude Drugs, General Rules for Preparations, and General Tests for their conformity to the Japanese Pharmacopoeia. (See the General Notices 5.)

Crude Drugs and Related Drugs

lution as directed under Liquid Chromatography ⟨2.01⟩ according to the following conditions, and determine the peak areas, A_T and A_S, of loganin in each solution.

$$\text{Amount (mg) of loganin} = M_S \times A_T/A_S \times 1/2$$

M_S: Amount (mg) of loganin for assay taken, calculated on the basis of the content obtained by qNMR

Operating conditions—

Detector: An ultraviolet absorption photometer (wavelength: 238 nm).

Column: A stainless steel column 4.6 mm in inside diameter and 15 cm in length, packed with octadecylsilanized silica gel for liquid chromatography (5 μm in particle diameter).

Column temperature: A constant temperature of about 50°C.

Mobile phase: A mixture of water, acetonitrile and methanol (55:4:1).

Flow rate: 1.2 mL per minute (the retention time of loganin is about 25 minutes).

System suitability—

System performance: When the procedure is run with 10 μL of the standard solution under the above operating conditions, the number of theoretical plates and symmetry factor of the peak of loganin are not less than 5000 and not more than 1.5, respectively.

System repeatability: When the test is repeated 6 times with 10 μL of the standard solution under the above operating conditions, the relative standard deviation of the peak area of loganin is not more than 1.5%.

Goshuyuto Extract

呉茱萸湯エキス

Change the Assay (2) as follows:

Assay

(2) [6]-Gingerol—Weigh accurately about 0.5 g of the dry extract (or an amount of the viscous extract, equivalent to about 0.5 g of the dried substance), add exactly 50 mL of diluted methanol (7 in 10), shake for 30 minutes, filter, and use the filtrate as the sample solution. Separately, weigh accurately about 10 mg of [6]-gingerol for assay, dissolve in methanol to make exactly 100 mL. Pipet 5 mL of this solution, add methanol to make exactly 50 mL, and use this solution as the standard solution. Perform the test with exactly 10 μL each of the sample solution and standard solution as directed under Liquid Chromatography ⟨2.01⟩ according to the following conditions, and determine the peak areas, A_T and A_S, of [6]-gingerol in each solution.

$$\text{Amount (mg) of [6]-gingerol} = M_S \times A_T/A_S \times 1/20$$

M_S: Amount (mg) of [6]-gingerol for assay taken, calculated on the basis of the content obtained by qNMR

Operating conditions—

Detector, column, column temperature and mobile phase: Proceed as directed in the operating conditions in (1).

Flow rate: 1.0 mL per minute (the retention time of [6]-gingerol is about 14 minutes).

System suitability—

System performance: When the procedure is run with 10 μL of the standard solution under the above operating conditions, the number of theoretical plates and the symmetry factor of the peak of [6]-gingerol are not less than 5000 and not more than 1.5, respectively.

System repeatability: When the test is repeated 6 times with 10 μL of the standard solution under the above operating conditions, the relative standard deviation of the peak area of [6]-gingerol is not more than 1.5%.

Hachimijiogan Extract

八味地黄丸エキス

Change the Assay (1) as follows:

Assay **(1)** Loganin—Weigh accurately about 0.5 g of the dry extract (or an amount of the viscous extract, equivalent to about 0.5 g of the dried substance), add exactly 50 mL of diluted methanol (1 in 2), shake for 15 minutes, filter, and use the filtrate as the sample solution. Separately, weigh accurately about 10 mg of loganin for assay, dissolve in diluted methanol (1 in 2) to make exactly 100 mL, and use this solution as the standard solution. Perform the test with exactly 10 μL each of the sample solution and standard solution as directed under Liquid Chromatography ⟨2.01⟩ according to the following conditions, and determine the peak areas, A_T and A_S, of loganin in each solution.

$$\text{Amount (mg) of loganin} = M_S \times A_T/A_S \times 1/2$$

M_S: Amount (mg) of loganin for assay taken, calculated on the basis of the content obtained by qNMR

Operating conditions—

Detector: An ultraviolet absorption photometer (wavelength: 238 nm).

Column: A stainless steel column 4.6 mm in inside diameter and 15 cm in length, packed with octadecylsilanized silica gel for liquid chromatography (5 μm in particle diameter).

Column temperature: A constant temperature of about 50°C.

Mobile phase: A mixture of water, acetonitrile and methanol (55:4:1).

Flow rate: 1.2 mL per minute (the retention time of loganin is about 25 minutes).

System suitability—

System performance: When the procedure is run with 10 μL of the standard solution under the above operating conditions, the number of theoretical plates and symmetry factor of the peak of loganin are not less than 5000 and not more than 1.5, respectively.

The JP Drugs are to be tested according to the provisions given in the pertinent monographs, General Notices, General Rules for Crude Drugs, General Rules for Preparations, and General Tests for their conformity to the Japanese Pharmacopoeia. (See the General Notices 5.)

Supplement I, JP XVIII   *Crude Drugs and Related Drugs*   2913

System repeatability: When the test is repeated 6 times with 10 μL of the standard solution under the above operating conditions, the relative standard deviation of the peak area of loganin is not more than 1.5%.

Hangekobokuto Extract

半夏厚朴湯エキス

Change the Assay (3) as follows:

Assay

(3) [6]-Gingerol—Weigh accurately about 0.5 g of the dry extract (or an amount of the viscous extract, equivalent to about 0.5 g of the dried substance), add exactly 50 mL of diluted methanol (7 in 10), shake for 15 minutes, filter, and use the filtrate as the sample solution. Separately, weigh accurately about 10 mg of [6]-gingerol for assay, dissolve in methanol to make exactly 100 mL. Pipet 5 mL of this solution, add methanol to make exactly 50 mL, and use this solution as the standard solution. Perform the test with exactly 10 μL each of the sample solution and standard solution as directed under Liquid Chromatography <2.01> according to the following conditions, and determine the peak areas, A_T and A_S, of [6]-gingerol in each solution.

$$\text{Amount (mg) of [6]-gingerol} = M_S \times A_T/A_S \times 1/20$$

M_S: Amount (mg) of [6]-gingerol for assay taken, calculated on the basis of the content obtained by qNMR

Operating conditions—

Detector: An ultraviolet absorption photometer (wavelength: 282 nm).

Column: A stainless steel column 4.6 mm in inside diameter and 15 cm in length, packed with octadecylsilanized silica gel for liquid chromatography (5 μm in particle diameter).

Column temperature: A constant temperature of about 30°C.

Mobile phase: A mixture of water, acetonitrile and phosphoric acid (620:380:1).

Flow rate: 1.0 mL per minute (the retention time of [6]-gingerol is about 15 minutes).

System suitability—

System performance: When the procedure is run with 10 μL of the standard solution under the above operating conditions, the number of theoretical plates and the symmetry factor of the peak of [6]-gingerol are not less than 5000 and not more than 1.5, respectively.

System repeatability: When the test is repeated 6 times with 10 μL of the standard solution under the above operating conditions, the relative standard deviation of the peak area of [6]-gingerol is not more than 1.5%.

Keishibukuryogan Extract

桂枝茯苓丸エキス

Change the Assay (3) as follows:

Assay

(3) Amygdalin—Weigh accurately about 0.5 g of the dry extract (or an amount of the viscous extract, equivalent to about 0.5 g of the dried substance), add exactly 50 mL of diluted methanol (1 in 2), shake for 15 minutes, filter, and use the filtrate as the sample solution. Separately, weigh accurately about 10 mg of amygdalin for assay, dissolve in diluted methanol (1 in 2) to make exactly 50 mL, and use this solution as the standard solution. Perform the test with exactly 10 μL each of the sample solution and standard solution as directed under Liquid Chromatography <2.01> according to the following conditions, and determine the peak areas, A_T and A_S, of amygdalin in each solution.

$$\text{Amount (mg) of amygdalin} = M_S \times A_T/A_S$$

M_S: Amount (mg) of amygdalin for assay taken

Operating conditions—

Detector: An ultraviolet absorption photometer (wavelength: 210 nm).

Column: A stainless steel column 4.6 mm in inside diameter and 15 cm in length, packed with octadecylsilanized silicagel for liquid chromatography (5 μm in particle diameter).

Column temperature: A constant temperature of about 45°C.

Mobile phase: A mixture of 0.05 mol/L sodium dihydrogen phosphate TS and methanol (5:1).

Flow rate: 0.8 mL per minute (the retention time of amygdalin is about 12 minutes).

System suitability—

System performance: When the procedure is run with 10 μL of the standard solution under the above operating conditions, the number of theoretical plates and the symmetry factor of the peak of amygdalin are not less than 5000 and not more than 1.5, respectively.

System repeatability: When the test is repeated 6 times with 10 μL of the standard solution under the above operating conditions, the relative standard deviation of the peak area of amygdalin is not more than 1.5%.

Leonurus Herb

ヤクモソウ

Change the Description as follows (No effect to English text):

The JP Drugs are to be tested according to the provisions given in the pertinent monographs, General Notices, General Rules for Crude Drugs, General Rules for Preparations, and General Tests for their conformity to the Japanese Pharmacopoeia. (See the General Notices 5.)

Magnolia Bark

コウボク

Change the origin/limits of content as follows:

Magnolia Bark is the bark of the trunk of *Magnolia obovata* Thunberg (*Magnolia hypoleuca* Siebold et Zuccarini), *Magnolia officinalis* Rehder et E. H. Wilson or *Magnolia officinalis* Rehder et E. H. Wilson var. *biloba* Rehder et E. H. Wilson (*Magnoliaceae*).

It contains not less than 0.8% of magnolol.

Maoto Extract

麻黄湯エキス

Change the Assay (2) as follows:

Assay

(2) Amygdalin—Weigh accurately about 0.5 g of the dry extract (or an amount of the viscous extract, equivalent to about 0.5 g of the dried substance), add exactly 50 mL of diluted methanol (1 in 2), shake for 15 minutes, and filter. Pipet 5 mL of the filtrate, flow through in a column packed with 2 g of polyamide for column chromatography, then elute with water to make exactly 20 mL, and use this effluent as the sample solution. Separately, weigh accurately about 10 mg of amygdalin for assay, dissolve in diluted methanol (1 in 2) to make exactly 50 mL, and use this solution as the standard solution. Perform the test with exactly 10 μL each of the sample solution and standard solution as directed under Liquid Chromatography <2.01> according to the following conditions, and determine the peak areas, A_T and A_S, of amygdalin in each solution.

$$\text{Amount (mg) of amygdalin} = M_S \times A_T/A_S \times 4$$

M_S: Amount (mg) of amygdalin for assay taken

Operating conditions—

Detector: An ultraviolet absorption photometer (wavelength: 210 nm).

Column: A stainless steel column 4.6 mm in inside diameter and 15 cm in length, packed with octadecylsilanized silica gel for liquid chromatography (5 μm in particle diameter).

Column temperature: A constant temperature of about 45°C.

Mobile phase: A mixture of 0.05 mol/L sodium dihydrogen phosphate TS and methanol (5:1).

Flow rate: 0.8 mL per minute (the retention time of amygdalin is about 12 minutes).

System suitability—

System performance: When the procedure is run with 10 μL of the standard solution under the above operating conditions, the number of theoretical plates and the symmetry factor of the peak of amygdalin are not less than 5000 and

not more than 1.5, respectively.

System repeatability: When the test is repeated 6 times with 10 μL of the standard solution under the above operating conditions, the relative standard deviation of the peak area of amygdalin is not more than 1.5%.

Mukoi-Daikenchuto Extract

無コウイ大建中湯エキス

Change the Assay (2) as follows:

Assay

(2) [6]-Shogaol—Weigh accurately about 0.5 g of Mukoi-Daikenchuto Extract, add exactly 50 mL of diluted methanol (3 in 4), shake for 15 minutes, centrifuge, and use the supernatant liquid as the sample solution. Separately, weigh accurately about 10 mg of [6]-shogaol for assay, dissolve in diluted methanol (3 in 4) to make exactly 100 mL. Pipet 10 mL of this solution, add diluted methanol (3 in 4) to make exactly 50 mL, and use this solution as the standard solution. Perform the test with exactly 20 μL each of the sample solution and standard solution as directed under Liquid Chromatography <2.01> according to the following conditions, and determine the peak areas, A_T and A_S, of [6]-shogaol in each solution.

$$\text{Amount (mg) of [6]-shogaol} = M_S \times A_T/A_S \times 1/10$$

M_S: Amount (mg) of [6]-shogaol for assay taken, calculated on the basis of the content obtained by qNMR

Operating conditions—

Detector: An ultraviolet absorption photometer (wavelength: 225 nm).

Column: A stainless steel column 4.6 mm in inside diameter and 15 cm in length, packed with octylsilanized silica gel for liquid chromatography (5 μm in particle diameter).

Column temperature: A constant temperature of about 50°C.

Mobile phase: Dissolve 0.1 g of oxalic acid dihydrate in 600 mL of water, and add 400 mL of acetonitrile.

Flow rate: 1.0 mL per minute (the retention time of [6]-shogaol is about 30 minutes).

System suitability—

System performance: When the procedure is run with 20 μL of the standard solution under the above operating conditions, the number of theoretical plates and the symmetry factor of the peak of [6]-shogaol are not less than 5000 and not more than 1.5, respectively.

System repeatability: When the test is repeated 6 times with 20 μL of the standard solution under the above operating conditions, the relative standard deviation of the peak area of [6]-shogaol is not more than 1.5%.

The JP Drugs are to be tested according to the provisions given in the pertinent monographs, General Notices, General Rules for Crude Drugs, General Rules for Preparations, and General Tests for their conformity to the Japanese Pharmacopoeia. (See the General Notices 5.)

Supplement I, JP XVIII　　　　　　　　　　　　　　*Crude Drugs and Related Drugs*　　2915

Nutmeg

ニクズク

Change the Japanese commonly used name as follows (No effect to English text):

Peach Kernel

トウニン

Change the Assay as follows:

Assay Weigh accurately 0.5 g of ground Peach Kernel, add 40 mL of diluted methanol (9 in 10), heat immediately under a reflux condenser for 30 minutes, and cool. Filter the mixture, add diluted methanol (9 in 10) to make exactly 50 mL. Pipet 5 mL of this solution, add water to make exactly 10 mL, and use this solution as the sample solution. Separately, weigh accurately about 10 mg of amygdalin for assay, dissolve in diluted methanol (1 in 2) to make exactly 50 mL, and use this solution as the standard solution.

Perform the test with exactly 10 μL each of the sample solution and standard solution as directed under Liquid Chromatography <2.01> according to the following conditions, and determine the peak areas, A_T and A_S, of amygdalin in each solution.

$$\text{Amount (mg) of amygdalin} = M_S \times A_T/A_S \times 2$$

M_S: Amount (mg) of amygdalin for assay taken

Operating conditions—

Detector: An ultraviolet absorption photometer (wavelength: 210 nm).

Column: A stainless steel column 4.6 mm in inside diameter and 15 cm in length, packed with octadecylsilianized silica gel for liquid chromatography (5 μm in particle diameter).

Column temperature: A constant temperature of about 45°C.

Mobile phase: A mixture of 0.05 mol/L sodium dihydrogen phosphate TS and methanol (5:1).

Flow rate: 0.8 mL per minute (the retention time of amygdalin is about 12 minutes).

System suitability—

System performance: When the procedure is run with 10 μL of the standard solution under the above operating conditions, the number of theoretical plates and the symmetry factor of the peak of amygdalin are not less than 5000 and not more than 1.5, respectively.

System repeatability: When the test is repeated 6 times with 10 μL of the standard solution under the above operating conditions, the relative standard deviation of the peak area of amygdalin is not more than 1.5%.

Powdered Peach Kernel

トウニン末

Change the Assay as follows:

Assay Weigh accurately 0.5 g of Powdered Peach Kernel, add 40 mL of diluted methanol (9 in 10), heat immediately under a reflux condenser for 30 minutes, and cool. Filter the mixture, add diluted methanol (9 in 10) to make exactly 50 mL. Pipet 5 mL of this solution, add water to make exactly 10 mL, and use this solution as the sample solution. Separately, weigh accurately about 10 mg of amygdalin for assay, dissolve in diluted methanol (1 in 2) to make exactly 50 mL, and use this solution as the standard solution. Perform the test exactly with 10 μL each of the sample solution and standard solution as directed under Liquid Chromatography <2.01> according to the following conditions, and determine the peak areas, A_T and A_S, of amygdalin in each solution.

$$\text{Amount (mg) of amygdalin} = M_S \times A_T/A_S \times 2$$

M_S: Amount (mg) of amygdalin for assay taken

Operating conditions—

Detector: An ultraviolet absorption photometer (wavelength: 210 nm).

Column: A stainless steel column 4.6 mm in inside diameter and 15 cm in length, packed with octadecylsilianized silica gel for liquid chromatography (5 μm in particle diameter).

Column temperature: A constant temperature of about 45°C.

Mobile phase: A mixture of 0.05 mol/L sodium dihydrogen phosphate TS and methanol (5:1).

Flow rate: 0.8 mL per minute (the retention time of amygdalin is about 12 minutes).

System suitability—

System performance: When the procedure is run with 10 μL of the standard solution under the above operating conditions, the number of theoretical plates and the symmetry factor of the peak of amygdalin are not less than 5000 and not more than 1.5, respectively.

System repeatability: When the test is repeated 6 times with 10 μL of the standard solution under the above operating conditions, the relative standard deviation of the peak area of amygdalin is not more than 1.5%.

Picrasma Wood

ニガキ

Add the following next to the Description as follows:

Identification To 0.1 g of pulverized Picrasma Wood add 5 mL of methanol, shake for 5 minutes, filter, and use the

The JP Drugs are to be tested according to the provisions given in the pertinent monographs, General Notices, General Rules for Crude Drugs, General Rules for Preparations, and General Tests for their conformity to the Japanese Pharmacopoeia. (See the General Notices 5.)

2916 *Crude Drugs and Related Drugs*

filtrate as the sample solution. Perform the test with the sample solution as directed under Thin-layer Chromatography <2.03>. Spot 2 μL of the sample solution on a plate of silica gel for thin-layer chromatography. Develop the plate with a mixture of ethyl acetate and hexane (20:1) to a distance of about 7 cm, and air-dry the plate. Examine under ultraviolet light (main wavelength: 365 nm): a blue-white fluorescent spot appears at an Rf value of about 0.35.

Powdered Picrasma Wood

ニガキ末

Add the following next to the Description as follows:

Identification To 0.1 g of Powdered Picrasma Wood add 5 mL of methanol, shake for 5 minutes, filter, and use the filtrate as the sample solution. Perform the test with the sample solution as directed under Thin-layer Chromatography <2.03>. Spot 2 μL of the sample solution on a plate of silica gel for thin-layer chromatography. Develop the plate with a mixture of ethyl acetate and hexane (20:1) to a distance of about 7 cm, and air-dry the plate. Examine under ultraviolet light (main wavelength: 365 nm): a blue-white fluorescent spot appears at an Rf value of about 0.35.

Plantago Herb

シャゼンソウ

Change the Description as follows (No effect to English text):

Prepared Glycyrrhiza

シャカンゾウ

Change the Description as follows:

Description Usually cut; in case with periderm external surface dark brown to dark red-brown and with longitudinal wrinkles; in case periderm fallen off, external surface light yellow-brown to brown and fibrous; on transversely cut surface light yellow-brown to brown, cortex and xylem almost distinctly defined, and exhibits radial structure; sometimes radial cleft observed.

Odor, fragrant; taste sweet, followed by slight bitterness.

Processed Ginger

カンキョウ

Change the Assay as follows:

Assay Weigh accurately about 1 g of pulverized Processed Ginger, place in a centrifuge tube, add 30 mL of the mobile phase, shake for 20 minutes, centrifuge, and separate the supernatant liquid. To the residue add 30 mL of the mobile phase, and repeat the extraction twice more. To the combined all extracts add the mobile phase to make exactly 100 mL, use this solution as the sample solution. Separately, weigh accurately about 5 mg of [6]-shogaol for assay, dissolve in the mobile phase to make exactly 100 mL, and use this solution as the standard solution. Perform the test with exactly 10 μL each of the sample solution and standard solution as directed under Liquid Chromatography <2.01> according to the following conditions, and determine the peak areas, A_T and A_S, of [6]-shogaol in each solution.

$$\text{Amount (mg) of [6]-shogaol} = M_S \times A_T/A_S$$

M_S: Amount (mg) of [6]-shogaol for assay taken, calculated on the basis of the content obtained by qNMR

Operating conditions—
Detector: An ultraviolet absorption photometer (wavelength: 225 nm).
Column: A stainless steel column 6 mm in inside diameter and 15 cm in length, packed with octadecylsilanized silica gel for liquid chromatography (5 μm in particle diameter).
Column temperature: A constant temperature of about 40°C.
Mobile phase: A mixture of acetonitrile and water (3:2).
Flow rate: Adjust so that the retention time of [6]-shogaol is about 14 minutes.
System suitability—
System performance: When the procedure is run with 10 μL of the standard solution under the above operating conditions, the number of theoretical plates and the symmetry factor of the peak of [6]-shogaol are not less than 5000 and not more than 1.5, respectively.
System repeatability: When the test is repeated 6 times with 10 μL of the standard solution under the above operating conditions, the relative standard deviation of the peak area of [6]-shogaol is not more than 1.5%.

Add the following:

Saikokeishikankyoto Extract

柴胡桂枝乾姜湯エキス

Saikokeishikankyoto Extract contains not less than 1.4 mg and not more than 5.6 mg of saikosaponin b_2, not less than 78 mg and not more than 234 mg of baicalin ($C_{21}H_{18}O_{11}$: 446.36), and not less than 15 mg and

The JP Drugs are to be tested according to the provisions given in the pertinent monographs, General Notices, General Rules for Crude Drugs, General Rules for Preparations, and General Tests for their conformity to the Japanese Pharmacopoeia. (See the General Notices 5.)

Supplement I, JP XVIII   *Crude Drugs and Related Drugs*   2917

not more than 45 mg of glycyrrhizic acid ($C_{42}H_{62}O_{16}$: 822.93), per extract prepared with the amount specified in the Method of preparation.

Method of preparation

	1)	2)
Bupleurum Root	6 g	6 g
Cinnamon Bark	3 g	3 g
Scutellaria Root	3 g	3 g
Oyster Shell	3 g	3 g
Processed Ginger	2 g	3 g
Glycyrrhiza	2 g	2 g
Trichosanthes Root	3 g	4 g

Prepare a dry extract or viscous extract as directed under Extracts, according to the prescription 1) or 2), using the crude drugs shown above.

Description The dry extract: Saikokeishikankyoto Extract is a light yellow-brown to brown powder. It has a characteristic odor and a hot, bitter and slightly sweet taste.

The viscous extract: Saikokeishikankyoto Extract is a black-brown viscous liquid. It has a characteristic odor and a bitter, hot and slightly sweet taste, followed by an astringent aftertaste.

Identification (1) Shake 1.0 g of the dry extract (or 3.0 g of the viscous extract) with 10 mL of water, add 10 mL of 1-butanol, and shake. Centrifuge this solution, and use the 1-butanol layer as the sample solution. Separately, dissolve 1 mg of saikosaponin b_2 for thin-layer chromatography in 1 mL of methanol, and use this solution as the standard solution. Perform the test with these solutions as directed under Thin-layer Chromatography <2.03>. Spot 5 µL of the sample solution and 2 µL of the standard solution on a plate of silica gel for thin-layer chromatography. Develop the plate with a mixture of ethyl acetate, ethanol (99.5) and water (8:2:1) to a distance of about 7 cm, and air-dry the plate. Spray evenly 4-dimethylaminobenzaldehyde TS for spraying on the plate, and heat the plate at 105°C for 5 minutes. Examine under ultraviolet light (main wavelength: 365 nm): one of the several spots obtained from the sample solution has the same color tone and Rf value with the yellow fluorescent spot from the standard solution (Bupleurum Root).

(2) Perform the test according to the following i) or ii) (Cinnamon Bark).

i) Put 10 g of dry extract (or 30 g of the viscous extract) in a 300-mL of hard-glass flask, add 100 mL of water and 1 mL of silicone resin, connect the apparatus for essential oil determination, and heat to boil under a reflux condenser. The graduated tube of the apparatus is to be previously filled with water to the standard line, and 2 mL of hexane is added to the graduated tube. After heating under reflux for 1 hour, separate the hexane layer, and use this solution as the sample solution. Separately, dissolve 1 mg of (E)-cinnamaldehyde for thin-layer chromatography in 1 mL of methanol, and use this solution as the standard solution. Perform the test with these solutions as directed under Thin-layer Chromatography <2.03>. Spot 20 µL of the sam-

ple solution and 2 µL of the standard solution on a plate of silica gel for thin-layer chromatography. Develop the plate with a mixture of hexane, diethyl ether and methanol (15:5:1) to a distance of about 7 cm, and air-dry the plate. Spray evenly 2,4-dinitrophenylhydrazine TS on the plate: one of the several spots obtained from the sample solution has the same color tone and Rf value with the yellow-orange to orange spot from the standard solution.

ii) Shake 2.0 g of dry extract (or 6.0 g of the viscous extract) with 10 mL of water, add 5 mL of hexane, and shake. Centrifuge this solution, and use the hexane layer as the sample solution. Separately, dissolve 1 mg of (E)-2-methoxycinnamaldehyde for thin-layer chromatography in 1 mL of methanol, and use this solution as the standard solution. Perform the test with these solutions as directed under Thin-layer Chromatography <2.03>. Spot 20 µL of the sample solution and 2 µL of the standard solution on a plate of silica gel for thin-layer chromatography. Develop the plate with a mixture of hexane and ethyl acetate (2:1) to a distance of about 7 cm, and air-dry the plate. Examine under ultraviolet light (main wavelength: 365 nm): one of the several spots obtained from the sample solution has the same color tone and Rf value with the blue-white fluorescent spot from the standard solution.

(3) Shake 1.0 g of the dry extract (or 3.0 g of the viscous extract) with 10 mL of water, add 25 mL of diethyl ether, and shake. Separate the diethyl ether layer, evaporate the solvent under low pressure (in vacuo), add 2 mL of diethyl ether to the residue, and use this solution as the sample solution. Separately, dissolve 1 mg of wogonin for thin-layer chromatography in 1 mL of methanol, and use this solution as the standard solution. Perform the test with these solutions as directed under Thin-layer Chromatography <2.03>. Spot 10 µL of the sample solution and 2 µL of the standard solution on a plate of silica gel for thin-layer chromatography. Develop the plate with a mixture of hexane and acetone (7:5) to a distance of about 7 cm, and air-dry the plate. Spray evenly iron (III) chloride-methanol TS on the plate: one of the several spots obtained from the sample solution has the same color tone and Rf value with the yellow-brown to grayish brown spot from the standard solution (Scutellaria Root).

(4) Shake 1.0 g of the dry extract (or 3.0 g of the viscous extract) with 10 mL of water, add 25 mL of diethyl ether, and shake. Separate the diethyl ether layer, evaporate the solvent under low pressure (in vacuo), add 2 mL of diethyl ether to the residue, and use this solution as the sample solution. Separately, dissolve 1 mg of [6]-shogaol for thin-layer chromatography in 1 mL of methanol, and use this solution as the standard solution. Perform the test with these solutions as directed under Thin-layer Chromatography <2.03>. Spot 20 µL of the sample solution and 5 µL of the standard solution on a plate of silica gel for thin-layer chromatography. Develop the plate with a mixture of ethyl acetate and hexane (1:1) to a distance of about 7 cm, and air-dry the plate. Spray evenly 4-dimethylaminobenzaldehyde TS for spraying on the plate, heat the plate at 105°C for 5 minutes, allow to cool, and spray water: one of the several

The JP Drugs are to be tested according to the provisions given in the pertinent monographs, General Notices, General Rules for Crude Drugs, General Rules for Preparations, and General Tests for their conformity to the Japanese Pharmacopoeia. (See the General Notices 5.)

2918　*Crude Drugs and Related Drugs*　　　　　　　　　　　　　　　　　*Supplement I, JP XVIII*

spots obtained from the sample solution has the same color tone and Rf value with the blue-green to grayish green spot from the standard solution (Processed Ginger).

(5) Shake 1.0 g of the dry extract (or 3.0 g of the viscous extract) with 10 mL of water, add 10 mL of 1-butanol, and shake. Centrifuge this solution, and use the 1-butanol layer as the sample solution. Separately, dissolve 1 mg of liquiritin for thin-layer chromatography in 1 mL of methanol, and use this solution as the standard solution. Perform the test with these solutions as directed under Thin-layer Chromatography $\langle 2.03 \rangle$. Spot 1 μL each of the sample solution and standard solution on a plate of silica gel for thin-layer chromatography. Develop the plate with a mixture of ethyl acetate, methanol and water (20:3:2) to a distance of about 7 cm, and air-dry the plate. Spray evenly dilute sulfuric acid on the plate, heat the plate at 105°C for 5 minutes, and examine under ultraviolet light (main wavelength: 365 nm): one of the several spots obtained from the sample solution has the same color tone and Rf value with the yellow to yellow-green fluorescent spot from the standard solution (Glycyrrhiza).

Purity (1) Heavy metals $\langle 1.07 \rangle$—Prepare the test solution with 1.0 g of the dry extract (or an amount of the viscous extract, equivalent to 1.0 g of the dried substance) as directed under the Extracts (4), and perform the test (not more than 30 ppm).

(2) Arsenic $\langle 1.11 \rangle$—Prepare the test solution with 0.67 g of the dry extract (or an amount of the viscous extract, equivalent to 0.67 g of the dried substance) according to Method 3, and perform the test (not more than 3 ppm).

Loss on drying $\langle 2.41 \rangle$　The dry extract: Not more than 9.5% (1 g, 105°C, 5 hours).

The viscous extract: Not more than 66.7% (1 g, 105°C, 5 hours).

Total ash $\langle 5.01 \rangle$　Not more than 13.0%, calculated on the dried basis.

Assay (1) Saikosaponin b$_2$—Weigh accurately about 0.5 g of the dry extract (or an amount of the viscous extract, equivalent to about 0.5 g of the dried substance), add 20 mL of diethyl ether and 10 mL of water, and shake for 10 minutes. After centrifuging, remove the diethyl ether layer, then add 20 mL of diethyl ether, proceed in the same manner as described above, and remove the diethyl ether layer. To the aqueous layer add 10 mL of methanol, shake for 30 minutes, centrifuge, and separate the supernatant liquid. To the residue add 20 mL of diluted methanol (1 in 2), shake for 5 minutes, centrifuge, and separate the supernatant liquid. Combine all the supernatant liquids, add diluted methanol (1 in 2) to make exactly 50 mL, and use this solution as the sample solution. Separately, use saikosaponin b$_2$ standard TS for assay as the standard solution. Perform the test with exactly 10 μL each of the sample solution and standard solution as directed under Liquid Chromatography $\langle 2.01 \rangle$ according to the following conditions, and determine the peak areas, A_T and A_S, of saikosaponin b$_2$ in each solution.

$$\text{Amount (mg) of saikosaponin b}_2 = C_S \times A_T/A_S \times 50$$

C_S: Concentration (mg/mL) of saikosaponin b$_2$ in saikosaponin b$_2$ standard TS for assay

Operating conditions—

Detector: An ultraviolet absorption photometer (wavelength: 254 nm).

Column: A stainless steel column 4.6 mm in inside diameter and 15 cm in length, packed with octadecylsilanized silica gel for liquid chromatography (5 μm in particle diameter).

Column temperature: A constant temperature of about 40°C.

Mobile phase: A mixture of 0.05 mol/L sodium dihydrogen phosphate TS and acetonitrile (5:3).

Flow rate: 1.0 mL per minute.

System suitability—

System performance: When the procedure is run with 10 μL of the standard solution under the above operating conditions, the number of theoretical plates and the symmetry factor of the peak of saikosaponin b$_2$ are not less than 5000 and not more than 1.5, respectively.

System repeatability: When the test is repeated 6 times with 10 μL of the standard solution under the above operating conditions, the relative standard deviation of the peak area of saikosaponin b$_2$ is not more than 1.5%.

(2) Baicalin—Weigh accurately about 0.1 g of the dry extract (or an amount of the viscous extract, equivalent to about 0.1 g of the dried substance), add exactly 50 mL of diluted methanol (7 in 10), shake for 15 minutes, filter, and use the filtrate as the sample solution. Separately, weigh accurately about 10 mg of Baicalin RS (separately determine the water $\langle 2.48 \rangle$ by coulometric titration, using 10 mg), and dissolve in methanol to make exactly 100 mL. Pipet 5 mL of this solution, add diluted methanol (7 in 10) to make exactly 10 mL, and use this solution as the standard solution. Perform the test with exactly 10 μL each of the sample solution and standard solution as directed under Liquid Chromatography $\langle 2.01 \rangle$ according to the following conditions, and determine the peak areas, A_T and A_S, of baicalin in each solution.

$$\text{Amount (mg) of baicalin (C}_{21}\text{H}_{18}\text{O}_{11})$$

$$= M_S \times A_T/A_S \times 1/4$$

M_S: Amount (mg) of Baicalin RS taken, calculated on the anhydrous basis

Operating conditions—

Detector: An ultraviolet absorption photometer (wavelength: 277 nm).

Column: A stainless steel column 4.6 mm in inside diameter and 15 cm in length, packed with octadecylsilanized silica gel for liquid chromatography (5 μm in particle diameter).

Column temperature: A constant temperature of about 40°C.

Mobile phase: A mixture of diluted phosphoric acid (1 in 200) and acetonitrile (19:6).

The JP Drugs are to be tested according to the provisions given in the pertinent monographs, General Notices, General Rules for Crude Drugs, General Rules for Preparations, and General Tests for their conformity to the Japanese Pharmacopoeia. (See the General Notices 5.)

Supplement I, JP XVIII *Crude Drugs and Related Drugs* 2919

Flow rate: 1.0 mL per minute.

System suitability—

System performance: When the procedure is run with 10 μL of the standard solution under the above operating conditions, the number of theoretical plates and the symmetry factor of the peak of baicalin are not less than 5000 and not more than 1.5, respectively.

System repeatability: When the test is repeated 6 times with 10 μL of the standard solution under the above operating conditions, the relative standard deviation of the peak area of baicalin is not more than 1.5%.

(3) Glycyrrhizic acid—Perform the test according to the following i) or ii).

i) Weigh accurately about 0.5 g of the dry extract (or an amount of the viscous extract, equivalent to about 0.5 g of the dried substance), add exactly 50 mL of diluted methanol (1 in 2), shake for 15 minutes, filter, and use the filtrate as the sample solution. Separately, weigh accurately about 10 mg of Glycyrrhizic Acid RS (separately determine the water <2.48> by coulometric titration, using 10 mg), dissolve in diluted methanol (1 in 2) to make exactly 100 mL, and use this solution as the standard solution. Perform the test with exactly 10 μL each of the sample solution and standard solution as directed under Liquid Chromatography <2.01> according to the following conditions, and determine the peak areas, A_T and A_S, of glycyrrhizic acid in each solution.

Amount (mg) of glycyrrhizic acid ($C_{42}H_{62}O_{16}$)
$$= M_S \times A_T/A_S \times 1/2$$

M_S: Amount (mg) of Glycyrrhizic Acid RS taken, calculated on the anhydrous basis

Operating conditions—

Detector: An ultraviolet absorption photometer (wavelength: 254 nm).

Column: A stainless steel column 4.6 mm in inside diameter and 15 cm in length, packed with octadecylsilanized silica gel for liquid chromatography (5 μm in particle diameter).

Column temperature: A constant temperature of about 40°C.

Mobile phase: Dissolve 3.85 g of ammonium acetate in 720 mL of water, and add 5 mL of acetic acid (100) and 280 mL of acetonitrile.

Flow rate: 1.0 mL per minute.

System suitability—

System performance: Dissolve 5 mg of monoammonium glycyrrhizinate for resolution check in 20 mL of dilute ethanol. When the procedure is run with 10 μL of this solution under the above operating conditions, the resolution between the peak having the relative retention time of about 0.9 to glycyrrhizic acid and the peak of glycyrrhizic acid is not less than 1.5. Dissolve 1 mg of (E)-cinnamaldehyde for thin-layer chromatography and 1 mg of baicalein for resolution check in 50 mL of methanol. To 2 mL of this solution add 2 mL of the standard solution. When the procedure is run with 10 μL of this solution under the above operating conditions, two peaks other than glycyrrhizic acid are ob-

served with the resolutions between the peak of glycyrrhizic acid and each of the two peaks being not less than 1.5.

System repeatability: When the test is repeated 6 times with 10 μL of the standard solution under the above operating conditions, the relative standard deviation of the peak area of glycyrrhizic acid is not more than 1.5%.

ii) Weigh accurately about 0.5 g of the dry extract (or an amount of the viscous extract, equivalent to about 0.5 g of the dried substance), add 20 mL of diethyl ether and 10 mL of water, and shake for 10 minutes. After centrifuge, remove the diethyl ether layer, add 20 mL of diethyl ether, proceed in the same manner as described above, and remove the diethyl ether layer. To the aqueous layer add 10 mL of methanol, shake for 30 minutes, centrifuge, and separate the supernatant liquid. To the residue add 20 mL of diluted methanol (1 in 2), shake for 5 minutes, centrifuge, and take the supernatant liquid. Combine these supernatant liquids, add diluted methanol (1 in 2) to make exactly 50 mL, and use this solution as the sample solution. Separately, weigh accurately about 10 mg of Glycyrrhizic Acid RS (separately determine the water <2.48> by coulometric titration, using 10 mg), dissolve in diluted methanol (1 in 2) to make exactly 100 mL, and use this solution as the standard solution. Perform the test with exactly 10 μL each of the sample solution and standard solution as directed under Liquid Chromatography <2.01> according to the following conditions, and determine the peak areas, A_T and A_S, of glycyrrhizic acid in each solution.

Amount (mg) of glycyrrhizic acid ($C_{42}H_{62}O_{16}$)
$$= M_S \times A_T/A_S \times 1/2$$

M_S: Amount (mg) of Glycyrrhizic Acid RS taken, calculated on the anhydrous basis

Operating conditions—

Proceed as directed in the operating conditions in i).

System suitability—

System repeatability: Proceed as directed in the system suitability in i).

System performance: Dissolve 5 mg of monoammonium glycyrrhizinate for resolution check in 20 mL of dilute ethanol. When the procedure is run with 10 μL of this solution under the above operating conditions, the resolution between the peak having the relative retention time of about 0.9 to glycyrrhizic acid and the peak of glycyrrhizic acid is not less than 1.5.

Containers and storage Containers—Tight containers.

The JP Drugs are to be tested according to the provisions given in the pertinent monographs, General Notices, General Rules for Crude Drugs, General Rules for Preparations, and General Tests for their conformity to the Japanese Pharmacopoeia. (See the General Notices 5.)

Senna Leaf

センナ

Change the Description and Identification (2) as follows (No effect to English text for Description):

Identification

(2) To 2 g of pulverized Senna Leaf add 20 mL of a mixture of tetrahydrofuran, methanol and dilute hydrochloric acid (16:4:1), shake for 5 minutes, filter, and use the filtrate as the sample solution. Separately, dissolve 1 mg of Sennoside A RS or sennoside A for thin-layer chromatography in 1 mL of a mixture of tetrahydrofuran and water (7:3), and use this solution as the standard solution. Perform the test with these solutions as directed under Thin-layer Chromatography <2.03>. Spot 5 μL each of the sample solution and standard solution on a plate of silica gel for thin-layer chromatography. Develop the plate with a mixture of 1-propanol, ethyl acetate, water and acetic acid (100) (40:40:30:1) to a distance of about 7 cm, and air-dry the plate. Examine under ultraviolet light (main wavelength: 365 nm): one of the several spots obtained from the sample solution has the same color tone and Rf value with the red to dark red fluorescent spot from the standard solution.

Powdered Senna Leaf

センナ末

Change the Identification (2) as follows:

Identification

(2) To 2 g of Powdered Senna Leaf add 20 mL of a mixture of tetrahydrofuran, methanol and dilute hydrochloric acid (16:4:1), shake for 5 minutes, filter, and use the filtrate as the sample solution. Separately, dissolve 1 mg of Sennoside A RS or sennoside A for thin-layer chromatography in 1 mL of a mixture of tetrahydrofuran and water (7:3), and use this solution as the standard solution. Perform the test with these solutions as directed under Thin-layer Chromatography <2.03>. Spot 5 μL each of the sample solution and standard solutions on a plate of silica gel for thin-layer chromatography. Develop the plate with a mixture of 1-propanol, ethyl acetate, water and acetic acid (100) (40:40:30:1) to a distance of about 7 cm, and air-dry the plate. Examine under ultraviolet light (main wavelength: 365 nm): one of the several spots obtained from the sample solution has the same color tone and Rf value with the red to dark red fluorescent spot from the standard solution.

Shimbuto Extract

真武湯エキス

Change the Assay (2) as follows:

Assay

(2) [6]-gingerol—Weigh accurately about 0.5 g of Shimbuto Extract, add exactly 50 mL of diluted methanol (7 in 10), shake for 15 minutes, filter, and use the filtrate as the sample solution. Separately, weigh accurately about 10 mg of [6]-gingerol for assay, dissolve in methanol to make exactly 100 mL. Pipet 5 mL of this solution, add methanol to make exactly 50 mL, and use this solution as the standard solution. Perform the test with exactly 10 μL each of the sample solution and standard solution as directed under Liquid Chromatography <2.01> according to the following conditions, and determine the peak areas, A_T and A_S, of [6]-gingerol in each solution.

$$\text{Amount (mg) of [6]-gingerol} = M_S \times A_T/A_S \times 1/20$$

M_S: Amount (mg) of [6]-gingerol for assay taken, calculated on the basis of the content obtained by qNMR

Operating conditions—

Detector: An ultraviolet absorption photometer (wavelength: 282 nm).

Column: A stainless steel column 4.6 mm in inside diameter and 15 cm in length, packed with octadecylsilanized silica gel for liquid chromatography (5 μm in particle diameter).

Column temperature: A constant temperature of about 30°C.

Mobile phase: A mixture of water, acetonitrile and phosphoric acid (620:380:1).

Flow rate: 1.0 mL per minute (the retention time of [6]-gingerol is about 15 minutes).

System suitability—

System performance: When the procedure is run with 10 μL of the standard solution under the above operating conditions, the number of theoretical plates and the symmetry factor of the peak of [6]-gingerol are not less than 5000 and not more than 1.5, respectively.

System repeatability: When the test is repeated 6 times with 10 μL of the standard solution under the above operating conditions, the relative standard deviation of the peak area of [6]-gingerol is not more than 1.5%.

Sinomenium Stem and Rhizome

ボウイ

Change the origin/limits of content as follows:

Sinomenium Stem and Rhizome is the climbing stem and rhizome of *Sinomenium acutum* Rehder et E. H. Wilson (*Menispermaceae*), usually cut transver-

Supplement I, JP XVIII   *Crude Drugs and Related Drugs*   2921

sely.

Tokakujokito Extract

桃核承気湯エキス

Change the Assay (1) as follows:

Assay

(1) Amygdalin—Weigh accurately about 0.5 g of Tokakujokito Extract, add exactly 50 mL of diluted methanol (1 in 2), shake for 15 minutes, and filter. Pipet 5 mL of the filtrate, elute through a column prepared previously with 2 g of polyamide for column chromatography using water to make exactly 20 mL of effluent , and use this solution as the sample solution. Separately, weigh accurately about 10 mg of amygdalin for assay, dissolve in diluted methanol (1 in 2) to make exactly 50 mL, and use this solution as the standard solution. Perform the test with exactly 10 μL each of the sample solution and standard solution as directed under Liquid Chromatography $\langle 2.01 \rangle$ according to the following conditions, and determine the peak areas, A_T and A_S, of amygdalin in each solution.

$$\text{Amount (mg) of amygdalin} = M_S \times A_T/A_S \times 4$$

M_S: Amount (mg) of amygdalin for assay taken

Operation conditions—

Detector: An ultraviolet absorption photometer (wavelength: 210 nm).

Column: A stainless steel column 4.6 mm in inside diameter and 15 cm in length, packed with octadecylsilanized silica gel for liquid chromatography (5 μm in particle diameter).

Column temperature: A constant temperature of about 45°C.

Mobile phase: A mixture of 0.05 mol/L sodium dihydrogen phosphate TS and methanol (5:1).

Flow rate: 0.8 mL per minute (the retention time of amygdalin is about 12 minutes).

Systemic suitability—

System performance: When the procedure is run with 10 μL of the standard solution under the above operating conditions, the number of theoretical plates and the symmetry factor of the peak of amygdalin are not less than 5000 and not more than 1.5, respectively.

System repeatability: When the test is repeated 6 times with 10 μL of the standard solution under the above operating conditions, the relative standard deviation of the peak area of amygdalin is not more than 1.5%.

Turmeric

ウコン

Change the Description as follows (No effect to English text):

Uncaria Hook

チョウトウコウ

Change the Assay as follows:

Assay Weigh accurately about 0.2 g of moderately fine powder of Uncaria Hook, transfer into a glass-stoppered centrifuge tube, add 30 mL of a mixture of methanol and dilute acetic acid (7:3), shake for 30 minutes, centrifuge, and separate the supernatant liquid. To the residue add two 10-mL portions of a mixture of methanol and dilute acetic acid (7:3), proceed in the same manner, and combine all of the supernatant liquid. To the combined liquid add a mixture of methanol and dilute acetic acid (7:3) to make exactly 50 mL, and use this solution as the sample solution. Separately, weigh accurately about 5 mg of rhynchophylline for assay, and dissolve in a mixture of methanol and dilute acetic acid (7:3) to make exactly 100 mL. Pipet 1 mL of this solution, add a mixture of methanol and dilute acetic acid (7:3) to make exactly 10 mL, and use this solution as the standard solution (1). Separately, dissolve 1 mg of hirsutine in 100 mL of a mixture of methanol and dilute acetic acid (7:3), and use this solution as the standard solution (2). Perform the test with exactly 20 μL each of the sample solution and standard solutions (1) and (2) as directed under Liquid Chromatography $\langle 2.01 \rangle$ according to the following conditions. Determine the peak areas, A_{Ta} and A_{Tb}, of rhynchophylline and hirsutine obtained from the sample solution, and the peak area, A_S, of rhynchophylline from the standard solution (1).

Amount (mg) of total alkaloids (rhynchophylline and hirsutine)
$$= M_S \times (A_{Ta} + 1.405A_{Tb})/A_S \times 1/20$$

M_S: Amount (mg) of rhynchophylline for assay taken

Operating conditions—

Detector: An ultraviolet absorption photometer (wavelength: 245 nm).

Column: A stainless steel column 4.6 mm in inside diameter and 25 cm in length, packed with octadecylsilanized silica gel for liquid chromatography (5 μm in particle diameter).

Column temperature: A constant temperature of about 40°C.

Mobile phase: Dissolve 3.85 g of ammonium acetate in 200 mL of water, add 10 mL of acetic acid (100) and water to make 1000 mL, and add 350 mL of acetonitrile.

Flow rate: Adjust so that the retention time of rhyn-

The JP Drugs are to be tested according to the provisions given in the pertinent monographs, General Notices, General Rules for Crude Drugs, General Rules for Preparations, and General Tests for their conformity to the Japanese Pharmacopoeia. (See the General Notices 5.)

2922 *Crude Drugs and Related Drugs*

chophylline is about 17 minutes.

System suitability—

System performance: Dissolve 5 mg of rhynchophylline for assay in 100 mL of a mixture of methanol and dilute acetic acid (7:3). To 5 mL of this solution add 1 mL of ammonia solution (28), and warm at about 50°C for 2 hours or heat under a reflux condenser for 10 minutes. After cooling, to 1 mL of the solution so obtained add a mixture of methanol and dilute acetic acid (7:3) to make 5 mL. When the procedure is run with 20 μL of this solution under the above operating conditions, the peak of isorhynchophylline appears in addition to the peak of rhynchophylline, and the resolution between these peaks is not less than 1.5.

System repeatability: When the test is repeated 6 times with 20 μL of the standard solution (1) under the above operating conditions, the relative standard deviation of the peak areas of rhynchophylline is not more than 1.5%.

Add the following:

Yokukansankachimpihange Extract

抑肝散加陳皮半夏エキス

Yokukansankachimpihange Extract contains not less than 0.6 mg and not more than 2.4 mg of saikosaponin b_2, not less than 10 mg and not more than 30 mg of glycyrrhizic acid ($C_{42}H_{62}O_{16}$: 822.93), and not less than 18 mg and not more than 72 mg of hesperidin, per extract prepared with the amount specified in the Method of preparation.

Method of preparation

	1)	2)
Japanese Angelica Root	3 g	3 g
Uncaria Hook	3 g	3 g
Cnidium Rhizome	3 g	3 g
Atractylodes Rhizome	4 g	—
Atractylodes Lancea Rhizome	—	4 g
Poria Sclerotium	4 g	4 g
Bupleurum Root	2 g	2 g
Glycyrrhiza	1.5 g	1.5 g
Citrus Unshiu Peel	3 g	3 g
Pinellia Tuber	5 g	5 g

Prepare a dry extract or viscous extract as directed under Extracts, according to the prescription 1) or 2), using the crude drugs shown above.

Description The dry extract: Yokukansankachimpihange Extract is a grayish brown to reddish yellow-brown powder. It has a characteristic odor, and has a sweet and slightly hot taste at first, later bitter.

The viscous extract: Yokukansankachimpihange Extract is a brown viscous liquid. It has a characteristic odor, and has a bitter and slightly sweet taste.

Identification (1) Shake 2.0 g of the dry extract (or 6.0 g

of the viscous extract) with 10 mL of water, then add 10 mL of diethyl ether, shake, and centrifuge. Separate the diethyl ether layer, add 10 mL of sodium hydroxide TS, and shake. Centrifuge this solution, and use the diethyl ether layer as the sample solution. Separately, use (Z)-ligustilide TS for thin-layer chromatography as the standard solution. Perform the test with these solutions as directed under Thin-layer Chromatography <2.03>. Spot 10 μL each of the sample solution and standard solution on a plate of silica gel for thin-layer chromatography. Develop the plate with a mixture of butyl acetate and hexane (2:1) to a distance of about 7 cm, and air-dry the plate. Examine under ultraviolet light (main wavelength: 365 nm): one of the several spots obtained from the sample solution has the same color tone and *R*f value with the blue-white fluorescent spot from the standard solution (Japanese Angelica Root; Cnidium Rhizome).

(2) Shake 2.0 g of the dry extract (or 6.0 g of the viscous extract) with 20 mL of water and 2 mL of ammonia TS, add 20 mL of diethyl ether, and shake. Separate the diethyl ether layer, evaporate the solvent under low pressure (in vacuo), add 1 mL of methanol to the residue, and use this solution as the sample solution. Separately, dissolve 1 mg each of rhyncophyllin for thin-layer chromatography and hirsutine for thin-layer chromatography in 1 mL of methanol, and use this solution as the standard solution. Perform the test with these solutions as directed under Thin-layer Chromatography <2.03>. Spot 10 μL of the sample solution and 2 μL of the standard solution on a plate of silica gel with fluorescent indicator for thin-layer chromatography. Develop the plate with a mixture of ethyl acetate, 1-propanol, water and acetic acid (100) (7:5:4:1) to a distance of about 7 cm, and air-dry the plate. Examine under ultraviolet light (main wavelength: 254 nm): at least one of the several spots obtained from the sample solution has the same color tone and *R*f value with one of the two dark violet spots from the standard solution (Uncaria Hook).

(3) For preparation prescribed Atractylodes Rhizome— Shake 1.0 g of the dry extract (or 3.0 g of the viscous extract) with 10 mL of water, add 25 mL of diethyl ether, and shake. Separate the diethyl ether layer, evaporate the solvent under low pressure (in vacuo), add 2 mL of diethyl ether to the residue, and use this solution as the sample solution. Separately, dissolve 1 mg of atractylenoide III for thin-layer chromatography in 2 mL of methanol, and use this solution as the standard solution. Perform the test with these solutions as directed under Thin-layer Chromatography <2.03>. Spot 5 μL each of the sample solution and standard solution on a plate of silica gel for thin-layer chromatography. Develop the plate with a mixture of hexane and ethyl acetate (2:1) to a distance of about 7 cm, and air-dry the plate. Spray evenly 1-naphthol-sulfuric acid TS on the plate, heat the plate at 105°C for 5 minutes, and allow to cool: one of the several spots obtained from the sample solution has the same color tone and *R*f value with the red to red-purple spot from the standard solution (Atractylodes Rhizome).

(4) For preparation prescribed Atractylodes Lancea

The JP Drugs are to be tested according to the provisions given in the pertinent monographs, General Notices, General Rules for Crude Drugs, General Rules for Preparations, and General Tests for their conformity to the Japanese Pharmacopoeia. (See the General Notices 5.)

Supplement I, JP XVIII *Crude Drugs and Related Drugs* 2923

Rhizome—Shake 2.0 g of the dry extract (or 6.0 g of the viscous extract) with 10 mL of water, add 25 mL of hexane, and shake. Separate the hexane layer, evaporate the solvent under low pressure (in vacuo), add 2 mL of hexane to the residue, and use this solution as the sample solution. Perform the test with the sample solution as directed under Thin-layer Chromatography <2.03>. Spot 20 μL of the sample solution on a plate of silica gel with fluorescent indicator for thin-layer chromatography. Develop the plate with a mixture of hexane and acetone (7:1) to a distance of about 7 cm, and air-dry the plate. Examine under ultraviolet light (main wavelength: 254 nm): a dark purple spot is observed at an Rf value of about 0.5. The spot shows a green-brown color after being sprayed evenly 4-dimethylaminobenzaldehyde TS for spraying, heated at 105°C for 5 minutes, and allowed to cool (Atractylodes Lancea Rhizome).

(5) Shake 1.0 g of the dry extract (or 3.0 g of the viscous extract) with 10 mL of water, add 10 mL of 1-butanol, and shake. Centrifuge this solution, and use the 1-butanol layer as the sample solution. Separately, dissolve 1 mg of saikosaponin b_2 for thin-layer chromatography in 1 mL of methanol, and use this solution as the standard solution. Perform the test with these solutions as directed under Thin-layer Chromatography <2.03>. Spot 10 μL of the sample solution and 2 μL of the standard solution on a plate of silica gel for thin-layer chromatography. Develop the plate with a mixture of ethyl acetate, ethanol (99.5) and water (8:2:1) to a distance of about 7 cm, and air-dry the plate. Spray evenly 4-dimethylaminobenzaldehyde TS for spraying on the plate, heat the plate at 105°C for 5 minutes, and examine under ultraviolet light (main wavelength: 365 nm): one of the several spots obtained from the sample solution has the same color tone and Rf value with the yellow fluorescent spot from the standard solution (Bupleurum Root).

(6) Shake 1.0 g of the dry extract (or 3.0 g of the viscous extract) with 10 mL of water, add 10 mL of 1-butanol, and shake. Centrifuge this solution, and use the 1-butanol layer as the sample solution. Separately, dissolve 1 mg of liquiritin for thin-layer chromatography in 1 mL of methanol, and use this solution as the standard solution. Perform the test with these solutions as directed under Thin-layer Chromatography <2.03>. Spot 1 μL each of the sample solution and standard solution on a plate of silica gel for thin-layer chromatography. Develop the plate with a mixture of ethyl acetate, methanol and water (20:3:2) to a distance of about 7 cm, and air-dry the plate. Spray evenly dilute sulfuric acid on the plate, heat the plate at 105°C for 5 minutes, and examine under ultraviolet light (main wavelength: 365 nm): one of the several spots obtained from the sample solution has the same color tone and Rf value with the yellow-green fluorescent spot from the standard solution (Glycyrrhiza).

(7) Shake 1.0 g of the dry extract (or 3.0 g of the viscous extract) with 10 mL of water, add 10 mL of 1-butanol, centrifuge, and use the 1-butanol layer as the sample solution. Separately, dissolve 1 mg of hesperidin for thin-layer chromatography in 1 mL of methanol, and use this solution as the standard solution. Perform the test with these solutions as directed under Thin-layer Chromatography <2.03>. Spot

20 μL of the sample solution and 10 μL of the standard solution on a plate of silica gel for thin-layer chromatography. Develop the plate with a mixture of ethyl acetate, acetone, water and acetic acid (100) (10:6:3:1) to a distance of about 7 cm, and air-dry the plate. Spray evenly 2,6-dibromo-N-chloro-1,4-benzoquinone monoimine TS on the plate, and expose the plate to ammonia vapor: one of the several spots from the sample solution has the same color tone and Rf value with the blue spot from the standard solution (Citrus Unshiu Peel).

Purity (1) Heavy metals <1.07>—Prepare the test solution with 1.0 g of the dry extract (or an amount of the viscous extract, equivalent to 1.0 g of the dried substance) as directed under Extracts (4), and perform the test (not more than 30 ppm).

(2) Arsenic <1.11>—Prepare the test solution with 0.67 g of the dry extract (or an amount of the viscous extract, equivalent to 0.67 g of the dried substance) according to Method 3, and perform the test (not more than 3 ppm).

Loss on drying <2.41> The dry extract: Not more than 10.0% (1 g, 105°C, 5 hours).

The viscous extract: Not more than 66.7% (1 g, 105°C, 5 hours).

Total ash <5.01> Not more than 9.0%, calculated on the dried basis.

Assay (1) Saikosaponin b_2—Weigh accurately about 0.5 g of the dry extract (or an amount of the viscous extract, equivalent to about 0.5 g of the dried substance), add 20 mL of diethyl ether and 10 mL of water, and shake for 10 minutes. After centrifugation, remove the diethyl ether layer, then add 20 mL of diethyl ether, proceed in the same manner as described above, and remove the diethyl ether layer. To the aqueous layer add 10 mL of methanol, shake for 30 minutes, centrifuge, and separate the supernatant liquid. To the residue add 20 mL of diluted methanol (1 in 2), shake for 5 minutes, then centrifuge, and separate the supernatant liquid. Combine all the supernatant liquids, add diluted methanol (1 in 2) to make exactly 50 mL, and use this solution as the sample solution. Separately, use saikosaponin b_2 standard TS for assay as the standard solution. Perform the test with exactly 10 μL each of the sample solution and standard solution as directed under Liquid Chromatography <2.01> according to the following conditions, and determine the peak areas, A_T and A_S, of saikosaponin b_2 in each solution.

$$\text{Amount (mg) of saikosaponin } b_2 = C_S \times A_T/A_S \times 50$$

C_S: Concentration (mg/mL) of saikosaponin b_2 in saikosaponin b_2 standard TS for assay

Operation conditions—

Detector: An ultraviolet absorption photometer (wavelength: 254 nm).

Column: A stainless steel column 4.6 mm in inside diameter and 15 cm in length, packed with octadecylsilanized silica gel for liquid chromatography (5 μm in particle diame-

---

The JP Drugs are to be tested according to the provisions given in the pertinent monographs, General Notices, General Rules for Crude Drugs, General Rules for Preparations, and General Tests for their conformity to the Japanese Pharmacopoeia. (See the General Notices 5.)

2924 *Crude Drugs and Related Drugs*

Supplement I, JP XVIII

ter).

Column temperature: A constant temperature of about 40°C.

Mobile phase: A mixture of 0.05 mol/L sodium dihydrogen phosphate TS and acetonitrile (5:3).

Flow rate: 1.0 mL per minute.

Systemic suitability—

System performance: When the procedure is run with 10 μL of the standard solution under the above operating conditions, the number of theoretical plates and the symmetry factor of the peak of saikosaponin b$_2$ are not less than 5000 and not more than 1.5, respectively.

System repeatability: When the test is repeated 6 times with 10 μL of the standard solution under the above operating conditions, the relative standard deviation of the peak area of saikosaponin b$_2$ is not more than 1.5%.

(2) Glycyrrhizic acid—Weigh accurately about 0.5 g of the dry extract (or an amount of the viscous extract, equivalent to about 0.5 g of the dried substance), add 20 mL of diethyl ether and 10 mL of water, and shake for 10 minutes. After centrifugation, remove the diethyl ether layer, then add 20 mL of diethyl ether, proceed in the same manner as above, and remove the diethyl ether layer. To the aqueous layer add 10 mL of methanol, shake for 30 minutes, then centrifuge, and separate the supernatant liquid. To the residue add 20 mL of diluted methanol (1 in 2), shake for 5 minutes, centrifuge, and take the supernatant liquid. Combine the supernatant liquids, add diluted methanol (1 in 2) to make exactly 50 mL, and use this solution as the sample solution. Separately, weigh accurately about 10 mg of Glycyrrhizic Acid RS (separately determine the water ⟨2.48⟩ by coulometric titration, using 10 mg), dissolve in diluted methanol (1 in 2) to make exactly 100 mL, and use this solution as the standard solution. Perform the test with exactly 10 μL each of the sample solution and standard solution as directed under Liquid Chromatography ⟨2.01⟩ according to the following conditions, and determine the peak areas, A_T and A_S, of glycyrrhizic acid in each solution.

Amount (mg) of glycyrrhizic acid ($C_{42}H_{62}O_{16}$)
= $M_S \times A_T/A_S \times 1/2$

M_S: Amount (mg) of Glycyrrhizic Acid RS taken, calculated on the anhydrous basis

Operation conditions—

Detector: An ultraviolet absorption photometer (wavelength: 254 nm).

Column: A stainless steel column 4.6 mm in inside diameter and 15 cm in length, packed with octadecylsilanized silica gel for liquid chromatography (5 μm in particle diameter).

Column temperature: A constant temperature of about 40°C.

Mobile phase: Dissolve 3.85 g of ammonium acetate in 720 mL of water, and add 5 mL of acetic acid (100) and 280 mL of acetonitrile.

Flow rate: 1.0 mL per minute.

Systemic suitability—

System performance: Dissolve 5 mg of monoammonium glycyrrhizinate for resolution check in 20 mL of dilute ethanol. When the procedure is run with 10 μL of this solution under the above operating conditions, the resolution between the peak having the relative retention time about 0.9 to glycyrrhizic acid and the peak of glycyrrhizic acid is not less than 1.5.

System repeatability: When the test is repeated 6 times with 10 μL of the standard solution under the above operating conditions, the relative standard deviation of the peak area of glycyrrhizic acid is not more than 1.5%.

(3) Hesperidin—Weigh accurately about 0.1 g of the dry extract (or an amount of the viscous extract, equivalent to about 0.1 g of dried substance), add exactly 50 mL of diluted tetrahydrofuran (1 in 4), shake for 30 minutes, centrifuge, and use the supernatant liquid as the sample solution. Separately, weigh accurately about 10 mg of hesperidin for assay, previously dried in a desiccator (silica gel) for 24 hours, dissolve in methanol to make exactly 100 mL. Pipet 10 mL of this solution, add diluted tetrahydrofuran (1 in 4) to make exactly 100 mL, and use this solution as the standard solution. Perform the test with exactly 10 μL each of the sample solution and standard solution as directed under Liquid Chromatography ⟨2.01⟩ according to the following conditions, and determine the peak areas, A_T and A_S, of hesperidin in each solution.

Amount (mg) of hesperidin = $M_S \times A_T/A_S \times 1/20$

M_S: Amount (mg) of hesperidin for assay taken

Operating conditions—

Detector: An ultraviolet absorption photometer (wavelength: 285 nm).

Column: A stainless steel column 4.6 mm in inside diameter and 15 cm in length, packed with octadecylsilanized silica gel for liquid chromatography (5 μm in particle diameter).

Column temperature: A constant temperature of about 40°C.

Mobile phase: A mixture of water, acetonitrile and acetic acid (100) (82:18:1).

Flow rate: 1.0 mL per minute.

System suitability—

System performance: Dissolve 1 mg each of hesperidin for assay and naringin for thin-layer chromatography in diluted methanol (1 in 2) to make 100 mL. When the procedure is run with 10 μL of this solution under the above operating conditions, naringin and hespeidin are eluted in this order with the resolution between these peaks being not less than 1.5.

System repeatability: When the test is repeated 6 times with 10 μL of the standard solution under the above operating conditions, the relative standard deviation of the peak area of hesperidin is not more than 1.5%.

Containers and storage Containers—Tight containers.

The JP Drugs are to be tested according to the provisions given in the pertinent monographs, General Notices, General Rules for Crude Drugs, General Rules for Preparations, and General Tests for their conformity to the Japanese Pharmacopoeia. (See the General Notices 5.)

Infrared
Reference Spectra

Add the following spectra:

Anastrozole

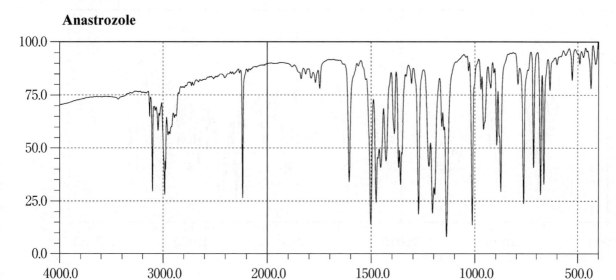

Budesonide

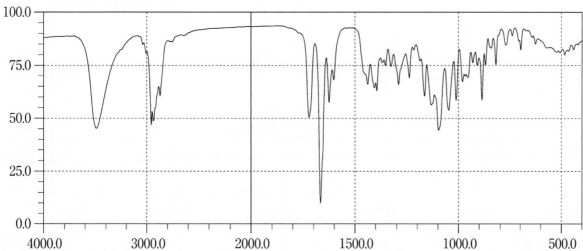

Croscarmellose Sodium

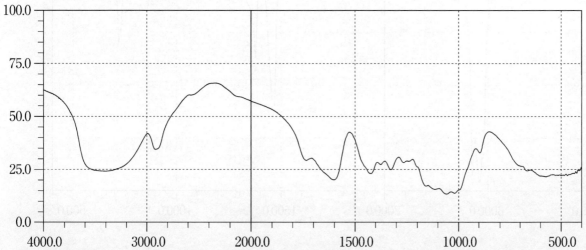

The JP Drugs are to be tested according to the provisions given in the pertinent monographs, General Notices, General Rules for Crude Drugs, General Rules for Preparations, and General Tests for their conformity to the Japanese Pharmacopoeia. (See the General Notices 5.)

Oxybutynin Hydrochloride

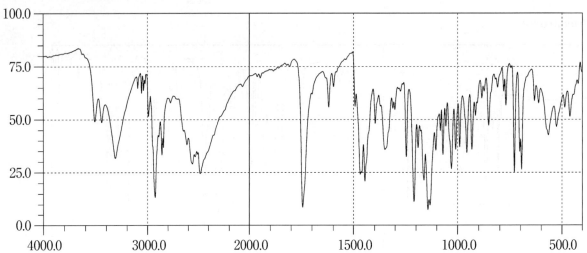

White Petrolatum

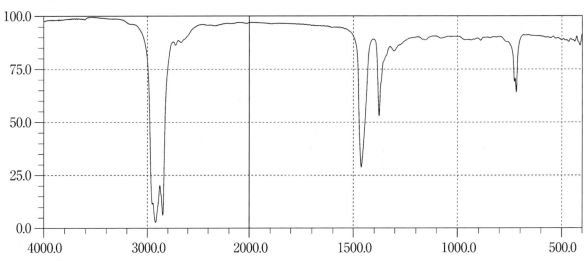

Yellow Petrolatum

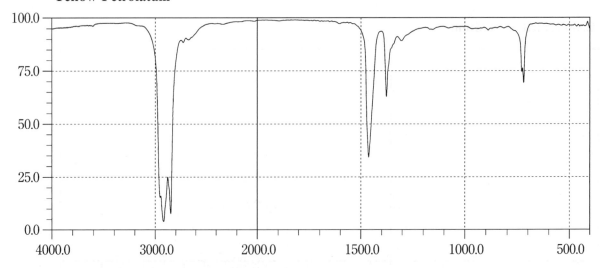

The JP Drugs are to be tested according to the provisions given in the pertinent monographs, General Notices, General Rules for Crude Drugs, General Rules for Preparations, and General Tests for their conformity to the Japanese Pharmacopoeia. (See the General Notices 5.)

Temozolomide

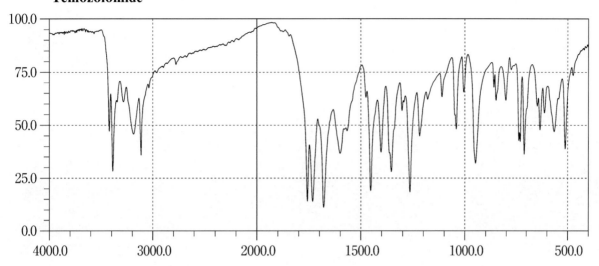

Ultraviolet-visible Reference Spectra

Add the following spectra:

Anastrozole

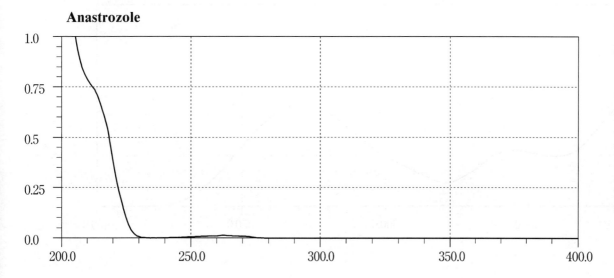

Budesonide

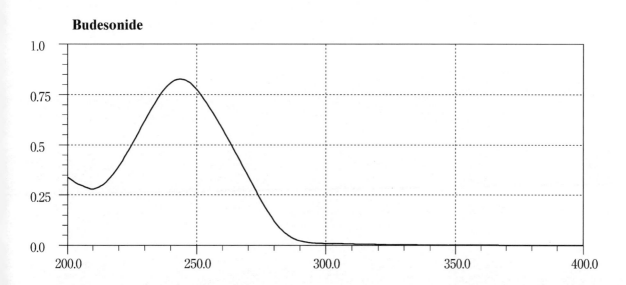

Oxybutynin Hydrochloride

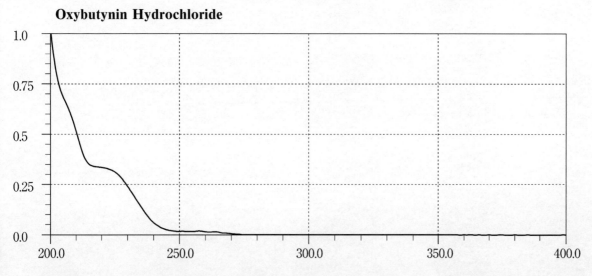

Temozolomide

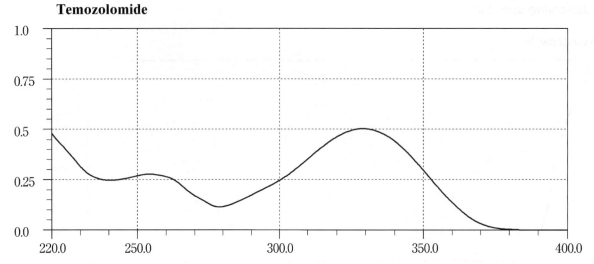

General Information

GENERAL INFORMATION

The General Information describes reference information and reference test methods necessary to assure the quality of medicines, which is attached to the JP. Therefore, the General Information is positioned as important information supplementing the JP although it should not be taken as indicating standards for conformity of drugs, except in the case specified when the drugs are granted approval based on the Law on Securing Quality, Efficacy and Safety of Products Including Pharmaceuticals and Medical Devices. Combination use of the General Information and the JP can contribute to improve quality of the JP and user's convenience.

The general information is classified into the following categories according to their contents, and each general information is individually numbered.

An individual number consists of three blocks. The left block indicates the category number and the central block indicates the number in the category. The figures in right block consist of the first two digits from the left indicating the JP at the recent revision (or new preparation, if not revised) and the third digit indicating as follows: 0 for major revision, 1 for supplement I, 2 for supplement II, and 3 for partial revision. For citation between the general information, the number corresponding to the general information is indicated in angle brackets 〈 〉.

> G0. Basic Concepts on Pharmaceutical Quality
> G1. Physics and Chemistry
> G2. Solid-state Properties
> G3. Biotechnological/Biological Products
> G4. Microorganisms
> G5. Crude Drugs
> G6. Drug Formulation
> G7. Containers and Package
> G8. Reference Standards
> GZ. Others

The salient points of the revision in this volume are as follows:

1. "G9. Pharmaceutical Excipients" was newly added to the category of the general information.

2. The following were newly prepared.
(1) Instrumental Measurement of Coloration of Liquids 〈G1-4-181〉
(2) Control Strategies and Change Control Concepts at Each Stage of Chromatography Lifecycle (Change Control in Chromatography Lifecycle) 〈G1-5-181〉
(3) Measurement of Powder Flow Properties by Shear Cell Methods 〈G2-5-181〉
(4) Biorisk Management of the Handling of Microorganisms in Microbial Tests 〈G4-11-181〉

(5) Functionality-related Characteristics of Excipients Relevant to Preparations 〈G9-1-181〉

3. The following were revised.
(1) Concept on Impurities in Chemically Synthesized Drug Substances and Drug Products 〈G0-3-181〉
(2) System Suitability 〈G1-2-181〉
(3) On the Scientific Names of Crude Drugs listed in the JP 〈G5-1-181〉
(4) Tablet Friability Test 〈G6-5-181〉
(5) Quality Control of Water for Pharmaceutical Use 〈GZ-2-181〉

4. The following was deleted.
(1) Near Infrared Spectrometry 〈G1-3-161〉

G0 Basic Concepts on Pharmaceutical Quality

Concept on Impurities in Chemically Synthesized Drug Substances and Drug Products
〈G0-3-181〉

Change the following as follows:

1. Classification of impurities found in chemically synthesized pharmaceuticals and the guidance to comply with for their control

Impurities found in chemically synthesized pharmaceuticals are roughly classified into organic impurities, inorganic impurities and residual solvents. Those impurities in new drug substances and products are controlled by the following guidelines agreed upon at the International Council for Harmonization of Technical Requirements for Pharmaceuticals for Human Use (hereinafter referred to as "ICH"). More specifically, "Impurities in New Drugs Substances (PAB/PCD Notification No. 877 dated September 25, 1995)" (hereinafter referred to as "ICH Q3A Guideline")[1] on specifications for organic impurities in drug substances applies to applications for marketing approval after April 1, 1997, while "Impurities in New Drug Products (PAB/PCD Notification No. 539 dated June 23, 1997" (hereinafter referred to as "ICH Q3B Guideline")[2] on specifications for organic impurities in drug products applies to applications for marketing approval after April 1, 1999. Meanwhile, specifications for inorganic impurities were specified by Japanese pharmacopoeial standards and known safety data.

2931

Now "Guideline for Elemental Impurities (PFSB/ELD Notification No. 4 dated September 30, 2015)" (hereinafter referred to as "ICH Q3D Guideline") applies to applications for marketing approval after April 1, 2017. In regard to residual solvents, "Impurities: Guideline for Residual Solvents (PAB/ELD Notification No. 307 dated March 30, 1998)" (hereinafter referred to as "ICH Q3C Guideline") applies to applications for marketing approval after April 1, 2000. Especially in regard to DNA-reactive impurities, "Assessment and control of DNA reactive (mutagenic) impurities in pharmaceuticals to limit potential carcinogenic risk (PSEHB/ELD Notification No. 3 dated November 10, 2015)" applies to applications for marketing approval after January 15, 2016. Although ICH Q3A guideline does not cover optical enantiomers, a type of organic impurities, "Specifications: Test Procedures and Acceptance Criteria for New Drug Substances and New Drug Products: Chemical Substances (PMSB/ELD Notification No. 568 dated May 1, 2001)" (hereinafter referred to as "ICH Q6A Guideline"), which was published subsequently, provides that enantiomers are impurities that should be controlled and, if measurable, should be controlled in accordance with the principle of the ICH Q3A guideline.

Control of impurities in accordance with the guidelines mentioned above is expected also for pharmaceuticals other than new drug substances and new drug products. Their applications for marketing (or applications for partial changes) are subject to those guidelines when necessary. The General Notices of the JP 17th Edition states that residual solvents of all JP-listed drugs, in principle, have to be controlled in accordance with specification "Residual Solvents" in General Tests unless otherwise specified in the individual monograph. In regard to elemental impurities, their tests and control methods have been added stepwise as introduction into the JP. In the JP 18th Edition, the provision regarding elemental impurities based on the ICH Q3D guideline was provided in the Paragraph 34 of General Notices, and also the General Test "Elemental Impurities ⟨2.66⟩" and General Information "Control of Elemental Impurities in Drug Products" were integrated to provide the General Test "Elemental Impurities ⟨2.66⟩" that reflects the revision of the ICH Q3D guideline.

2. The concept of ICH Q3A and Q3B guidelines for the control of organic impurities

ICH Q3A and Q3B guidelines require setting acceptance criteria for organic impurities based on the information gained from development stages for new drugs. Concerning impurities in drug substances, ICH Q3A guideline refers to the items to be examined from chemical and safety perspectives. ICH Q3B guideline complements Q3A guideline, and has the same basic concept as Q3A. Chemical aspects to be examined include classification and identification of impurities, their reporting method, specification settings and analytical methods. Safety aspects include specific guidelines for qualifying the safety of impurities that were not present, or were present at substantially lower levels, in batches of a drug substance used in safety and clinical studies.

Qualification of the safety is the process of acquiring and evaluating data that establishes the biological safety of an individual impurity or a given impurity profile at the level(s) specified. The applicant should describe a rationale for establishing impurity acceptance criteria that includes safety considerations in attachments when applicated for approval. The level of any impurities present in a new drug substance that has been adequately tested in safety and/or clinical studies would be considered qualified.

Identified impurities, unidentified impurities and total impurities are specified based on the data obtained according to the guidelines. The threshold of unspecified impurities in a drug substance is determined depending on the daily intake of the drug substance. When the maximum daily dosage is not more than 2 g, it is set at 0.10%. The establishment of individual specifications is required for impurities at a level greater than 0.10%.

In regard to drug products, the ICH Q3B guideline cover the degradation products of drug substances or reaction products between the drug substance and additive/primary packaging. Therefore, even if organic impurities other than degradation products (e.g., by-products and synthetic intermediates) in the drug substance are found as impurities in the drug product, they need not be monitored or specified since they have already been controlled as the drug substance specifications. However, degradation products elevated in the drug product need to be monitored and specified.

3. Principles for controlling organic impurities in the articles listed in the JP

Conventionally in the JP, specified impurities, unspecified impurities and total impurities are specified in accordance with ICH Q3A and Q3B guidelines for pharmaceutical products, whose impurities have been controlled by those guidelines, in the process listing in the JP. (However, this shall not apply to the long-term listed pharmaceutical products which had existed in the JP before these guidelines were applicable. However, when a new application is filed for those JP-listed pharmaceutical products, control of impurities in accordance with ICH Q3A and Q3B guidelines may be required, if necessary.) In order to specify the impurities, analysis data during development submitted from the drafting company and impurity analysis data from commercial production batches after consistent manufacturing is achieved should be assessed. Safety evaluation is not required again for the process listing in the JP since it has been performed at the time of approval.

ICH Q3A and Q3B guidelines cover impurities in the drug substances manufactured by chemical syntheses and the drug products manufactured with those drug substances. Similarly, the following types of products are not covered in the JP: biological/biotechnological products, peptides, oligonucleotides, radiopharmaceuticals, fermentation products and semi-synthetic products derived therefrom, herbal products and crude products of animal or plant origin.

When organic impurities assessed in accordance with the

Supplement I, JP XVIII   *General Information*   2933

principles of ICH Q3A and Q3B guidelines are listed as JP tests of purity, the operational rationality of the JP is considered and its own modification is added. (i) Except in exceptional circumstances, impurity reference standards are not established. In order to identify an impurity using liquid chromatography, the relative retention time of the impurity to the drug substance is used for identification. (ii) When only unidentified impurities in highly pure pharmaceutical products (not more than 0.1%) are specified, it is generally exempted to set acceptance criteria for total impurities. (iii) When acceptance criteria set based only on actual measured values result in many impurities with slightly different acceptance criteria, consideration can be given so that the purity test consists of a small number of representative acceptance criteria, if possible. (iv) Chemical structural information and the chemical name of the impurities are not disclosed. Those measures enable impurity control without impurity reference standards, and can simplify system suitability tests for highly pure pharmaceutical products.

Meanwhile, the method to identify impurities by use of relative retention time is column-dependent and analysis becomes difficult when appropriate columns are not available. Therefore, the JP 17th Edition also allows the use of the analysis method with impurity reference standards when designing purity tests for a drug substance. In addition, the JP adopted a policy to disclose chemical names and structure formulas as the information on impurities including, in principle, optical enantiomers.

As mentioned in the ICH Q3A guideline, there are cases where the structure determination of impurities is incomplete. Therefore, the chemical structures disclosed in the section Others of monographs include structures that have been determined by NMR, etc., as well as chemically reasonable structures that are estimated from synthetic pathways, etc. At that time, if the stereochemistry is not confirmed, the structure of the relevant part is described using wavy lines, and the hydrogen bonded to the relevant carbon is not described (except when it is essential to show the structure). Furthermore, the chemical name does not include the distinction between *R*-form and *S*-form, and *E*-form and *Z*-form.

The JP-specific consideration may be given to purity tests for organic impurities in drug products in the process listing in the JP. Also in the JP, impurities derived from the products of the reaction between the drug substance and additive/primary packaging are specified as impurities in the drug product. Those impurities are formulation-dependent and may not be formed in different formulations. Since the JP is an official compendium that allows a wide variety of formulations, when it is not appropriate to specify impurities uniformly in the individual monograph, they are subject to the specifications at the time of approval, along with the statement "Being specified separately when the drug is granted approval based on the Law."

When the specifications for impurities are reviewed for a new entry of a pharmaceutical product in an individual monograph of the JP, acceptance criteria for impurities may be included in the review according to the following concepts. ICH Q6A guideline point out: Data available upon the marketing application are limited and it has to be taken into consideration that the limited data may influence the design of acceptance criteria. Regarding impurities, since impurity profiles gained during the manufacturing stages may sometimes be different from that gained from development stage, it is stated that changes in impurity profiles at the manufacturing stage should be considered as appropriate. According to this concept, for impurities which should be specified in the process listing in the JP, not only information from development stage but also information about impurity profiles if there are changes at the manufacturing stage, and information at the stage after the product manufacturing becomes stable (hereinafter referred to as the "stable production stage") should be taken into consideration.

However, it is undesirable to remove impurities that are present at substantially lower levels, or become undetectable at the stable production stage indiscriminately from the list of candidate compounds to be specified. JP-listed drugs are accepted as drugs by conformance to the specifications in the individual monograph. However, generic drugs, whose manufacturing methods are not necessarily the same as that of the drug substance used for JP monograph, may have different impurity profiles and contain such impurities. Providing information in the process listing in the JP based on the detection results during development stage may result in encompassing impurities found in drug substances and drug products distributed as JP drugs.

Therefore, before the removal of impurities that are present at substantially lower levels or become undetectable at the stable production stage from the JP specification list, the need to establish specifications should be fully examined based on ICH Q3A and Q3B guidelines with respect to safety.

For a drug substance that was approved by the method to identify its impurities with impurity reference materials, it is desirable also in the individual JP monograph, in principle, to establish specifications and test methods appropriately so that the specified impurity becomes identifiable. In regard to impurity control during the manufacturing process, impurities can be controlled by establishing an appropriate control strategy including release testing, in-process tests and process parameters control.

4. References
1) ICH: Guideline for Q3A, Impurities in New Drug Substances.
2) ICH: Guideline for Q3B, Impurities in New Drug Products.

G1 Physics and Chemistry

Change the following as follows:

System Suitability ⟨G1-2-181⟩

In order to ensure the reliability on the results of drug analyses, it is essential to verify that the test method to be applied to the test, including the method prescribed in the Japanese Pharmacopoeia (JP), can give the results adequate for its intended use using the analytical system in the laboratory in which the test is to be performed, then to carry out system suitability testing for confirming that the analytical system maintains the state suitable for the quality test.

1. Definition and role of system suitability

"System Suitability" is the concept for ensuring that the performance of the analytical system is as suitable for the analysis of the drug as was at the time when the verification of the test method was performed using the system. Usually, system suitability testing should be carried out at every series of drug analysis. The test procedures and acceptance criteria of system suitability testing must be prescribed in the test methods of drugs. The results of drug analyses are not acceptable unless the requirements of system suitability have been met.

System suitability testing is an integral part of test methods using analytical instruments, and based on the concept that the equipments, electronic data processing systems, analytical operations, samples to be analyzed and operators constitute an integral system that can be evaluated, when the test procedures and acceptance criteria of system suitability testing are prescribed in the test methods.

2. Points to consider in setting system suitability

Parameters of system suitability testing to be prescribed in the test method depend on the intended use and type of analytical method. Since system suitability testing is to be carried out in a routine manner, it is preferable to select the parameters necessary for ensuring that the analytical system maintains the state suitable for the analysis of the drug and to prescribe its test procedure able to carry out easily and rapidly.

For example, in the case of quantitative purity tests using liquid chromatography or gas chromatography, the evaluation of parameters such as "System performance" (to confirm the ability to analyze target substance specifically), "System repeatability" (to confirm that the degree of variation in the analytical results of target substance in replicate injections is within the allowable limit) and "Test for required detectability" (to confirm the linearity of chromatographic response around the specification limit) are usually required. However, in the area percentage method, if the influence of a matrix is evaluated and appropriate confirmation of detection is established, such as using a solution with the lowest concentration level that should be controlled in consideration of the property of an analyte, the specifica-

tion of system repeatability may not be necessary.

The specifications of system suitability in chromatography should be in accordance with Chromatography ⟨2.00⟩ or Liquid Chromatography ⟨2.01⟩. The followings are supplements to the section of system suitability prescribed in "Liquid Chromatography ⟨2.01⟩".

2.1. System repeatability of HPLC and GC

2.1.1. Allowable limit of system repeatability

It is described in the section of system suitability in "Liquid Chromatography ⟨2.01⟩" that "In principle, total number of replicate injections should be 6", and "The allowable limit of "System repeatability" should be set at an appropriate level based on the data when suitability of the method for the evaluation of quality of the drug was verified, and the precision necessary for the quality test". Based on the above description, an allowable limit of system repeatability for 6 replicate injections should be set in consideration with the following descriptions. However, in the case that the test method prescribed in the JP monograph is used for the test, the allowable limit of system repeatability prescribed in the monograph should be applied.

(i) Assay for drug substance (for drug substance with the content nearby 100%): An adequate allowable limit should be set at the level that the chromatographic system is able to give the precision suitable for the evaluation of variation in the content of active ingredient within and among the batches of drug substance. For example, the allowable limit of "not more than 1.0%" is usually recommended for the drug substances whose width of content specification are not more than 5%, as is in the case of content specification of 98.0 – 102.0% which is often observed in the assay using liquid chromatography.

(ii) Assay for drug products: An adequate allowable limit should be set considering the width of content specification of the drug product and the allowable limit prescribed in the assay of drug substance (when the drug product is analyzed by a method with the same chromatographic conditions as those used for the analysis of drug substance).

(iii) Purity test for related substances: An adequate allowable limit should be set considering the concentration of active ingredients in the solution used for the system suitability testing. In the case that a solution with active ingredient concentration of 0.5 – 1.0% is used for the test of system repeatability, an allowable limit of "not more than 2.0%" is usually recommended.

Recommendations for allowable limits described above should not be applicable to gas chromatography.

2.1.2. Method for decreasing the number of replicate injections without losing the quality of system repeatability testing

It is described in the section of system suitability in "Liquid Chromatography ⟨2.01⟩" that "In principle, total number of replicate injections should be 6. However, in the case that a long time is necessary for one analysis, such as the analysis using the gradient method, or the analysis of samples containing late eluting components, it may be acceptable to decrease the number of replicate injections by adopt-

Supplement I, JP XVIII *General Information* 2935

ing new allowable limit of "System repeatability" which can guarantee a level of "System repeatability" equivalent to that at 6 replicate injections." In consideration of the above description, a method for decreasing the number of replicate injections without losing the quality of system repeatability testing is described below. By utilizing this method, if necessary, one can set the test for system repeatability with reduced number of replicate injections and can change the number once being set.

The following table shows the allowable limits to be attained in the test at 3 – 5 replicate injections ($n = 3 - 5$) to keep the quality test equivalent to that of test at $n = 6$.

However, it should be kept in mind that decrease in the number of replicate injections results in increase in the weight of each injection and it becomes more important to maintain the equipment in a suitable state.

Table Allowable limits to be attained in the test at 3 – 5 replicate injections ($n = 3 - 5$) to keep the quality of test equivalent to that of test at $n = 6^*$

		Allowable limit (RSD)					
Allowable limit prescribed in the test of $n = 6$		1.0%	2.0%	3.0%	4.0%	5.0%	10.0%
Allowable limit to be attained	$n = 5$	0.88%	1.76%	2.64%	3.52%	4.40%	8.81%
	$n = 4$	0.72%	1.43%	2.15%	2.86%	3.58%	7.16%
	$n = 3$	0.47%	0.95%	1.42%	1.89%	2.37%	4.73%

* The probability for inadequate analytical systems to meet the requirements of system suitability testing, is supposed to be 5%.

Delete the following monograph:

Near Infrared Spectrometry
⟨G1-3-161⟩

Add the following:

Instrumental Measurement of Coloration of Liquids ⟨G1-4-181⟩

This test is harmonized with the European Pharmacopoeia and the U.S. Pharmacopeia.

The parts of the text that are not harmonized among the targeted texts for the harmonization are marked with symbols (♦ ♦), and the texts that are uniquely specified by the JP other than the targeted texts for the harmonization are marked with symbols (◇ ◇).

Information on the harmonization with the European Pharmacopoeia and the U.S. Pharmacopeia is available on the website of the Pharmaceuticals and Medical Devices Agency.

1. Principle

The observed color of an object depends primarily on its light absorbing characteristics. However a variety of conditions such as light-source differences, spectral energy of the illuminant, visual sensitivity of the observer, size differences, background differences and directional differences affect the perception of color. Hue, lightness or brightness and saturation are three attributes of the color. Instrumental measurement under defined conditions allows numerical expression of a color. The base of any instrumental measurement of color is that the human eye has been shown to detect color via three types of receptors.

Instrumental methods for measurement of color provide more objective data than the subjective viewing of colors by a small number of individuals. With adequate maintenance and calibration, instrumental methods can provide accurate, precise and consistent measurements of color that do not drift with time. Through extensive color matching experiments with human subjects having normal color vision, distribution coefficients (weighting factors) have been measured for each wavelength within the wavelength range of the visible spectrum, giving the relative amount of stimulation of each receptor type caused by the light of that wavelength. The International Commission on Illumination (CIE) has developed models taking into account the light source and the angle at which the observer is looking at the target (field of view). In a visual test for color of solution, there are requirements that lead to the use of a 2° angle and diffuse daylight. The mean sensitivity of the human eye is represented by the distribution coefficients $\bar{x}_\lambda$, $\bar{y}_\lambda$ and $\bar{z}_\lambda$ (Fig. 1).

For any color, the amount of stimulation of each receptor type is defined by the set of tristimulus values (X, Y and Z).

The relationship between the distribution coefficients and the tristimulus values (X, Y and Z) is given by the following equations, expressed in terms of integrals. ◇According to the definition in Japanese Industrial Standard Z 8120, the short wavelength limit of the visible light wavelength range can generally be considered to be between 360 – 400 nm and the long wavelength limit is between 760 – 830 nm.◇

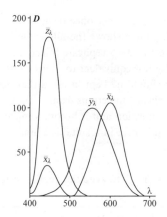

Fig. 1 Mean sensitivity of the human eye represented by distribution coefficients, CIE 2° standard observer (*D*: distribution coefficient; λ: wavelength in nm)

$$X = k \int_0^\infty f_\lambda \bar{x}_\lambda S_\lambda d\lambda$$

$$Y = k \int_0^\infty f_\lambda \bar{y}_\lambda S_\lambda d\lambda$$

$$Z = k \int_0^\infty f_\lambda \bar{z}_\lambda S_\lambda d\lambda$$

$$k = 100 / \int_0^\infty \bar{y}_\lambda S_\lambda d\lambda$$

k: normalising constant characterizing the stimulation of one receptor type and the used illumination
S_λ: relative spectral power distribution of the illuminant
$\bar{x}_\lambda$, $\bar{y}_\lambda$ and $\bar{z}_\lambda$: color matching distribution coefficients for CIE 2° Standard Observer
f_λ: spectral transmittance T_λ of the material
λ: wavelength (nm)

In practical calculations of tristimulus values, the integration is approximated by a summation, as follows:

$$X = k \sum_\lambda T_\lambda \bar{x}_\lambda S_\lambda \Delta\lambda$$

$$Y = k \sum_\lambda T_\lambda \bar{y}_\lambda S_\lambda \Delta\lambda$$

$$Z = k \sum_\lambda T_\lambda \bar{z}_\lambda S_\lambda \Delta\lambda$$

$$k = \frac{100}{\sum_\lambda S_\lambda \bar{y}_\lambda \Delta\lambda}$$

The tristimulus values can be used to calculate the CIE Lab color space coordinates: L^* (lightness or brightness), a^* (red-green) and b^* (yellow-blue); these are defined by:

$$L^* = 116 f(Y/Y_n) - 16$$
$$a^* = 500 [f(X/X_n) - f(Y/Y_n)]$$
$$b^* = 200 [f(Y/Y_n) - f(Z/Z_n)]$$

Where

$f(X/X_n) = (X/X_n)^{1/3}$ if $X/X_n > (6/29)^3$,

otherwise,

$f(X/X_n) = 841/108 (X/X_n) + 4/29$;
$f(Y/Y_n) = (Y/Y_n)^{1/3}$ if $Y/Y_n > (6/29)^3$,

otherwise,

$f(Y/Y_n) = 841/108 (Y/Y_n) + 4/29$;
$f(Z/Z_n) = (Z/Z_n)^{1/3}$ if $Z/Z_n > (6/29)^3$,

otherwise,

$f(Z/Z_n) = 841/108 (Z/Z_n) + 4/29$.

X_n, Y_n and Z_n, are the tristimulus values of *purified water*.

In the spectrophotometric method, transmittance values are obtained at discrete wavelengths throughout the visible spectrum. These values are then used to calculate the tristimulus values through the use of weighting factors $\bar{x}_\lambda$, $\bar{y}_\lambda$ and $\bar{z}_\lambda$ for a 2° Standard Observer and CIE standard illuminant C (see the International Commission on Illumination publication, CIE).

2. Spectrophotometric method

Operate a suitable spectrophotometer according to the instructions of the manufacturer and determine the transmittance *T* at least from 400 nm to 700 nm, at intervals of not greater than 10 nm. Express the result as a percentage (%). Calculate the tristimulus values *X*, *Y*, and *Z* and the color co-ordinates L^*, a^* and b^*.

3. Determination of coloration

Calibrate the instrument as per the instrument manufacturer's recommendation. System performance tests are done prior to each measurement or at regular intervals, depending on the use of the apparatus. To this purpose, use certified reference materials (Certified filters or certified standard solutions recommended by the instrument's manufacturer.) within the measurement range.

Operate the apparatus according to the manufacturer's instructions and measure the test solution and standard solution(s) under the same conditions (e.g. path length of the cuvette, temperature).

For transmittance measurements *purified water* is used as standard and assigned a transmittance of 100.0% at all wavelengths throughout the visible spectrum.

Then the weighing factors $\bar{x}_\lambda$, $\bar{y}_\lambda$ and $\bar{z}_\lambda$ for CIE standard illuminant C are used to calculate the tristimulus values corresponding to color co-ordinates $L^* = 100$, $a^* = 0$ and $b^* = 0$.

Reference measurements can be made using the color co-ordinates of *purified water* or freshly prepared matching fluids for color, or using the respective color co-ordinates stored in the instrument manufacturer's database, provided the latter have been obtained under the same testing conditions.

If the test solution is turbid or hazy, it is filtered or centrifuged. If the test solution is not filtered or centrifuged, any haziness or turbidity is reported with the results. Air

Supplement I, JP XVIII   *General Information* 2937

bubbles are to be avoided and removed.

The instrumental method is used to compare two solutions in respect to their color or color difference, or a deviation from a defined color. Calculate the color difference between the test solution t and a matching fluid for color r as ΔE^*_{tr} using the following equation:

$$E^*_{tr} = \sqrt{(\Delta L^*)^2 + (\Delta a^*)^2 + (\Delta b^*)^2}$$

where ΔL^*, Δa^* and Δb^* are the differences in colour coordinates.

Instead of the color coordinates CIE *Lab*, the colour coordinates CIE *LCh* may be used.

4. Assessment of location within the $L^*a^*b^*$ color space

Instruments may provide information on the actual location of the test solution within the $L^*a^*b^*$ color space. Using appropriate algorithms, correspondence to matching fluids for color (such as "test solution equals matching fluid for color XY", "test solution close to matching fluid for color XY" or "test solution between matching fluids for color XY and XZ") can be obtained.

Add the following:

Control Strategies and Change Control Concepts at Each Stage of Chromatography Lifecycle (Change Control in Chromatography Lifecycle) ⟨G1-5-181⟩

Analytical methods (analytical procedures) for pharmaceuticals must be set to provide test results suitable for their purpose, which must be considered throughout the lifecycle of analytical procedures, from design to development, qualification and continuous verification. In the field of drug development, particularly in the fields of manufacturing control and quality control, the effort of systematic quality assurance by quality risk assessment is implemented throughout the lifecycle (General Information "Basic Concept of Quality Risk Management" ⟨G0-2-170⟩). Effort to apply similar approaches to control strategy at each stage of the life cycle of analytical procedures are described.[1)-4)]

Various chromatographic systems are widely used for the analysis of pharmaceuticals, their components and impurities. Under these circumstances, a guide for changing analytical conditions was presented in the internationally harmonized test methods using chromatography (Chromatography ⟨2.00⟩). However, there are various causes and timings for changing analysis conditions, and the positions of these factors in the overall lifecycle should be considered when change control of analytical condition is designed. Therefore, this general information describes the outline of the methodology for establishing control strategy at each stage of a chromatography lifecycle, aiming at the efficient control of analytical procedures, including changes of ana-

lytical methods. The methodology described below does not intend to newly add or mitigate regulatory requirements, but can be apprehended as the systematic documentation of the work that has been performed in laboratories. In addition, the concept of change control described in this General Information can be used as a reference for quality tests of pharmaceuticals in public testing institutions.

1. Analytical procedures that give test results suitable for the purpose of the test

Before designing and developing an analytical procedure, the purpose and goal (target profile) for the development of the analytical procedure are provisionally set and finalized in the latter stage of the development. When chromatography is used for quantitative analysis of active ingredients, etc., an analyte must be quantified with an accuracy and a precision within a certain range including the labeled amount in the presence of impurities or excipients. In addition, quantitative tests for impurities must be able to quantify impurities with an accuracy and a precision in the presence of various components presented in a sample within a range from the reporting threshold[5)] to 120% of the specification limit. As stated in section 5, for example, an analytical procedure may be changed or an analytical procedure itself may become unnecessary due to changes in impurity profiles, etc., however, the target profile of this analytical procedure can be the indicator whether the analytical performance characteristics are appropriate over the lifecycle. Here, the analytical performance characteristics are mainly characteristics evaluated by the "validation characteristics" described in General Information "Validation of Analytical Procedures" ⟨G1-1-130⟩. (In the test methods prescribed in the Japanese Pharmacopoeia, specifications and acceptance criteria in the monographs can be a target profile.)

2. Design and development of the draft procedure of chromatography

When the target profile of an analytical procedure is proposed, the draft of the analytical procedure is designed based on this profile, and the analytical procedure is established. In the process of the establishment, the implementation of risk assessment deepens the understanding of sources of variability in a series of analytical operations including analytical systems and their effect on reported values. Sources of variability are investigated using a method such as a characteristic diagram (Ishikawa diagram), and the root causes are identified and eliminated. At that time, the justification of various relevant validation characteristics proposed in the target profile, such as accuracy and precision, as well as specificity and linearity that affect the accuracy and precision, is confirmed. By a series of the confirmation of the justification, the target profile of the analytical procedure is reflected in key analytical performance characteristics[1)], and at the same time, it is possible to identify sources of variability and modify the analytical method from the results of those experiments. In addition, design of experiments (DOE), etc. can be used to clarify the relationship among the sources of variability and to study the degree of the variation that can occur when the analytical procedure is conducted under different conditions. Then, the sources of variability to be controlled and the acceptable ranges are clarified, and the analytical procedure is optimized. Appropriate experimental results obtained during the establishment of the analytical procedure could be used as a substitute for validation data.

Establish a control strategy based on the results of risk assessment. Control items may also include, for example, temperature, stability of sample solution, and number of replicates as well as the requirements of system suitability as described below.

System suitability testing is set as an appropriate check test to evaluate the effect of the sources of variability remaining in the analytical procedure that cannot be controlled as variable sources of variability(e.g., pH of mobile phase and column size) (General Information "System Suitability" ⟨G1-2-181⟩). Therefore, system suitability testing should be considered as a minimum control method during the qualification stage of analytical performance described below. System suitability testing should be set to focus on the analytical performance characteristics that can be affected and to ensure that the testing is considered to meet the requirements of the target profile. For system suitability testing, for example, resolution and a symmetry factor are set.

3. Preparatory stage for qualification

A control strategy for an analytical method is proposed by the clarification of the sources of variability and accumulated knowledge, and the analytical performance is ready to be qualified.

When a test method is already prescribed in the Japanese Pharmacopoeia, based on the test method, it is necessary to understand and examine beforehand to what extent additional sources of variability exist in the laboratory where the actual analysis is conducted and to what extent advance information has been already obtained. Additional sources of variability include, for example, samples, reagents, facilities, instruments, and the number of replicates that can occur with those variations. When applying a test method prescribed in the Japanese Pharmacopoeia, in many cases analysts do not have the knowledge and understanding obtained during the development of the analytical method. Therefore, the analysts should be aware of the potential risks due to additional sources of variability and should ensure that the above risks are appropriately reduced by the qualification of the analytical performance, etc. (Column information available on the Pharmaceuticals and Medical Devices Agency website may be useful as advance information.)

4. Qualification of analytical procedure performance

The purpose of qualification is to confirm that an analytical procedure constantly meets a target profile in a routinely used laboratory. For qualification testing, a protocol is prepared and the test is performed according to the procedure manual and appropriate control. As the result of the test, for example, when the variation of the reported values may

exceed the requirements in the target profile, examine whether the control strategy is optimized for the laboratory, identify the sources of variability, and the control strategy of the analytical method may be improved or revised. If an analytical method was developed in a routinely used laboratory, the qualification of analytical performance could be omitted.

Even when applying a test method prescribed in the Japanese Pharmacopoeia, different control strategies are required for different laboratories and instruments. For qualification in the laboratory where a test method prescribed in the Japanese Pharmacopoeia is performed, the process of the quality risk management of the analytical method should be considered to meet the intended target profiles of specifications and acceptance criteria in each monograph.

In the qualification when applying test methods prescribed in the Japanese Pharmacopoeia, it is not essential to perform the verification of the validity of validation characteristics again to the same extent when establishing the analytical procedures, however, it is necessary to confirm the qualification using appropriate validation characteristics listed in General Information "Validation of Analytical Procedures" ⟨G1-1-130⟩. The content of the implementation should consider the type of analytical procedures, related instruments, etc. In addition, consideration should be given to factors derived from test samples. For example, when applying a test method prescribed in the Japanese Pharmacopoeia, impurities that may differ depending on a drug substance or drug product can affect the "specificity" of the test method. When resolution is set in the system suitability testing, confirm the effect by the resolution, and if the specificity is reduced, examine the effect on the test result. If the analytical performance deteriorates, it will be necessary to examine the analytical conditions. In addition, since different excipients in drug products may affect interference with a substance to be analyzed (specificity), detection (detection limit), recovery (accuracy) and variation in quantitative values (precision), perform the qualification using system suitability testing and appropriate validation characteristics described in General Information "Validation of Analytical Procedures" ⟨G1-1-130⟩.

5. Continuous verification of Analytical Methods

1) Routine monitoring: At this stage, data on the performance of analytical procedures, such as analytical results, suitability for system suitability, deviations from specifications and specific trends, are collected and analyzed. If nonconformity to the system suitability, deviation from the specification, or a specific trend becomes clear, it is necessary to examine the cause and take corrective and preventive measures.

2) Change of analytical procedures: As with the manufacture of pharmaceuticals, analytical procedures may be changed for the activity of continual improvement and for analysis in different environments. When newly applying a test method prescribed in the Japanese Pharmacopoeia, it may be necessary to change the procedure according to

Supplement I, JP XVIII   *General Information*   2939

the current equipment or columns. Furthermore, it is expected that an analytical method will need to be changed as the result of routine monitoring described in 1). Depending on the extent of the change, the contents and amount of work for evaluating the effect of the change on the test results vary. Examples of possible changes are shown below.

① When an analytical procedure is changed within the acceptable range of the procedure evaluated at the time of the development of the analytical procedure, it is necessary to evaluate the effect on a case-by-case basis and confirm that the changed procedure always meets the target profile. (However, this does not apply when such acceptable range has not been examined at the time of the development of the analytical method.) Even if the change of each condition is within the acceptable range, when multiple conditions are changed, it may be necessary to take similar measures as the following ②.

② When an analytical procedure is changed beyond the acceptable range of variability of the procedure evaluated at the time of the development of the analytical method, risk assessment is required. In addition, if the acceptable range of changes has not been examined by quality risk management at the time of the development of the analytical method, risk assessment is required when changing the analytical conditions. When conducting risk assessment, consider which analytical performance characteristics (validation characteristics) can be affected by the change. Then, qualification is performed to confirm that the analytical performance does not deviate from the target profile (refer to 4). Specifically, verify using validation characteristics that may be affected by the change among validation characteristics listed in General Information "Validation of Analytical Procedures" *⟨G1-1-130⟩*. When validation characteristics that may be affected by a change are set as one item of system suitability testing, the validation characteristics may be verified by using the system suitability testing. Further, when changing a column size and the composition of a mobile phase in chromatography, verify analytical performance appropriately, referring to "Adjustment of Chromatographic Conditions" in Chromatography *⟨2.00⟩*.

③ When a laboratory is changed or a test method prescribed in the Japanese Pharmacopoeia is newly applied, the analytical performance characteristics may be affected by the change in analytical instruments, analysts, reagents, etc., so perform risk assessment and appropriate qualification (refer to 3 and 4). On the other hand, when updating analytical equipment or columns or replacing analysts in a same laboratory, at least perform system suitability testing with the changed analytical system to confirm that the same results are obtained before and after the change.

④ When changing to a new analytical procedure or technology, qualification must be performed during the development of the new analytical procedure (refer to 2, 3 and 4) to demonstrate that the new procedure meets the target profile.

⑤ When a change that affects a target profile (e.g., changes in specifications, changes to methods for determining the amount of a new analyte, such as impurities that were not considered in the original target profile) is required, it may be necessary to review the current analytical procedure and qualification to update the target profile and assess whether the analytical procedure meets the requirements of the new target profile (refer to 1, 2, 3 and 4).

The extent of work to confirm whether a change in an analytical method gives a test result suitable for the purpose depends on ① risk associated with the change, ② knowledge obtained about the analytical procedure, and ③ control strategies. Whatever changes are made, perform more or less risk assessment to ensure that the changed analytical procedure provides the results that meet the purpose of the test method (i.e., within the range specified in the target profile).

6. References
1) G.P. Martin, et al., Pharmacopeial Forum 39 (5), 2013
2) Proposed New USP General Chapter: The Analytical Procedure Lifecycle ⟨1220⟩, Pharmacopeial Forum 43 (1), 2017
3) K.L. Barnett, et al., Pharmacopeial Forum 42 (5), 2016
4) E. Kovacs, et al., Pharmacopeial Forum 42 (5), 2016
5) ICH: Guideline for Q3A (R2), Impurities in New Drug Substances.

G2   Solid-state Properties

Add the following:

Measurement of Powder Flow Properties by Shear Cell Methods
⟨G2-5-181⟩

In the manufacturing of pharmaceuticals, a large number of processes involve powder transfer and feeding such as putting raw materials into a mixer and filling a powder into the mortar of a tableting machine. Since powder flowability is related to preparation characteristics such as mass and content uniformity, it greatly affects the product quality. It is important to evaluate powder flow properties in the design of formulations, processes and pharmaceutical production equipment. Since shear cell methods are among the most important methods for measuring powder flow properties and can be performed under a wide variety of stress conditions, parameters useful for predicting various powder behaviors during the manufacturing of pharmaceuticals, such as an angle of critical state line, unconfined yield strength and flow factor, can be determined.

1. Principle

A powder in a hopper, etc. may not immediately flow due to adhesion/coagulation of particles and interference to the mutual motion by complex surface shape when shear stresses are applied from the outside. When a sufficiently large shear stress is attained, the powder suddenly starts to flow. In addition, powder flow under quasi-static conditions such as flow in a bin strongly depends on the consolidation stresses. Consolidation is an operation to apply a load to a powder bed to reduce the bulk volume to change the bulk density or the void fraction of the powder bed. The shear cell methods are the tests to determine the flow properties of a powder in the process of transition from a static state to a non-static state when the powder is sheared by applying a normal stress. In other words, a maximum shear stress immediately before fail and a dynamic friction force in a steady-state flow are measured.

Powder flowability under compressed conditions is governed by three factors: the degree of consolidation (bulk density or void fraction, ε), normal stress (σ) and shear stress (τ). A three dimensional representation of the applied normal stress, shear stress and void fraction is called the Roscoe condition diagram (Fig. 1), and the shear cell methods are test methods to obtain the Roscoe condition diagram or yield loci which constitute the Roscoe condition diagram.

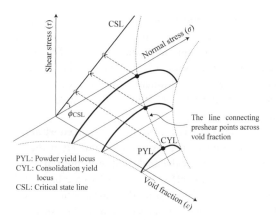

Fig. 1 Roscoe condition diagram

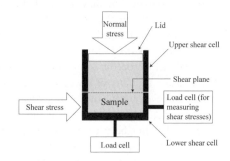

Fig. 2 Example of translational shear cell

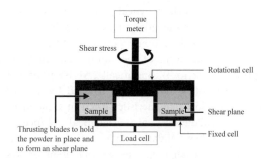

Fig. 3 Example of rotational shear cell

2. Apparatus

The shear cell methods can be performed under constant load or constant volume conditions. In both conditions, apparatuses typically consist of a shear cell, weights or a press machine for applying normal stress to a sample, a mechanism for shearing a sample, and load cells for measuring normal stresses and shear stresses.

2.1. Shear cell

Many shear cells have the structure which can make a shear plane somewhere in a powder bed by shearing a powder filled in a container dividable into two parts, upper and lower cells, while applying a normal stress. In the constant load conditions, a lid that fits within an upper cell is free to move up and down when a shear stress is applied, and the volume of the powder container changes. In the constant volume conditions, the position of the lid is fixed by pressing the lid with a press machine, etc.

The shear cells are classified into two types according to the motion that provides a shear stress; translational or rotational.

2.1.1. Translational shear cell

In the translational shear cell, one of the upper and lower cells is fixed and the other is moved horizontally (translationally) to apply a shear stress to the powder bed filled in the two cells. The shear plane forms at the boundary between the powder contained in the lower cell and the powder contained in the upper ring cell. Some translational shear cells are cylindrical (Fig. 2), and others are sandwiching a sample between two plates on top and bottom and with no side walls. The representative example of the former is the Jenike shear cell, and that of the latter is a parallel-plate cell.

2.1.2. Rotational shear cell

In the rotational shear cell, one of the upper and lower cells is fixed, and the other is rotated to apply a shear stress to the powder bed filled in the two cells. Some rotational shear cells are cylindrical and others are annular (Fig. 3). Any rotational shear cells usually have surface features that prevent the powder from sliding at the cell surface. Several blades are radially attached on the side of the shear cell where it contacts the sample, so that the powder is hold in place by the thrusting blades. A shear plane forms in the powder bed directly under the blades when the shear cell is rotated.

2.2. Other components

A load cell is a device using a spring, a piezoelectric element, etc. to detect a load or torque and converts the applied force into an electrical signal. The load cells and weights for applying a normal stress to a sample must be regularly calibrated with standards with measurement

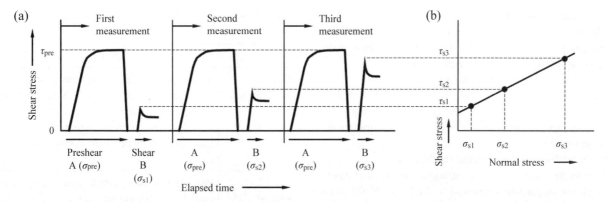

Fig. 4 Plots of shear stress versus time during the test procedure (a) and corresponding powder yield locus (b)

traceability.

3. Measurement

A temperature of 20 ± 5°C and a relative humidity of 50 ± 10% are recommended as measurement environment. A fresh powder samples should be used for each test. However, this does not apply to samples clearly having no consolidation history or rare samples, if the description of their reuse is recorded. Gently fill the shear cell with a sample of powder using a spatula or a sieve with an opening size larger than the maximum particle size of the sample. At this time, care should be taken not to form cavities in the powder bed. The surface of the filled sample is leveled with a spatula, etc. Under the constant load conditions, first the powder sample is consolidated (preshear) in order to perform a test with a desired constant void fraction during one measurement.

The test procedure under constant load conditions using the Jenike shear cell, etc. is shown in Fig. 4 by a pattern diagram. Prior to a test, the powder sample is sheared with applying a preconsolidation stress (σ_{pre}) until a shear stress reaches a steady value (τ_{pre}) for preshear (Fig. 4 (a) A). Under the constant load conditions, the volume of powder can decrease or increase during the preshear and becomes constant when a steady-state is achieved. In other words, the void fraction of the powder bed where the shear stress became constant under certain normal stress conditions is uniquely determined by the powder flow properties. In the following main test, measurements are performed on the sample having this void fraction. After the shear stress is reduced to zero, the normal stress acting on the sample is decreased from σ_{pre} to a new value (σ_{sx}, $x = 1, 2, 3\cdots$) for the next step of the test procedure (Fig. 4 (a) B). When the shear stress is gradually increased, the maximum shear stress measured immediately before the consolidated powder starts to flow is τ_{sx} ($x = 1, 2, 3\cdots$). The A-B procedure is repeated at 3 to 5 points of σ_{sx} which is less than the normal stress at preshear (σ_{pre}), and the powder yield locus (PYL, Fig. 4 (b)) is obtained by plotting the results.

On the other hand, under the constant volume conditions, shear stresses are continuously measured with progressively changing a normal stress while the void fraction is kept at a specified value by a press machine, etc. con-

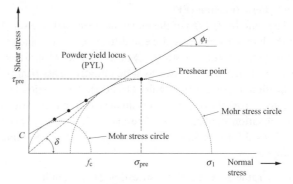

Fig. 5 Graphical representation of various parameters obtainable from PYL

trolling the lid position. Since the void fraction is constant under the constant volume conditions, the consolidation yield locus (CYL) in Fig. 1 is obtained during the process of consolidation failure. The PYL and CYL share a preshear point and are combined to form a single yield locus (YL).

4. Data analysis

Shear stresses can be measured in both states where a powder is not flowing (static state) and where a powder is flowing (dynamic state).

The approximate line connecting the points (σ_{sx}, τ_{sx}) shown in Fig. 4 (b) represents the relationship between the shear stress and normal stress immediately before the consolidated powder sample starts to fail, namely, the relationship in a static state, and is referred to as a PYL. Further, the point (σ_{pre}, τ_{pre}), where the shear stress τ_{pre} reached constant by applying the preshear normal stress σ_{pre}, is added to Fig. 4 (b) (Fig. 5). This point is measured in a dynamic state and is called a preshear point. Next, two circles having a center on the normal stress axis are drawn: The first is a circle passing through the preshear point and tangential to the PYL (the larger semicircle in Fig. 5). The second is a circle passing through the origin and tangential to the PYL (the smaller semicircle in Fig. 5). The circles having a center on the normal stress axis and tangential to a PYL are called the Mohr stress circles.

Various parameters that describe powder flowability can be obtained from a PYL and Mohr stress circles.

4.1. Shearing cohesion (C)

The failure shear stress at zero normal stress, normally obtained by extrapolation of the PYL. An indication of the intrinsic strength of an unconfined powder.

4.2. Angle of internal friction (φ_i)

The angle formed by the PYL and the σ axis. The inclination (tan φ_i) of the PYL indicates the internal friction between the powder particles under the consolidation conditions measured.

4.3. Effective angle of internal friction (δ)

The angle formed by the straight line which passes through the origin and tangential to the larger Mohr stress circle in Fig. 5, and the σ axis. The angle may be used as a relative indication of the internal friction when the powder flow is in a steady-state.

4.4. Flow function (FF)

The ratio (σ_1/f_c: ff_c) of the maximum principal stress (σ_1) of the larger Mohr stress circle and the maximum principal stress (uniaxial collapse stress: f_c) of the smaller Mohr stress circle in Fig. 5 may be used as a quantitative classification indication of powder flowability (Table 1). A regression line obtained from the σ_1-f_c relationship measured under various consolidation conditions for one material, which is called FF, is used for powder flow analysis such as when designing a hopper.

Table 1 General classification of flowability

ff_c	Flowability
< 1	Not flowing
1 – 2	Very cohesive, difficult-flowing
2 – 4	Cohesive, slightly difficult-flowing
4 – 10	Easy-flowing
10 <	Free-flowing

It should be noted that even a same powder shows different flowability if the degree of consolidation is different because the above parameters can be determined from Fig. 5 where the measurements were performed with a sample having one specified void fraction.

On the other hand, the critical state line (CSL) in Fig. 1 is obtained by projecting the preshear points (black circles in the figure), which are determined from several samples having a different void fraction, onto the σ-τ plane, and is a straight line passing through the origin. Since the CSL shows the normal stress-shear stress relationship in a dynamic state, it reflects the powder flow properties without depending on the type of apparatus used for measurement. The angle formed by the CSL and the σ axis is called the angle of critical state line (φ_{CSL}); the smaller the value, the higher the flowability.

5. Report of results

Measurements under the same conditions are repeated an appropriate number of times according to the variation in the obtained values, and the average value is reported along with the items listed in Table 2.

Table 2 Examples of items to be described in the report of results

Item	Content
General information	Measurement date/time, name of operator, sample name, apparatus used (type, model/manufacturing company) and type of cells, measurement method (constant load method or constant volume method), etc.
Sample-related information	Particle size and particle size distribution, method of particle size measurement, bulk density, water content, conditions for drying, etc.
Measurement conditions	Temperature and relative humidity during measurements, size of cells used, sample amount, preconsolidation conditions, shear rate, etc.
Results	Normal stress and shear stress of each measurement in the main test, σ-τ plot showing yield locus, various parameters obtained by the analysis of angle of critical state line, etc.
Other special notes	Descriptions when the measurement conditions such as the preconsolidation stress and the number of measurements are changed from the normal setting, or when the sample is reused, etc.

G4 Microorganisms

Add the following:

Biorisk Management of the Handling of Microorganisms in Microbial Tests ⟨G4-11-181⟩

This general information describes basic requirements in the safe handling of microorganisms to be considered in performing the microbial tests in the General Tests (4.02 Microbial Assay for Antibiotics, 4.05 Microbiological Examination of Non-sterile Products, 4.06 Sterility Test), the Test for Crude Drugs (5.02 Microbial Limit Test for Crude Drugs and Preparations containing Crude Drugs and Preparations containing Crude Drugs as Main Ingredient), the tests in the General Information G3 Biotechnological/Biological products (Basic Requirements for Viral Safety of Biotechnological/Biological Products listed in Japanese Pharmacopoeia ⟨G3-13-141⟩ and Mycoplasma Testing for Cell Substrates used for the Production of Biotechnological/Biological Products ⟨G3-14-170⟩) and the tests in General Information G4 Microorganisms (Preser-

Supplement I, JP XVIII *General Information* 2943

vatives-Effectiveness Tests <*G4-3-170*>, Rapid Microbial Methods <*G4-6-170*>, Rapid Identification of Microorganisms Based on Molecular Biological Method <*G4-7-160*>, Rapid Counting of Microbes using Fluorescent Staining <*G4-8-152*> and Disinfection and Decontamination Methods <*G4-9-170*>).

In the work of handling microorganisms, it is required to manage accurately biorisk generated by performing tests. Since risks while handling microorganisms vary depending on the characteristics of microorganisms and the contents of work handled, it is necessary to perform risk assessment for each work to identify, analyze and evaluate the risks, to protect workers handling microorganisms and also to reduce risks in laboratory biosafety and biosecurity. In the practice, a responsible person and a person in charge related to biorisk management should be assigned in the organization, and rules and plans for the operation should be established by them. In order to reduce risk, measures for laboratory biosafety should be performed by combining four elements: safety control, personal protective equipment, safety equipment, and physical containment facilities/equipment. The established risk management method should be updated through continuous risk reviews[1].

The basic concept necessary for biorisk management in the handling of microorganisms is shown below.

1. Explanation of terms

The definitions of terms used in this general information are as follows.

1.1. Laboratory: Facilities/equipment that handle microorganisms for the purpose of performing experiments for inspection, testing, studies, etc.

1.2. Biohazard: A disaster caused by organisms and biological products.

1.3. Classification of microbiological risk level: A classification of the risk of microorganisms to workers handling microorganisms and related persons.

1.4. Laboratory Biosafety: Risk mitigation measures according to biohazard risks are called biosafety. The purpose is to prevent the unintentional exposure, spread and accidental leaks of pathogens or toxins. Among them, laboratory biosafety should be performed by combining four elements, safety control, personal protective equipment, safety equipment and physical containment facilities/equipment.

1.5. Laboratory Biosafety Level (BSL): BSLs are classified from BSL1 to BSL4 by combining the four elements that practice laboratory biosafety, and risk mitigation measures according to each BSL should be constructed.

1.6. Biosecurity: Biosecurity means prevention and control in laboratories in order to protect unauthorized access, loss, theft, overuse, misuse, diversion and intentional release of Valuable Biological Materials which need protection/monitoring.

1.7. Biorisk: Biorisk is the merged risk of laboratory biosafety and biosecurity, and includes all probability and chance where harmful events (accidental infection, unauthorized access, loss, theft, overuse, misuse, diversion or intentional release) will occur.

1.8. Biorisk Management: Biorisk management consists of three elements: risk assessment, risk mitigation and performance.

1.9. Worker handling microorganisms: A person who handles microorganisms directly in a laboratory and a person who enters a laboratory to maintain laboratory facilities.

1.10. Related person: A person who has a possibility of infection, such as a laboratory user who contact with a worker handling microorganisms, a colleague or a housemate of a worker handling microorganisms.

1.11. Good Microbiological Technique (GMT): Standard techniques for the safe handling of microorganisms. It includes the preparation of educational programs for acquiring technology, standard work procedures and rules.

1.12. Personal Protective Equipment (PPE): A set of tools worn by individuals to protect workers handling microorganisms against exposure of biohazardous substances. For example, masks, respiratory protection tools, goggles, gloves, protective clothing, shoe covers, etc.

1.13. Safety Equipment: A set of apparatus, instruments, and devices that protects workers handling microorganisms from exposure to biohazardous substances. For example, electric pipettes, sealed containers, biological safety cabinets, etc. A biological safety cabinet is to protect workers, laboratory environment and work materials from exposure to infectious aerosols. There are mainly two types, an opened type which isolates the inside and outside by air barrier and a sealed glove box type.

1.14. Physical containment facilities/equipment: Physical containment facilities/equipment are classified into 4, physical containment level P1, P2, P3, and P4. The object of the facilities/equipment is to provide workers with safe handling of hazardous substance according to the classification of the risk level.

1.15. Controlled area: An area where biorisk management is required. The area includes not only laboratories for handling microorganisms, but also waste treatment facilities/equipment, wastewater treatment facilities/equipment, air conditioning machine rooms, etc. that have biohazard risk.

2. Risk assessment in handling microorganisms

The following risks accompanying the handling of microorganisms in each execution plan of tests should be evaluated.

2.1. Risks concerning with laboratory biosafety

2.1.1. Risks due to the characteristics of microorganisms

(i) Risks based on the classification of microbiological risk level

Microorganisms have a different extent of harm to humans depending on their species or strain. Considering the symptoms of workers handling microorganisms when infected with microorganisms and impact on related persons, microorganisms are classified to the microbiological risk levels 1 to 4 (Table 1) in descending order of the risk. The classification of individual microbiological risk level differs according to country/region, target (human or livestock), presence of therapeutics or prophylaxis, minimum infective dose, route of infection, amount used, work contents, etc. Microorganisms that do not exist in Japan are often classified as high risk levels, when it is handled in Japan.

(ii) Risks due to the routes of microbial infection and exposure

Consider both the infectious route of microorganisms used and the supposed exposure to workers according to handling methods. In natural infection, oral cavity, nasal cavity and ocular mucosa are likely to be routes of infection, and contact with mucosa, oral infection, droplet infection, aerial infection, presence of insect vectors, etc. should be considered. In laboratory infection, attention should be paid to needle-stick infection, infection from skin wounds, and infection caused by contact with contaminants such as laboratory tools.

(iii) Risk due to host sensitivity

The different risks of susceptibility of workers handling microorganisms to microorganism should be considered. As a preventive measure for infection, vaccination can provide resistance to workers handling microorganisms and reduce the risk of infection.

(iv) Risks by using microorganisms specified in relevant laws and regulations

When using, possessing, storing and transporting microbial species, strains and toxins specified by the laws[2-5], comply with the relevant laws. For general matters, refer to the laws, notices and administrative communications that describe them in detail.

2.1.2. Risks from handling operations

(i) Risks due to the form and amount of microorganisms handled

Pipetting and other laboratory operations often generate droplets and aerosol, and aerosol containing microorganisms have a high risk of being diffused extensively by air currents. Take into account that as the amount of microorganisms and toxins handled increases, the associated risks increase.

(ii) Risks due to the skill of workers handling microorganisms

Consider that work by persons who do not have sufficient knowledge about microorganisms to be handled or who have not received sufficient education and training on how to handle microorganisms appropriately becomes to be high risk.

(iii) Risk due to the shape of tools handled

Considering that using glassware for work increases not only the risk of contamination due to breakage but also the risk of infection through wounds caused by breakages, examine the purpose when using glassware.

(iv) Risks accompanying work contents

Consider that opening containers containing liquid or a powder, handling liquid using a pipette or pipetter, stirring liquid with a vortex mixer or transporting a supernatant after centrifugation to another container may increase the risk of generating aerosol.

(v) Risks in each work process

If there are multiple work processes, consider that the risk varies depending on the work contents of each process.

(vi) Risks on accepting/dispensing microorganisms

Consider new risks arising from the acceptance and dispensation of microorganisms, strains and toxins.

(vii) Risks on transporting microorganisms

When transporting samples containing microorganisms, consider that the risk (impact on external) differs between transporting within controlled areas and transporting to the outside of controlled areas.

(viii) Risk of infectious wastes

All tools and samples contaminated with microorganisms during work should be handled as infectious waste having the risk of infection until they are decontaminated (disinfection or sterilization) to inactivate microorganisms.

(ix) Risks in case of emergency

Consider emergency response when workers handling microorganisms are exposed to microorganisms, contamination of facilities/equipment, leakage of microorganisms to the outside of facilities, etc.

2.2. Risks concerning with biosecurity

When entrance management to microorganism handling facilities and a storage management method of microorganisms are not properly carried out, illegal access to microorganisms, loss, theft, overuse, misuse, diversion, intentional release, etc. become risks in biosecurity.

3. Risk mitigation measures in handling microorganisms

For each risk clarified by evaluation, necessary measures should be taken to reduce the risk to workers handling microorganisms and related persons. The following contents are necessary.

3.1. Establishment of biorisk management system

Institutions that possess and handle microorganisms are required to establish a management organization for biorisk management regardless of the number of workers handling microorganisms[6-8].

- Clarify roles, authorities, and responsibilities in the management organization.
- Assign a responsible person for biorisk management.
- Assign a person in charge of biorisk management.
- Establish rules and plans for biorisk management.

The contents to be performed include the following.

- Reduce risks in laboratory biosafety.
- Reduce risks in biosecurity.
- Carry out education and training for biorisk.
- Establish and carry out a maintenance plan for facilities/equipment in controlled areas.
- Comply with relevant laws and regulations.

3.2. Mitigation of risks concerning with laboratory biosafety

There are four main elements in risk mitigation measures concerning handling microorganisms: safety control, personal protective equipment, safety instruments/devices and physical containment facilities/equipment. Reduce risks by performing laboratory biosafety measures (Table 2) that combine the four elements according to biorisk[9].

(i) Safety Management

Safety management includes all related matters and requires the following:

- Establish rules for various items necessary for the safe

Supplement I, JP XVIII *General Information* 2945

handling of microorganisms.
- Prepare standard operation procedures based on good microbiological technique (GMT).
- Continue education and training in order to learn good microbiological technique (GMT).
- If there are effective preventive measures such as vaccines against microorganisms to be used for the health management of workers handling microorganisms, introduce a system to utilize the vaccination history of workers handling microorganisms.
- Establish emergency measures.
- Carry out education and training for biorisk.

(ii) Personal protective equipment

Use appropriate personal protective equipment (PPE) during work to reduce the risk of microbial exposure. Select the appropriate personal protective equipment (PPE) according to the characteristics and infectious routes of microorganisms to be handled, and work contents.

(iii) Safety equipment

Use an electric pipette, etc., so that workers handling microorganisms do not contact with microorganisms directly. Use non-leaking tools/devices made of materials that are not easily damaged. When disposing sharp tools such as injection needles, dispose them in containers (such as needle collection containers) that do not allow them to penetrate.

Microorganisms should be handled in biological safety cabinets, etc. to reduce the risks of exposure to microorganisms contained in aerosol generated and their spread to workplaces. For samples with high risk of aerosol infection, use a centrifuge applied with measures to confine aerosol. Safety equipments used in a biological safety cabinet should be taken out after decontamination in the biological safety cabinet.

Microorganisms (including bacterial spores and fungal spores) should not be handled in a clean-bench etc. where containment capability is not guaranteed.

(iv) Physical containment facilities/equipment

Define a risk level by risk assessment based on the characteristics of microorganisms and work contents, and use necessary physical containment facilities/equipment. For facilities/equipment there are requirements specified for each containment level[10,11], and facilities/equipment being physical containment level 3 (P3) or higher are required to take effective measures to prevent workers handling microorganisms from exposure by aerosol containing microorganisms generated during work and to prevent leakage to surrounding areas.

(v) Risk mitigation at the time of accepting/dispensing microorganisms

Comply with the relevant laws[2-5] when accepting and dispensing microorganisms. When accepting new microorganisms in an institution, the institution should define a laboratory biosafety level (BSL) by assessing the microbiological risks, and determine in advance necessary items such as measures for emergency and exposure. Before dispensing, check the laboratory biosafety of the recipient. For general matters, refer to the laws, notices, and administrative communications, etc. that describe them in detail.

(vi) Risk mitigation on transporting microorganisms

When transporting microbial samples, take appropriate measures to prevent leakage even when transporting within controlled areas. When transporting outside the controlled areas, it is fundamental to apply triple packaging that prevents the sample from leaking[12]. Comply with the laws[2-5] when transporting outside facilities.

(vii) Risk mitigation of infectious wastes

Inactivate infectious wastes absolutely by disinfectants suitable for target microorganisms or by autoclaving. Inactivation treatment should be completed within a controlled area.

(viii) Risk mitigation in case of emergency

Document appropriate measures in preparation for emergency such as microbial exposure or leakage. The measures should include communication methods, maintenance of a communication network, specific measures, stockpiling of necessary devices/tools, and education/training for them. Establish an organization framework to implement them.

3.3. Mitigation of risks concerning with biosecurity

Mitigation of the risk in biosecurity should include the following[13]:

(i) Access controls for workers handling microorganisms
- ID management
- Registration management of workers handling microorganisms
- locking
- Entry/exit management

(ii) Inventory control of microorganisms
- Storage and acceptance/dispense management of microorganisms

3.4. Education and training for biorisk

To improve the skills of workers handling microorganisms, perform educational training for understanding risks in handling microorganism and seafty measures for them. The characteristics of microorganisms, risks due to work, acquisition and training of good microbiological technique (GMT), emergency response, etc. are important. The education/training should be repeated.

3.5. Compliance with relevant laws and regulations

Regarding the handling of specified microorganisms, etc. in the laws[2-5], comply with the relevant laws regarding possession, management and transport of microorganisms and toxins. For general matters, refer to the laws, notices, and administrative communications, etc. that describe them in detail.

4. Review and update of biorisk management

In order to evaluate that biorisk management is functioning effectively, risk assessment, mitigation and performance are periodically reviewed and the management plan is updated. For example, the Plan-Do-Check-Action (PDCA) cycle is a method of appropriate management.

5. References

1) The Japanese Pharmacopoeia Eighteenth Edition, General information "Basic Concept of Quality Risk Management <G0-2-170>"

2) Law No. 114, 1998, "Act on the Prevention of Infectious Diseases and Medical Care for Patients with Infecti-

ous Diseases" (April 1, 1999 enforcement).

3) Law No. 166, 1950, "Act on Domestic Animal Infectious Disease Control" (Jun 1, 1951 enforcement).

4) Law No. 151, 1950, "Plant Protection Act" (May 4, 1950 enforcement).

5) Law No. 97, 2003, "Act on the Conservation and Sustainable Use of Biological Diversity through Regulations on the Use of Living Modified Organisms" (February 19, 2004 enforcement).

6) CEN (European Committee for Standardization). CWA (CEN Workshop Agreement) 15793" Laboratory biorisk management", Sep. 2011.

7) ISO/DIS 35001: 2019, Biorisk management for laboratories and other related organisations.

8) CEN (European Committee for Standardization). CWA (CEN Workshop Agreement) 16393 "Laboratory biorisk management-Guideline for the implementation of CWA 15793: 2008", Jan. 2012.

9) WHO, Laboratory biosafety manual Third Edition, 2004. ISBN 92-4-154650-6.

10) February 1, 1961, Ministry of Health, Labour and Welfare Ordinance No. 2 "Regulations for Buildings and Facilities for Pharmacies", Article 8 "Buildings and Facilities of Manufacturing Sites for Manufacturers of Specified Biological Drugs"

11) December 24, 2004, Ministry of Health, Labour and Welfare Ordinance No. 179 "Ministerial Ordinance on Standards for Manufacturing Control and Quality Control of Pharmaceuticals and Quasi-drugs" Chapter 2 Section 4 "Manufacturing Management and Quality Control of Biological Drugs".

12) WHO, Guidance on regulations for the Transport of Infectious Substances 2013-2014.

13) WHO, Biorisk management: Laboratory biosecurity guidance, 2006.

Supplement I, JP XVIII *General Information*

Table 1 Classification of microbiological risk level

Microbiological risk level	criteria
1	There is no or low risk for workers handling microorganisms and related persons. A microorganism that is unlikely to cause human and animal disease (those that do not cause disease to healthy humans).
2	Moderate risk for workers handling microorganisms and low risk for related persons. It can cause disease if it infects humans or animals, but it is unlikely to cause serious health damage to workers handling microorganisms and related persons. There are effective treatments and preventive measures, and low risk of spread to related persons. Many people already have acquired immunity to it and the infection can be easily prevented.
3	High risk for workers handling microorganisms, low risk for related persons. Infection with humans or animals causes serious disease, but is usually less likely to be transmitted from infected persons to related persons. There are effective treatments and preventive measures.
4	High risk to workers handling microorganisms and related persons. Infecting humans or animals can cause serious disease, and transmission from infected persons to related persons can occur directly or indirectly. Usually there is no effective treatment or preventive measures.

Table 2 Classification of laboratory biosafety Level (BSL) and measures

BSL classification	Safety management	Personal protective equipment	Safety equipment	Facility/ equipment (physical containment level)
BSL1	GMT and management system (management organization, handling procedures, education/ training)	Personal protective equipment	Safety equipment	P1 (Basic laboratory)
BSL2	Standard microbial handling procedures corresponding to the microbiological risk level 2, in addition to the requirements of BSL1	In addition to the requirements of BSL1, personal protective equipment complying with the microbiological risk level 2	Safety equipment complying with the microbiological risk level 2, in addition to the requirements of BSL1	P2 (Basic laboratory complying with the microbiological risk level 2)
BSL3	Dedicated standard microbial handling procedures corresponding to the microbiological risk level 3, in addition to BSL2 requirements	In addition to the requirements of BSL2, dedicated personal protective equipment complying with the microbiological risk level 3	Dedicated safety equipment complying with the microbiological risk level 3, In addition to BSL2 requirements	P3 (physical containment laboratory)
BSL4	Dedicated standard microbial handling procedures corresponding to the microbiological risk level 4, in addition to the requirements of BSL3	In addition to the requirements of BSL3, dedicated personal protective equipment complying with the microbiological risk level 4	Dedicated safety equipment complying with the microbiological risk level 4, in addition to the requirements of BSL3	P4 (high grade physical containment laboratory)

Comprehensive risk management methods are classified from BSL1 to BSL4 according to each microbiological risk level, and measures are added and strengthened in order according to newly generated and concerned risks as the BSL value increases. In particular, BSL3 and BSL4 require the use of dedicated good microbiological technique, personal protective equipment and safety equipment.

G5   Crude Drugs

On the Scientific Names of Crude Drugs listed in the JP ⟨G5-1-181⟩

Change the following as follows:

Scientific Names used in the JP and Those being used Taxonomically

Crude Drug	Scientific names used in the JP = Scientific names being used taxonomically (Combined notation, Standard form for author or authors) / Scientific names that are different from those written in JP but identical to them taxonomically or being regarded as identical, and typical sub-classified groups belonging to their species. The names marked with "*" are those being written together in JP.	Family
Akebia Stem モクツウ	*Akebia quinata* Decaisne = *Akebia quinata* (Thunb. ex Houtt.) Decne.	Lardizabalaceae
	Akebia trifoliata Koidzumi = *Akebia trifoliata* (Thunb.) Koidz.	
	Interspecific hybrid between above species	
Clove チョウジ Clove Oil チョウジ油	*Syzygium aromaticum* Merrill et L. M. Perry = *Syzygium aromaticum* (L.) Merr. & L. M. Perry	Myrtaceae
	* *Eugenia caryophyllata* Thunberg = *Eugenia caryophyllata* Thunb. *Eugenia caryophyllus* (Spreng.) Bullock & S. G. Harrison	
Gardenia Fruit サンシシ	*Gardenia jasminoides* J. Ellis	Rubiaceae
	Gardenia jasminoides J. Ellis f. *longicarpa* Z. W. Xie & M. Okada	
Glehnia Root and Rhizome ハマボウフウ	*Glehnia littoralis* F. Schmidt ex Miquel = *Glehnia littoralis* F. Schmidt ex Miq.	Umbelliferae
Magnolia Bark コウボク	*Magnolia obovata* Thunberg = *Magnolia obovata* Thunb.	Magnoliaceae
	* *Magnolia hypoleuca* Siebold et Zuccarini = *Magnolia hypoleuca* Siebold & Zucc.	
	Magnolia officinalis Rehder et E. H. Wilson	
	Magnolia officinalis Rehder et E. H. Wilson var. *biloba* Rehder et E. H. Wilson	
Sinomenium Stem and Rhizome ボウイ	*Sinomenium acutum* Rehder et E. H. Wilson = *Sinomenium acutum* (Thunb.) Rehder & E. H. Wilson	Menispermaceae

G6 Drug Formulation

Tablet Friability Test ⟨G6-5-181⟩

Change the following as follows:

This test is harmonized with the European Pharmacopoeia and the U.S. Pharmacopeia.

Information on the harmonization with the European Pharmacopoeia and the U.S. Pharmacopeia is available on the website of the Pharmaceuticals and Medical Devices Agency.

The Tablet Friability Test is a method to determine the friability of compressed uncoated tablets. The test procedure presented in this chapter is generally applicable to most compressed tablets. Measurement of tablets friability supplements other physical strength test, such as tablet crushing strength.

Apparatus

Use a drum, with an internal diameter between 283.0 and 291.0 mm and a depth between 36.0 and 40.0 mm, of transparent synthetic polymer with polished internal surfaces, and subject to minimum static build-up (see Fig. 1 for a typical apparatus). One side of the drum is removable. The tablets are tumbled at each turn of the drum by a curved projection with an inside radius between 75.5 and 85.5 mm that extends from the middle of the drum to the outer wall. The outer diameter of the central ring is between 24.5 and 25.5 mm. The drum is attached to the horizontal axis of a device that rotates between 24 and 26 rpm. Thus, at each turn the tablets roll or slide and fall onto the drum wall or onto each other.

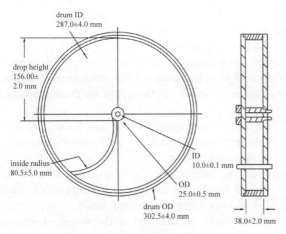

Fig. 1 Tablet friability apparatus

Procedure

For tablets with a unit mass equal to or less than 650 mg, take a sample of *n* whole tablets corresponding as near as possible to 6.5 g. For tablets with a unit mass of more than 650 mg, take a sample of 10 whole tablets. The tablets should be carefully dedusted prior to testing. Accurately weigh the tablet sample, and place the tablets in the drum. Rotate the drum 100 times, between 24 and 26 rpm and remove the tablets. Remove any loose dust from the tablets as before, and accurately weigh.

Generally, the test is run once. If obviously cracked, cleaved, or broken tablets are present in the tablet sample after tumbling, the sample fails the test. If the results are difficult to interpret or if the mass loss is greater than the targeted value, the test should be repeated twice and the mean of the three tests determined. A mass loss from a single test or a mean mass loss from the three tests of not more than 1.0% is considered acceptable for most products. Typically, in case of effervescent and chewable tablets the friability specifications may be different.

If tablet size or shape causes irregular tumbling, adjust the drum base so that the base forms an angle of about 10° with the horizontal and the tablets no longer bind together when lying next to each other, which prevents them from falling freely.

In the case of hygroscopic tablets, an appropriate humidity environment is required for testing.

Drums with dual scooping projections, or apparatus with more than one drum, designed for the running of multiple samples at the same time, are also permitted.

G9 Pharmaceutical Excipients

Add the following:

Functionality-Related Characteristics of Excipients Relevant to Preparations ⟨G9-1-181⟩

Functionality-Related Characteristics (FRC) of excipients are the physical and chemical properties of excipients which are closely relevant to the improvement of the usefulness of active pharmaceutical ingredients and preparations in the manufacturing process, storage, and use of the preparations.

As described in the General Rules for Preparations [1] General Notices for Preparations (6), excipients "must be pharmacologically inactive and harmless in the administered amount", and play roles "to increase the utility of the active substance(s) and preparation, to make formulation process easier, to keep the product quality, to improve the usability, and so forth." In the monographs of excipients, specifications and test methods are prescribed for the main purpose of identifying substances and ensuring qualities.

FRC may be effective parameters for excipients to play the above roles, however, no criteria are set for the test methods since the FRC required for excipients depend on the purpose of the use and the formula of preparations and

2950   *General Information*   *Supplement I, JP XVIII*

are different from the quality characteristics that are directly related to the safety and stability of excipients. In addition, the test methods of FRC described in this section do not limit the application of other appropriate test methods.

The FRC of Yellow Petrolatum and White Petrolatum, and the recommended test method for reference are shown below.

Yellow Petrolatum, White Petrolatum: Test method for consistency

Yellow Petrolatum and White Petrolatum are purified mixtures of hydrocarbons obtained from petroleum, and are generally used as the base of semi-solid preparations such as ointments. Ointments are defined in the [3] General Rules for Preparations 11.4. Ointments (3) as to "have a suitable viscosity for application to the skin", and their hardness/softness, one of the rheological properties of the dosage form, can be shown by measuring the consistency as a characteristic parameter. The test method to determine the consistency of Yellow Petrolatum and White Petrolatum according to Method 2 under Rheological Measurements for Semi-solid Preparations <6.16> is as follows.

(i) Apparatus   Perform the test using a standard cone or an optional cone. The containers for the test are flat-bottom metal cylinders that are 100 ± 6 mm in diameter and not less than 65 mm in height.

(ii) Procedure   Place the required number of empty containers in an oven, and bring them and a quantity of test substance in a container with a cover to a temperature of 82 ± 2.5°C, pour the Yellow Petrolatum or White Petrolatum into one or more of the containers, filling to within 6 mm of the rim. Cool to 25 ± 2.5°C over a period of not less than 16 hours, protected from drafts. Two hours before the test, place the containers in a water bath at 25 ± 0.5°C. If the room temperature is below 23.5°C or above 26.5°C, adjust the temperature of the cone to 25 ± 0.5°C by placing it in the water bath. Without disturbing the surface of the substance under test, place the container on the penetrometer table, and lower the cone until the tip just touches the top surface of the test substance at a spot 25 mm to 38 mm from the edge of the container. Adjust the zero setting and quickly release the plunger, then hold it free for 5 seconds. Secure the plunger, and read the total penetration from the scale. Make three or more trials, each so spaced that there is no overlapping of the areas of penetration. Where the penetration exceeds 20 mm, use a separated container of the test substance for each trial. Read the penetration to the nearest 0.1 mm. Calculate the average of the three or more readings.

GZ   Others

Quality Control of Water for Pharmaceutical Use *<GZ-2-181>*

Change 4.5 Physicochemical Monitoring and below as follows:

4.5.   Physicochemical Monitoring

Physicochemical monitoring of a pharmaceutical water processing system is usually performed using conductivity and TOC as the indicators. By monitoring conductivity, total amounts of inorganic salts present in the water can be estimated, and by monitoring TOC, total amount of organic compounds present in the water can be estimated. Normally, Conductivity Measurements <2.51> and Test for Total Organic Carbon <2.59> specified in the General Tests, Processes and Apparatus of the JP should be applied to these physicochemical monitoring. However, since tests for monitoring are performed in the situations different from those for judging pass/fail to the acceptance criteria prescribed in the monographs, supplements necessary to cover the situations to which the JP general tests cannot be applied, are described below.

To adopt the monitoring using conductivity and TOC as the indicators for inorganic and organic impurities at individual facility, appropriate alert and action levels for each indicator, and countermeasures against unexpected apparatus failures should be established.

4.5.1.   Monitoring of Conductivity

Measurement of conductivity for monitoring is usually conducted continuously using an in-line apparatus with a flow-through type or pipe-insertion type cell. Alternatively, offline batch testing may be performed using a dip type cell with water specimens taken at appropriate locations of the pharmaceutical water processing system.

(1)   On-line or in-line measurement

Usually, it is somewhat difficult to control the temperature exactly in in-line conductivity monitoring. Therefore, the following approach can be applied for the monitoring at any temperature.

(i)   Determine the temperature and the conductivity of the water specimens using a non-temperature-compensated conductivity reading.

(ii)   From the Table 3, find the temperature value equal to or just lower than the measured temperature. Adopt the corresponding conductivity value on this table as the allowable conductivity at the measured temperature.

(iii)   If the observed conductivity is not greater than the allowable conductivity adopted above, the water tested meets the requirement for monitoring conductivity. If the observed conductivity exceeds the allowable conductivity, off-line measurement is performed.

Supplement I, JP XVIII

Table 3 Allowable Conductivity for Different Temperatures*

Temperature (°C)	Allowable Conductivity (μS·cm^{-1})	Temperature (°C)	Allowable Conductivity (μS·cm^{-1})
0	0.6		
5	0.8	55	2.1
10	0.9	60	2.2
15	1.0	65	2.4
20	1.1	70	2.5
25	1.3	75	2.7
30	1.4	80	2.7
35	1.5	85	2.7
40	1.7	90	2.7
45	1.8	95	2.9
50	1.9	100	3.1

* Applicable only to non-temperature-compensated conductivity measurements.

(2) Off-line Measurement

(i) Measure the conductivity of the water specimen, by transferring it into a container and agitating it vigorously in order to attain equilibrium between the water specimen and the atmosphere on absorbing/desorbing carbon dioxide.

(ii) Transfer a sufficient amount of water to be tested into a suitable container, and stir the water specimen. Adjust the temperature to 25 ± 1°C, and begin agitating the water specimen vigorously, while observing the conductivity periodically. When the change in conductivity becomes not greater than 0.1 μS·cm^{-1} per 5 minutes, adopt the observed value as the conductivity (25°C) of the water specimen.

(iii) If the conductivity of the water specimen at 25°C obtained above is not greater than 2.1 μS·cm^{-1}, the water tested meets the requirement for monitoring conductivity. If the observed value exceeds 2.1 μS·cm^{-1}, it should be judged that the water tested does not meet the requirement for monitoring conductivity.

4.5.2. TOC Monitoring

The acceptance criterion of TOC is specified as "not greater than 0.50 mg/L (500 ppb)" in the monographs of *Purified Water* and *Water for Injection*. However it is recommended for each facility preparing pharmaceutical water to conduct the operation control of a pharmaceutical water processing system through TOC monitoring on produced water based on its own alert and action levels for TOC determined individually. The following are the recommended action levels for TOC.

• Action Level: ≤ 300 ppb (in-line)

≤ 400 ppb (off-line)

The Quality Standards for Drinking Water provided under the Article 4 of the Japanese Water Supply Law require that TOC of tap water (*Water*) should be "not greater than 3 mg/L (3 ppm)". Taking the above recommended action

levels into consideration, it is also recommended for each facility to conduct quality control of source water through TOC monitoring based on its own alert and action levels for TOC determined individually.

The JP specifies Test for Total Organic Carbon <2.59>, and normally, TOC measurement should be conducted using an apparatus which meets the requirements described in the JP method. However, if a TOC apparatus conforms to the apparatus suitability test requirements described in "< 643> TOTAL ORGANIC CARBON" of the USP, or those described in the "*Methods of Analysis 2.2.44.* TOTAL ORGANIC CARBON IN WATER FOR PHARMACEUTICAL USE" of the EP, the apparatus can be used for the monitoring of a pharmaceutical water processing system, if sufficiently pure water not contaminated with ionic organic substances, or organic substances having nitrogen, sulfur, phosphorus or halogen atoms in their chemical structures, is used as the source water supplied to the system.

A TOC apparatus, characterized by calculating the amount of TOC from the difference in conductivity before and after the decomposition of organic substances without separating carbon dioxide from the sample solution, may be influenced negatively or positively, when applied to the water specimens containing ionic organic substances, or organic substances having nitrogen, sulfur, phosphorus or halogen atoms in their chemical structures. Therefore, the apparatus used for TOC monitoring should be selected appropriately in consideration of the purity of the water to be monitored and the contamination risk in the case of apparatus failure.

4.6. Temporary Storage of *Water for Injection*

In storing *Water for Injection* temporarily, adequate measures able to prevent microbial proliferation stringently, such as circulating it in a loop at a high temperature must be taken, and an appropriate storage time should also be established based on the validation studies, in consideration of the risks of contamination and quality deterioration.

5. Points to Consider for Assuring the Quality of Pharmaceutical Water in Containers

There are some specific points to consider for assuring the quality of pharmaceutical water in containers (*Purified Water in Containers, Sterile Purified Water in Containers* and *Sterile Water for Injection in Containers*), which are available as commercially products.

5.1. Methods for Preparing Sterile Pharmaceutical Water in Containers

The following two different preparation methods are described in the monographs of *Sterile Purified Water in Containers* and *Sterile Water for Injection in Containers*.

(i) Introduce *Purified Water* or *Water for Injection* into a hermetic container, seal up the container, then sterilize the product.

(ii) Make *Purified Water* or *Water for Injection* sterile by using a suitable method, introduce the sterilized water into a sterile hermetic container by applying aseptic manipulation, then seal up the container.

For assuring the sterility of pharmaceutical water

2952 *General Information*

products, only the validation of final sterilization process is required in the case of preparation method (i), whereas validations of all the processes are indispensable in the case of preparation method (ii), since the latter is based on the idea to assure the sterility of pharmaceutical water products by "aseptically" introducing *Purified Water* (or *Water for Injection*) treated in advance with filtration sterilization, etc. into a sterile hermetic container, and sealing it up.

5.2. Deterioration of Water Quality during the Storage in Containers

5.2.1. Inorganic impurities (Conductivity as the indicator)

The conductivity of pharmaceutical water in containers may increase to some higher levels due to the absorption of carbon dioxide from the atmosphere at the time of its preparation and that passed through plastic layer of the containers during storage, and also due to ionic substances released from the containers, even if the conductivity of *Purified Water* or *Water for Injection* used for its production is maintained at the level not more than $1.3 \mu S \cdot cm^{-1}$ (25°C). Particularly in the cases of pharmaceutical water products packed in small scale glass containers, it is necessary to pay attention to the change of conductivity during storage.

5.2.2. Organic impurities (Potassium Permanganate-reducing Substances or TOC as the indicator)

The JP specifies the classical test of potassium permanganate-reducing substances in the monographs of *Purified Water in Containers*, *Sterile Purified Water in Containers* and *Sterile Water for Injection in Containers* for controlling organic impurities in pharmaceutical water in containers. It forms a remarkable contrast to the specifications of *Purified Water* and *Water for Injection*, in which the JP requires to control organic impurities in pharmaceutical water in bulk based on the test of TOC (acceptance criterion: not more than 0.5 mg/L (500 ppb)). This is because that it is considered difficult to establish the specification of pharmaceutical water in containers for organic impurities based on the test of TOC from the facts that there were many cases of remarkable increases in TOC values after storage of water in containers. Particularly in the cases of pharmaceutical water products packed in small scale plastic containers, it is necessary to pay attention to the increase of materials released from containers during storage.

The test of potassium permanganate-reducing substances is retained in the specifications of pharmaceutical water in containers, not as the most suitable method for the test of organic impurities present in the water in containers, but as a counter measure for performing the test of the water in containers with the same test method despite of the material (glass, polyethylene, polypropylene, etc.) and the size (0.5 – 2000 mL) of the containers, and the duration of storage. Therefore, it is recommended to adopt the test of TOC as the alternative for the test of potassium permanganate-reducing substances, and to perform quality control of pharmaceutical water in containers based on TOC measurements under the responsibility of each manufacturer, if possible. In such cases, it is recommended to adopt the following values as the levels preferable to attain.

For products containing not more than 10 mL of water:
TOC   not greater than 1500 ppb
For products containing more than 10 mL of water:
TOC   not greater than 1000 ppb

As for the pharmaceutical water packed in the plastic containers made of polyethylene, polypropylene, etc., in addition to the concern for the release of materials such as monomer, oligomers, plasticizers, etc. from plastics, it is necessary to pay attention to the storage environment of the products to avoid the contaminations with low molecular volatile organics such as alcohol, or low molecular air pollutants such as nitrogen oxides, since these plastics have the properties of permeating various gases and water.

5.2.3. Microbial Limit (Total Aerobic Microbial Count)

For *Purified Water in Containers*, it is not required to assure the sterility, but it is necessary to produce it by using sanitary or aseptic processes in order to meet the acceptance criterion of "10^2 CFU/mL" for total aerobic microbial count throughout the period of their storages. It is also necessary to take special care against microbial contamination during its circulation. In addition, it is recommended to use them as soon as possible after opening their seals.

The acceptance criterion of "10^2 CFU/mL" for total aerobic microbial count of *Purified Water in Container* is at the same level as the action level for microbial count in the production of *Purified Water* (in bulk). However, different from the case of microbiological monitoring of *Purified Water*, Soybean-Casein Digest Agar Medium is used for the test of total aerobic microbial count of *Purified Water in Containers* to detect microorganisms contaminated from the surroundings during its storage.

5.3. Points to consider in the case that commercially available products of pharmaceutical water in containers are used for the manufacture or the tests of pharmaceutical products

It is allowable to use commercially available products of pharmaceutical water in containers (*Purified Water in Containers*, *Sterile Purified Water in Containers* and *Sterile Water for Injection in Containers*) for the manufacture of pharmaceutical products and products for clinical trial, and for the tests of pharmaceutical products. In such cases, it is necessary to consider the following points.

(i)   Use them soon after confirming their compliances to the requirements of the JP monograph from the test results at the time of its receipt or those offered from the supplier of the products.

(ii)   In the case that such products are used for manufacturing pharmaceutical products, it is necessary to perform process validation as a part of manufacturing process of pharmaceutical products. In the case that they are used for manufacturing products for clinical trial, it is necessary to confirm that the water doesn't give any adverse effects on the quality of the products.

(iii)   The products of sterile pharmaceutical water in containers should be used only once after opening their seals, and it must be avoided to use them again after storage.

(iv)   It is recommended to prepare a standard operation

practice (SOP) adequate for its intended use, considering that the contamination and quality deterioration of the water due to human and laboratory environmental origins might go on rapidly immediately after opening the product seal.

INDEX

A

Absorptive Cream, 815
Acacia, 1939
  Powdered, 1939
Acebutolol Hydrochloride, 399, 2845
Acemetacin, 399, 2845
  Capsules, 400
  Tablets, 401
Acetaminophen, 402, 2845
Acetazolamide, 403, 2845
Acetic Acid, 403, 2845
  Glacial, 404, 2845
Acetohexamide, 404, 2845
Acetylcholine Chloride for Injection,
  406, 2845
Acetylcysteine, 406, 2845
Acetylsalicylic Acid, 488
  Tablets, 488
Achyranthes Root, 1940, 2907
Aciclovir, 407, 2845
  for Injection, 410
  for Syrup, 412
  Granules, 408
  Injection, 409
  Ointment, 410
  Ophthalmic Ointment, 411
  Syrup, 411
  Tablets, 413
Aclarubicin Hydrochloride, 413, 2845
Acrinol
  and Zinc Oxide Oil, 415
  and Zinc Oxide Oil, Compound,
    416
  and Zinc Oxide Ointment, 416
  Hydrate, 414, 2845
Actinomycin D, 417
Adrenaline, 417, 2845
  Injection, 418
  Solution, 418
Adsorbed
  Diphtheria-Purified Pertussis-Teta-
    nus Combined Vaccine, 873
  Diphtheria-Tetanus Combined Tox-
    oid, 873
  Diphtheria Toxoid for Adult Use,
    873
  Hepatitis B Vaccine, 1106
  Purified Pertussis Vaccine, 1500
  Tetanus Toxoid, 1812
Afloqualone, 419, 2845
Agar, 1940
  Powdered, 1941
Ajmaline, 420
  Tablets, 420

Akebia Stem, 1941, 2907
Alacepril, 421, 2845
  Tablets, 422
L-Alanine, 423, 2845
Albumin Tannate, 424
Alcohol, 964
  Dehydrated, 965
  for Disinfection, 966
Aldioxa, 424, 2845
  Granules, 425
  Tablets, 426
Alendronate
  Sodium Hydrate, 426, 2845
  Sodium Injection, 428
  Sodium Tablets, 429
Alimemazine Tartrate, 430, 2845
Alisma Tuber, 1941
  Powdered, 1942
Allopurinol, 430, 2845
  Tablets, 431
Alminoprofen, 432
  Tablets, 433
Aloe, 1942
  Powdered, 1943
Alpinia Officinarum Rhizome, 1944
Alprazolam, 434, 2845
Alprenolol Hydrochloride, 434, 2845
Alprostadil, 435
  Alfadex, 438
  Injection, 436, 2845
Alum, 442
  Solution, 439
  Powder, Salicylated, 1670
Aluminum
  Acetylsalicylate, 489
  Monostearate, 440, 2845
  Potassium Sulfate Hydrate, 442,
    2845
  Silicate Hydrate with Silicon Dioxide,
    1944
  Silicate, Natural, 442, 2845
  Silicate, Synthetic, 443, 2845
Amantadine Hydrochloride, 444,
  2845
Ambenonium Chloride, 445, 2845
Amidotrizoic Acid, 445, 2845
Amikacin Sulfate, 446, 2845
  for Injection, 448
  Injection, 447
Aminophylline
  Hydrate, 448, 2846
  Injection, 449
Amiodarone Hydrochloride, 450,
  2846
  Tablets, 451
Amitriptyline Hydrochloride, 452,

2846
  Tablets, 453
Amlexanox, 453, 2846
  Tablets, 455
Amlodipine Besilate, 456, 2846
  Orally Disintegrating Tablets, 457
  Tablets, 458
Ammonia Water, 459, 2846
Amobarbital, 459, 2846
Amomum Seed, 1945
  Powdered, 1945
Amosulalol Hydrochloride, 460, 2846
  Tablets, 461
Amoxapine, 462, 2846
Amoxicillin
  Capsules, 464
  Hydrate, 463, 2846
Amphotericin B, 465
  for Injection, 466, 2868
  Syrup, 466
  Tablets, 467, 2868
Ampicillin
  Anhydrous, 467, 2846
  Hydrate, 468, 2846
  Sodium, 470, 2846
  Sodium and Sulbactam Sodium for
    Injection, 471, 2868
  Sodium for Injection, 471
Ampiroxicam, 473, 2846
  Capsules, 473
Amyl Nitrite, 474
Anastrozole, 2869
  Tablets, 2870
Anemarrhena Rhizome, 1945
Anesthamine, 971
Anesthetic Ether, 968
Angelica Dahurica Root, 1946
Anhydrous
  Ampicillin, 467, 2846
  Caffeine, 588, 2848
  Citric Acid, 768, 2851
  Dibasic Calcium Phosphate, 604,
    2848
  Ethanol, 965, 2880
  Lactose, 1233, 2857
  Sodium Sulfate, 2154
Antipyrine, 475, 2846
Apricot Kernel, 1946, 2907
  Water, 1947
Aprindine Hydrochloride, 476, 2846
  Capsules, 476
Aralia Rhizome, 1947
Arbekacin Sulfate, 477, 2846
  Injection, 479
Areca, 1948
Argatroban Hydrate, 479, 2846

2955

2956 Index

L-Arginine, 481, 2846
Hydrochloride, 481, 2846
Hydrochloride Injection, 482
Aromatic Castor Oil, 1976
Arotinolol Hydrochloride, 482, 2846
Arsenic Trioxide, 484
Arsenical Paste, 483
Artemisia
Capillaris Flower, 1948, 2907
Leaf, 1949, 2907
Ascorbic Acid, 484, 2846
and Calcium Pantothenate Tablets,
485
Injection, 484
Powder, 485
Asiasarum Root, 1949
Asparagus Root, 1950
L-Aspartic Acid, 487, 2846
Aspirin, 488, 2846
Aluminum, 489
Tablets, 488
Aspoxicillin Hydrate, 490, 2846
Astragalus Root, 1950
Atenolol, 491, 2846
Atorvastatin Calcium
Hydrate, 492, 2846
Tablets, 493
Atractylodes
Lancea Rhizome, 1951
Lancea Rhizome, Powdered, 1951
Rhizome, 1952
Rhizome, Powdered, 1952
Atropine Sulfate
Hydrate, 494
Injection, 495
Auranofin, 496, 2846
Tablets, 497
Azathioprine, 498, 2846
Tablets, 499
Azelastine Hydrochloride, 500, 2846
Granules, 501
Azelnidipine, 502, 2846
Tablets, 502
Azithromycin Hydrate, 504, 2846
Azosemide, 505, 2846
Tablets, 505
Aztreonam, 506, 2846
for Injection, 507

B

Bacampicillin Hydrochloride, 508,
2846
Bacitracin, 509, 2846
Baclofen, 510, 2846
Tablets, 511
Bakumondoto Extract, 1953
Bamethan Sulfate, 512, 2847
Barbital, 512, 2847
Barium Sulfate, 513, 2847
Bear Bile, 1955
Bearberry Leaf, 1955, 2908
Beclometasone Dipropionate, 514,

2847
Beef Tallow, 1956
Beeswax
White, 1956
Yellow, 1956
Bekanamycin Sulfate, 515, 2847
Belladonna
Extract, 1958
Root, 1957
Total Alkaloids, 1958
Benidipine Hydrochloride, 516, 2847
Tablets, 516
Benincasa Seed, 1959
Benoxinate Hydrochloride, 1458
Benserazide Hydrochloride, 518, 2847
Bentonite, 519
Benzalkonium Chloride, 519
Solution, 520
Solution 50, Concentrated, 520
Benzbromarone, 521, 2847
Benzethonium Chloride, 522
Solution, 522
Benzocaine, 971
Benzoic Acid, 523, 2847
Benzoin, 1960
Benzyl
Alcohol, 523, 2872
Benzoate, 525
Benzylpenicillin
Benzathine Hydrate, 525, 2847
Potassium, 527, 2847
Potassium for Injection, 528
Bepotastine Besilate, 529, 2847
Tablets, 530
Beraprost Sodium, 531
Tablets, 532
Berberine
Chloride Hydrate, 533, 2847
Tannate, 534
Betahistine Mesilate, 535, 2847
Tablets, 536
Betamethasone, 538, 2847
Dipropionate, 540, 2847
Sodium Phosphate, 541
Tablets, 539
Valerate, 542
Valerate and Gentamicin Sulfate
Cream, 543
Valerate and Gentamicin Sulfate
Ointment, 544
Betamipron, 545, 2847
Betaxolol Hydrochloride, 546, 2847
Bethanechol Chloride, 547, 2847
Bezafibrate, 548, 2847
Extended-release Tablets, 549
Bicalutamide, 549, 2847
Tablets, 2872
Bifonazole, 552, 2847
Biotin, 552, 2847
Biperiden Hydrochloride, 553, 2847
Biphasic Isophane Insulin Human (Ge-
netical Recombination) Injectable
Aqueous Suspension, 1159, 2886

Bisacodyl, 554, 2847
Suppositories, 554
Bismuth
Subgallate, 555, 2847
Subnitrate, 556
Bisoprolol Fumarate, 556, 2847
Tablets, 557
Bitter
Cardamon, 1960, 2908
Orange Peel, 1960
Tincture, 1961
Bleomycin
Hydrochloride, 559, 2847
Sulfate, 561, 2847
Bofutsushosan Extract, 1961
Boiogito Extract, 1966
Boric Acid, 562, 2847
Bromazepam, 563, 2847
Bromfenac Sodium
Hydrate, 563, 2847
Ophthalmic Solution, 565
Bromhexine Hydrochloride, 565,
2847, 2873
Bromocriptine Mesilate, 566, 2847
Bromovalerylurea, 567, 2847
Brotizolam, 568, 2847
Tablets, 568
Brown Rice, 1968
Bucillamine, 570, 2847
Tablets, 570
Bucumolol Hydrochloride, 572, 2848
Budesonide, 2873
Bufetolol Hydrochloride, 572, 2848
Buformin Hydrochloride, 573, 2848
Delayed-release Tablets, 574
Tablets, 575
Bumetanide, 576, 2848
Bunazosin Hydrochloride, 577, 2848
Bupivacaine Hydrochloride Hydrate,
577, 2848
Bupleurum Root, 1968
Bupranolol Hydrochloride, 578, 2848
Buprenorphine Hydrochloride, 579,
2848
Burdock Fruit, 1969, 2908
Burnt Alum, 441
Busulfan, 580, 2848
Butenafine Hydrochloride, 580, 2848
Cream, 581
Solution, 582
Spray, 583
Butropium Bromide, 583, 2848, 2875
Butyl Parahydroxybenzoate, 584,
2848, 2875
Byakkokaninjinto Extract, 1969

C

Cabergoline, 585, 2848
Cacao Butter, 1972
Cadralazine, 587, 2848
Tablets, 587
Caffeine

Supplement I, JP XVIII   *Index*   2957

and Sodium Benzoate, 590, 2848
Anhydrous, 588, 2848
Hydrate, 589, 2848
Calcitonin Salmon, 591
Calcium
Chloride Hydrate, 596, 2848
Chloride Injection, 596
Folinate, 597
Folinate Hydrate, 597, 2848
Gluconate Hydrate, 598, 2848
Hydroxide, 598, 2848
Lactate Hydrate, 599, 2848
Leucovorin, 597
Levofolinate Hydrate, 600, 2848
Oxide, 601
Pantothenate, 602, 2848
Paraaminosalicylate Granules, 604
Paraaminosalicylate Hydrate, 603,
2848
Polystyrene Sulfonate, 607, 2848
Sodium Edetate Hydrate, 608, 2848
Stearate, 609, 2848
Calumba, 1972
Powdered, 1972
Camellia Oil, 1972
Camostat Mesilate, 610, 2848
d-Camphor, 611
dl-Camphor, 611
Candesartan Cilexetil, 612, 2848
and Amlodipine Besylate Tablets,
615
and Hydrochlorothiazide Tablets,
618
Tablets, 613
Capsicum, 1973
and Salicylic Acid Spirit, 1975
Powdered, 1973
Tincture, 1974
Capsules, 622
Capsules
Acemetacin, 400
Amoxicillin, 464
Ampiroxicam, 473
Aprindine Hydrochloride, 476
Cefaclor, 641
Cefadroxil, 646
Cefalexin, 649
Cefdinir, 665
Cefixime, 673
Cinoxacin, 762
Clindamycin Hydrochloride, 776
Clofibrate, 783
Clorazepate Dipotassium, 797
Diltiazem Hydrochloride Extended-
release, 864
Doxifluridine, 898
Droxidopa, 906
Emedastine Fumarate Extended-
release, 922
Ethyl Icosapentate, 975
Flopropione, 1017
Fluconazole, 1019
Hypromellose, 622

Indometacin, 1153
Lansoprazole Delayed-release, 1242
Methotrexate, 1332
Nifedipine Extended-release, 1422
Nizatidine, 1432
Pilsicainide Hydrochloride, 1519
Pullulan, 622
Ribavirin, 1633
Rifampicin, 1640
Roxatidine Acetate Hydrochloride
Extended-release, 1657
Sodium Iodide (^{123}I), 1714
Sodium Iodide (^{131}I), 1714
Sulpiride, 1758
Tacrolimus, 1770
Temozolomide, 2900
Teprenone, 1804
Tranexamic Acid, 1851
Tranilast, 1854
Trientine Hydrochloride, 1870
Ubenimex, 1885
Captopril, 622, 2848
Carbamazepine, 623, 2848
Carbazochrome Sodium Sulfonate Hy-
drate, 624, 2848
Carbidopa Hydrate, 625, 2849
L-Carbocisteine, 626, 2849
Tablets, 626
Carbon Dioxide, 627
Carboplatin, 628
Injection, 629
Carboxymethylcellulose, 630
Calcium, 631
Sodium, 632
Cardamon, 1975, 2908
Carmellose, 630, 2849
Calcium, 631, 2849
Sodium, 632, 2849
Carmofur, 634, 2849
Carnauba Wax, 1975
Carteolol Hydrochloride, 635, 2849
Carumonam Sodium, 635, 2849
Carvedilol, 637, 2849
Tablets, 638
Cassia Seed, 1976
Castor Oil, 1976
Aromatic, 1976
Catalpa Fruit, 1976
Cefaclor, 640, 2849
Capsules, 641
Combination Granules, 642
Fine Granules, 644
Cefadroxil, 645, 2849
Capsules, 646
for Syrup, 647
Cefalexin, 647, 2849
Capsules, 649
Combination Granules, 650
for Syrup, 651
Cefalotin Sodium, 652, 2849
for Injection, 653
Cefatrizine Propylene Glycolate, 654,
2849

for Syrup, 655
Cefazolin Sodium, 656, 2849
for Injection, 657
Hydrate, 658, 2849
Cefbuperazone Sodium, 659, 2849
Cefcapene Pivoxil Hydrochloride
Fine Granules, 662
Hydrate, 660, 2849
Tablets, 663
Cefdinir, 664, 2849
Capsules, 665
Fine Granules, 666
Cefditoren Pivoxil, 667, 2849
Fine Granules, 668
Tablets, 668
Cefepime Dihydrochloride
for Injection, 671
Hydrate, 669, 2849
Cefixime
Capsules, 673
Fine Granules, 674
Hydrate, 672
Cefmenoxime Hydrochloride, 675,
2849
Cefmetazole Sodium, 677, 2849
for Injection, 678
Cefminox Sodium Hydrate, 678, 2849
Cefodizime Sodium, 679, 2849
Cefoperazone Sodium, 681, 2849
and Sulbactam Sodium for Injection,
683, 2878
for Injection, 682
Cefotaxime Sodium, 684, 2849
Cefotetan, 685, 2849
Cefotiam
Hexetil Hydrochloride, 687, 2849
Hydrochloride, 689, 2849
Hydrochloridefor Injection, 690
Cefozopran Hydrochloride, 691, 2849
for Injection, 692
Cefpiramide Sodium, 692, 2849
Cefpirome Sulfate, 694, 2849
Cefpodoxime Proxetil, 695, 2849
for Syrup, 696
Tablets, 697
Cefroxadine
for Syrup, 700
Hydrate, 698, 2849
Cefsulodin Sodium, 701, 2849
Ceftazidime
for Injection, 704
Hydrate, 702, 2850
CefteramPivoxil, 704, 2850
Fine Granules, 706
Tablets, 706
Ceftibuten Hydrate, 707, 2850
Ceftizoxime Sodium, 709, 2850
Ceftriaxone Sodium Hydrate, 710,
2850
Cefuroxime Axetil, 712, 2850
Celecoxib, 714, 2850
Cellacefate, 715, 2850
Cellulose

2958   *Index*   *Supplement I, JP XVIII*

Acetate Phthalate, 715
    Microcrystalline, 716, 2850
    Powdered, 719, 2850, 2878
Celmoleukin (Genetical Recombination), 719
Cetanol, 722
Cetirizine Hydrochloride, 723, 2850
    Tablets, 724
Cetotiamine Hydrochloride Hydrate, 725, 2850
Cetraxate Hydrochloride, 726, 2850
Chenodeoxycholic Acid, 727, 2850
Cherry Bark, 1977
Chloral Hydrate, 728
Chloramphenicol, 728, 2850
    and Colistin Sodium Methanesulfonate Ophthalmic Solution, 731
    Palmitate, 729, 2850
    Sodium Succinate, 730, 2850
Chlordiazepoxide, 732, 2850
    Powder, 733
    Tablets, 734
Chlorhexidine
    Gluconate Solution, 735
    Hydrochloride, 735, 2850
Chlorinated Lime, 736
Chlormadinone Acetate, 736, 2850
Chlorobutanol, 737
Chlorphenesin Carbamate, 738, 2850
    Tablets, 739
Chlorpheniramine Maleate, 740, 2850
    Injection, 741
    Powder, 741
    Tablets, 742
d-Chlorpheniramine Maleate, 743, 2850
Chlorpromazine Hydrochloride, 744, 2850
    Injection, 745
    Tablets, 745
Chlorpropamide, 747, 2850
    Tablets, 747
Cholecalciferol, 748
Cholesterol, 749
Chorionic Gonadotrophin, 1085
    for Injection, 1086
Chotosan Extract, 1977
Chrysanthemum Flower, 1980
Cibenzoline Succinate, 750, 2850
    Tablets, 750
Ciclacillin, 751, 2850
Ciclosporin, 752, 2850
Cilastatin Sodium, 753, 2850
Cilazapril
    Hydrate, 755, 2850
    Tablets, 755
Cilnidipine, 757, 2850
    Tablets, 758
Cilostazol, 759, 2850
    Tablets, 760
Cimetidine, 761, 2850
Cimicifuga Rhizome, 1980, 2908
Cinchocaine Hydrochloride, 846

Cinnamon
    Bark, 1981
    Bark, Powdered, 1981
    Oil, 1982
Cinoxacin, 762, 2850
    Capsules, 762
Ciprofloxacin, 763, 2850
    Hydrochloride Hydrate, 765, 2850
Cisplatin, 766
Cistanche Herb, 1982
Citicoline, 767, 2850
Citric Acid
    Anhydrous, 768, 2851
    Hydrate, 769, 2851
Citrus Unshiu Peel, 1983
Clarithromycin, 770, 2851
    for Syrup, 771
    Tablets, 772
Clebopride Malate, 773, 2851
Clemastine Fumarate, 774, 2851
Clematis Root, 1983
Clindamycin
    Hydrochloride, 775, 2851
    Hydrochloride Capsules, 776
    Phosphate, 777, 2851
    Phosphate Injection, 778
Clinofibrate, 779, 2851
Clobetasol Propionate, 779, 2851
Clocapramine Hydrochloride Hydrate, 780, 2851
Clofedanol Hydrochloride, 781, 2851
Clofibrate, 782, 2851
    Capsules, 783
Clomifene Citrate, 784, 2851
    Tablets, 784
Clomipramine Hydrochloride, 785, 2851
    Tablets, 786
Clonazepam, 787, 2851
    Fine Granules, 787
    Tablets, 788
Clonidine Hydrochloride, 789, 2851
Cloperastine
    Fendizoate, 790, 2851
    Fendizoate Tablets, 791
    Hydrochloride, 792, 2851
Clopidogrel
    Sulfate, 793, 2851
    Sulfate Tablets, 794
Clorazepate Dipotassium, 796, 2851
    Capsules, 797
Clotiazepam, 798, 2851
    Tablets, 798
Clotrimazole, 799, 2851
Clove, 1984, 2909
    Oil, 1984, 2909
    Powdered, 1984
Cloxacillin Sodium Hydrate, 800, 2851
Cloxazolam, 801, 2851
Cnidium
    Monnieri Fruit, 1985, 2909
    Rhizome, 1985

Rhizome, Powdered, 1986
Cocaine Hydrochloride, 802
Coconut Oil, 1986
Codeine Phosphate
    Hydrate, 803
    Powder, 1%, 804
    Powder, 10%, 805
    Tablets, 805
Cod Liver Oil, 803
Codonopsis Root, 1986
Coix Seed, 1987
    Powdered, 1987
Colchicine, 807
Colestimide, 808, 2851
    Granules, 809
    Tablets, 809
Colistin
    Sodium Methanesulfonate, 810, 2851
    Sulfate, 811
Compound
    Acrinol and Zinc Oxide Oil, 416
    Diastase and Sodium Bicarbonate Powder, 843
    Iodine Glycerin, 1171
    Methyl Salicylate Spirit, 1347
    Oxycodone and Atropine Injection, 1460
    Oxycodone Injection, 1460
    Phellodendron Powder for Cataplasm, 2098
    Rhubarb and Senna Powder, 2115
    Salicylic Acid Spirit, 1669
    Scopolia Extract and Diastase Powder, 2136
    Thianthol and Salicylic Acid Solution, 1820
Concentrated
    Glycerin, 1081, 2855
    Glycerol, 1081
Condurango, 1987
    Fluidextract, 1988
Copovidone, 812, 2851
Coptis Rhizome, 1988
    Powdered, 1989
Corn
    Oil, 1990
    Starch, 1738
Cornus Fruit, 1990, 2909
Cortisone Acetate, 814
Corydalis Tuber, 1991, 2909
    Powdered, 1992, 2910
Crataegus Fruit, 1993
Creams
    Absorptive, 815
    Betamethasone Valerate and Gentamicin Sulfate, 543
    Butenafine Hydrochloride, 581
    Hydrophilic, 815
    Ibuprofen Piconol, 1134
    Ketoconazole, 1222
    Lanoconazole, 1239
    Terbinafine Hydrochloride, 1806

Supplement I, JP XVIII   *Index*   2959

Cresol, 816
  Solution, 816
  Solution, Saponated, 816
Croconazole Hydrochloride, 817, 2851
Croscarmellose Sodium, 633, 2849, 2877
Crospovidone, 818, 2851
Crude Glycyrrhiza Extract, 2016
Curcuma Rhizome, 1993
Cyanamide, 819, 2851
Cyanocobalamin, 820
  Injection, 821
Cyclopentolate Hydrochloride, 821, 2851
Cyclophosphamide
  Hydrate, 822, 2851
  Tablets, 822
Cycloserine, 823, 2851
Cyperus Rhizome, 1994
  Powdered, 1994
Cyproheptadine Hydrochloride Hydrate, 824, 2851
L-Cysteine, 825, 2851
  Hydrochloride Hydrate, 826, 2851
L-Cystine, 826, 2851
Cytarabine, 827, 2852

D

Dactinomycin, 417
Daiokanzoto Extract, 1995
Daisaikoto Extract, 1996
Danazol, 828, 2852
Dantrolene Sodium Hydrate, 828, 2852
Daunorubicin Hydrochloride, 829, 2852
Deferoxamine Mesilate, 831, 2852
Dehydrated Alcohol, 965
Dehydrocholic Acid, 832, 2852
  Injection, 833, 2852
  Purified, 832, 2852
Demethylchlortetracycline Hydrochloride, 834, 2852
Dental
  Antiformin, 475
  Iodine Glycerin, 1172
  Paraformaldehyde Paste, 1479
  Phenol with Camphor, 1508
  Sodium Hypochlorite Solution, 475
  Triozinc Paste, 1877
Deslanoside, 835
  Injection, 836
Dexamethasone, 836, 2852
Dextran
  40, 837, 2852
  40 Injection, 838
  70, 839, 2852
  Sulfate Sodium Sulfur 5, 840, 2852
  Sulfate Sodium Sulfur 18, 840, 2852
Dextrin, 841, 2852

Dextromethorphan Hydrobromide Hydrate, 841, 2852
Diagnostic Sodium Citrate Solution, 1705
Diastase, 842
  and Sodium Bicarbonate Powder, 843
  and Sodium Bicarbonate Powder, Compound, 843
Diazepam, 843, 2852
  Tablets, 844
Dibasic
  Calcium Phosphate, Anhydrous, 604, 2848
  Calcium Phosphate Hydrate, 605, 2848
  Sodium Phosphate Hydrate, 1719, 2865
Dibekacin Sulfate, 845, 2852
  Ophthalmic Solution, 845
Dibucaine Hydrochloride, 846, 2852
Diclofenac Sodium, 846, 2852
  Suppositories, 847
Dicloxacillin Sodium Hydrate, 848
Diethylcarbamazine Citrate, 849, 2852
  Tablets, 849
Difenidol Hydrochloride, 850, 2852
Diflorasone Diacetate, 851, 2852
Diflucortolone Valerate, 852, 2852
Digenea, 1998
Digoxin, 853
  Injection, 854
  Tablets, 855
Dihydrocodeine Phosphate, 857
  Powder, 1%, 857
  Powder, 10%, 858
Dihydroergotamine Mesilate, 859
Dihydroergotoxine Mesilate, 860, 2852
Dilazep Hydrochloride Hydrate, 862, 2852
Diltiazem Hydrochloride, 863, 2852
  Extended-release Capsules, 864
Dilute
  Hydrochloric Acid, 1111, 2856
  Iodine Tincture, 1171
Diluted Opium Powder, 2082
Dimemorfan Phosphate, 865, 2852
Dimenhydrinate, 866
  Tablets, 866
Dimercaprol, 867, 2852
  Injection, 868
Dimorpholamine, 868, 2852
  Injection, 869
Dinoprost, 869
Dioscorea Rhizome, 1999
  Powdered, 1999
Diphenhydramine, 870, 2852
  and Bromovalerylurea Powder, 871
  Hydrochloride, 871, 2852
  , Phenol and Zinc Oxide Liniment, 872

  Tannate, 872, 2852
Diphtheria
  Antitoxin, Equine, Freeze-dried, 873
  -Purified Pertussis-Tetanus Combined Vaccine, Adsorbed, 873
  -Tetanus Combined Toxoid, Adsorbed, 873
  Toxoid, 873
  Toxoid for Adult Use, Adsorbed, 873
Dipyridamole, 874, 2852
Disodium Edetate Hydrate, 1706, 2864
Disopyramide, 875, 2852
Distigmine Bromide, 875, 2852
  Tablets, 876
Disulfiram, 877, 2852
Dobutamine Hydrochloride, 877, 2853
Docetaxel
  for Injection, 880
  Hydrate, 878, 2853
  Injection, 879
Dolichos Seed, 2000
Domperidone, 881, 2853
Donepezil Hydrochloride, 882, 2853
  Fine Granules, 883
  Tablets, 884
Dopamine Hydrochloride, 886, 2853
  Injection, 886
Doripenem
  for Injection, 889
  Hydrate, 887, 2853
Dorzolamide Hydrochloride, 891, 2853
  and Timolol Maleate Ophthalmic Solution, 893
  Ophthalmic Solution, 892
Doxapram Hydrochloride Hydrate, 95, 2853
Doxazosin Mesilate, 896, 2853
  Tablets, 897
Doxifluridine, 898, 2853
  Capsules, 898
Doxorubicin Hydrochloride, 899
  for Injection, 900
Doxycycline Hydrochloride
  Hydrate, 901, 2853
  Tablets, 903
Dried
  Aluminum Hydroxide Gel, 440, 2845
  Aluminum Hydroxide Gel Fine Granules, 440
  Aluminum Potassium Sulfate, 441
  Sodium Carbonate, 1701, 2864
  Sodium Sulfite, 1727, 2865
  Thyroid, 1825
  Yeast, 1924
Droperidol, 904, 2853
Droxidopa, 905, 2853
  Capsules, 906

2960 Index

Fine Granules, 906
Dydrogesterone, 907, 2853
Tablets, 908

E

Ebastine, 909, 2853
Orally Disintegrating Tablets, 909
Tablets, 911
Ecabet Sodium
Granules, 913
Hydrate, 912, 2853
Ecothiopate Iodide, 914, 2853
Edaravone, 915, 2853
Injection, 915
Edrophonium Chloride, 917, 2853
Injection, 918
Elcatonin, 919
Eleutherococcus Senticosus Rhizome, 2000
Emedastine Fumarate, 921, 2853
Extended-release Capsules, 922
Emorfazone, 923, 2853
Tablets, 924
Enalapril Maleate, 924, 2853
Tablets, 926
Enflurane, 927
Enoxacin Hydrate, 928, 2853
Entacapone, 928, 2853
Tablets, 930
Enviomycin Sulfate, 931, 2853, 2879
Epalrestat, 932, 2853
Tablets, 933
Eperisone Hydrochloride, 934, 2853
Ephedra Herb, 2001
Ephedrine Hydrochloride, 935, 2853
Injection, 935
Tablets, 937
Powder, 10%, 936
Epimedium Herb, 2001
Epinephrine, 417
Injection, 418
Solution, 418
Epirizole, 938, 2853
Epirubicin Hydrochloride, 939, 2853
Eplerenone, 940, 2853
Tablets, 941
Epoetin
Alfa (Genetical Recombination), 942
Beta (Genetical Recombination), 945, 2879
Ergocalciferol, 948
Ergometrine Maleate, 949
Injection, 949
Tablets, 950
Ergotamine Tartrate, 950
Eribulin Mesilate, 951, 2853
Erythromycin, 955, 2853
Delayed-release Tablets, 956
Ethylsuccinate, 956
Lactobionate, 957
Stearate, 958

Estazolam, 958, 2853
Estradiol Benzoate, 959
Injection (Aqueous Suspension), 960
Estriol, 960, 2853
Injection (Aqueous Suspension), 961
Tablets, 961
Etacrynic Acid, 962, 2853
Tablets, 963
Ethacridine Lactate, 414
Ethambutol Hydrochloride, 964, 2853
Ethanol, 964, 2880
Anhydrous, 965, 2880
for Disinfection, 966
Ethenzamide, 967, 2854
Ether, 967
Anesthetic, 968
Ethinylestradiol, 968
Tablets, 969
Ethionamide, 970, 2854
Ethosuximide, 970, 2854
Ethyl
Aminobenzoate, 971, 2854
L-Cysteine Hydrochloride, 973, 2854
Icosapentate, 974, 2854
Icosapentate Capsules, 975
Loflazepate, 976, 2854
Loflazepate Tablets, 978
Parahydroxybenzoate, 979, 2854, 2880
Ethylcellulose, 971, 2854
Ethylenediamine, 974, 2854
Ethylmorphine Hydrochloride Hydrate, 979
Etidronate Disodium, 980, 2854
Tablets, 981
Etilefrine Hydrochloride, 982, 2854
Tablets, 983
Etizolam, 984, 2854
Fine Granules, 984
Tablets, 985
Etodolac, 987, 2854
Etoposide, 987, 2854
Eucalyptus Oil, 2002
Eucommia Bark, 2002
Euodia Fruit, 2003
Exsiccated Gypsum, 2023
Extracts
Bakumondoto, 1953
Belladonna, 1958
Bofutsushosan, 1961
Boiogito, 1966
Byakkokaninjinto, 1969
Chotosan, 1977
Crude Glycyrrhiza, 2016
Daiokanzoto, 1995
Daisaikoto, 1996
Glycyrrhiza, 2015
Goreisan, 2017
Goshajinkigan, 2018, 2911
Goshuyuto, 2021, 2912

Hachimijiogan, 2024, 2912
Hangekobokuto, 2027, 2913
Hangeshashinto, 2028
Hochuekkito, 2032
Juzentaihoto, 2043
Kakkonto, 2046
Kakkontokasenkyushin'i, 2049
Kamikihito, 2052
Kamishoyosan, 2055
Keishibukuryogan, 2058, 2913
Maoto, 2070, 2914
Mukoi-Daikenchuto, 2075, 2914
Nux Vomica, 2079
Orengedokuto, 2084
Otsujito, 2087
Rikkunshito, 2116
Ryokeijutsukanto, 2119
Saibokuto, 2122
Saikokeishikankyoto, 2916
Saikokeishito, 2125
Saireito, 2128
Scopolia, 2135
Shakuyakukanzoto, 2143
Shimbuto, 2145, 2920
Shosaikoto, 2147
Shoseiryuto, 2150
Tokakujokito, 2160, 2921
Tokishakuyakusan, 2162
Unseiin, 2169
Yokukansan, 2173
Yokukansankachimpihange, 2922

F

Famotidine, 988, 2854
for Injection, 990
Injection, 989
Powder, 991
Tablets, 992
Faropenem Sodium
for Syrup, 994
Hydrate, 993, 2854
Tablets, 995
Felbinac, 996, 2854
Cataplasm, 997
Tape, 997
Felodipine, 998, 2854
Tablets, 999
Fenbufen, 1000, 2854
Fennel, 2003
Oil, 2004
Powdered, 2003
Fenofibrate, 1001, 2854
Tablets, 1002
Fentanyl Citrate, 1003, 2854
Ferrous Sulfate Hydrate, 1004, 2854
Fexofenadine Hydrochloride, 1004, 2854
Tablets, 1005
Filgrastim (Genetical Recombination), 1007
Injection, 1009
Fine Granules

Cefaclor, 644
Cefcapene Pivoxil Hydrochloride,
    662
Cefdinir, 666
Cefditoren Pivoxil, 668
Cefixime, 674
CefteramPivoxil, 706
Clonazepam, 787
Donepezil Hydrochloride, 883
Dried Aluminum Hydroxide Gel,
    440
Droxidopa, 906
Etizolam, 984
Haloperidol, 1091
Ifenprodil Tartrate, 1140
Irsogladine Maleate, 1191
Levofloxacin, 1257
Nifedipine, 1422
Nifedipine Delayed-release, 1420
Pravastatin Sodium, 1566
Precipitated Calcium Carbonate,
    594
Probucol, 1581
Quetiapine Fumarate, 1615
Risperidone, 1645
Sarpogrelate Hydrochloride, 1672,
    2898
Tranilast, 1855
Troxipide, 1878
Flavin Adenine Dinucleotide Sodium,
    1010, 2854
Flavoxate Hydrochloride, 1012, 2854
Flecainide Acetate, 1012, 2854
    Tablets, 1013
Flomoxef Sodium, 1014, 2854
    for Injection, 1016
Flopropione, 1017, 2854
    Capsules, 1017
Fluconazole, 1018, 2854
    Capsules, 1019
    Injection, 1020
Flucytosine, 1021, 2854
Fludiazepam, 1022, 2854
    Tablets, 1022
Fludrocortisone Acetate, 1023, 2854
Fluidextracts
    Condurango, 1988
    Platycodon, 2102
    UvaUrsi, 2171
Flunitrazepam, 1024, 2854
Fluocinolone Acetonide, 1025
Fluocinonide, 1026
Fluorescein Sodium, 1027
Fluorometholone, 1028, 2854
Fluorouracil, 1029, 2854
Fluphenazine Enanthate, 1030, 2854
Flurazepam Hydrochloride, 1030,
    2855
Flurbiprofen, 1031, 2855
Flutamide, 1032, 2855
Flutoprazepam, 1033, 2855
    Tablets, 1033
Fluvoxamine Maleate, 1034, 2855

Tablets, 1036
Foeniculated Ammonia Spirit, 2004
Folic Acid, 1037
    Injection, 1037
    Tablets, 1038
Formalin, 1039
    Water, 1039
Formoterol Fumarate Hydrate, 1040,
    2855, 2881
Forsythia Fruit, 2004
Fosfomycin
    Calcium Hydrate, 1040, 2855
    Calcium for Syrup, 1042
    Sodium, 1043, 2855
    Sodium for Injection, 1044
Fradiomycin Sulfate, 1045, 2855
Freeze-dried
    BCG Vaccine (for Percutaneous
        Use), 514
    Botulism Antitoxin, Equine, 563
    Diphtheria Antitoxin, Equine, 873
    Habu Antivenom, Equine, 1090
    Inactivated Tissue Culture Rabies
        Vaccine, 1625
    Live Attenuated Measles Vaccine,
        1301
    Live Attenuated Mumps Vaccine,
        1390
    Live Attenuated Rubella Vaccine,
        1662
    Mamushi Antivenom, Equine, 1296
    Smallpox Vaccine, 1696
    Smallpox Vaccine Prepared in Cell
        Culture, 1696
Fritillaria Bulb, 2005
Fructose, 1046, 2855
    Injection, 1046, 2855
Fudosteine, 1047, 2855
    Tablets, 1048
Furosemide, 1049, 2855
    Injection, 1050
    Tablets, 1050
Fursultiamine Hydrochloride, 1051,
    2855

G

Gabexate Mesilate, 1052, 2855
β-Galactosidase
    (Aspergillus), 1053, 2855
    (Penicillium), 1054, 2855
Gallium (⁶⁷Ga) Citrate Injection, 1055
Gambir, 2005
    Powdered, 2005
Gardenia Fruit, 2006, 2910
    Powdered, 2006
Gastrodia Tuber, 2007
Gatifloxacin
    Hydrate, 1055, 2855
    Ophthalmic Solution, 1057
Gefarnate, 1058, 2855
Gefitinib, 1059, 2855
Gelatin, 1060, 2855

Purified, 1062, 2855
Gentamicin Sulfate, 1064, 2855
    Injection, 1066
    Ointment, 1066
    Ophthalmic Solution, 1067
Gentian, 2007
    and Sodium Bicarbonate Powder,
        2008
    Powdered, 2008
Geranium Herb, 2009
    Powdered, 2009
Ginger, 2009, 2910
    Powdered, 2010, 2911
    Processed, 2109, 2916
Ginseng, 2011
    Powdered, 2012
Glacial Acetic Acid, 404, 2845
Glehnia Root and Rhizome, 2013,
    2911
Glibenclamide, 1067, 2855
Gliclazide, 1068, 2855
Glimepiride, 1069, 2855
    Tablets, 1070
Glucagon (Genetical Recombination),
    1072
Glucose, 1073, 2855
    Hydrate, 1074, 2855
    Injection, 1076
    Purified, 1075, 2855
L-Glutamic Acid, 1077, 2855
L-Glutamine, 1078, 2855
Glutathione, 1079, 2855
Glycerin, 1080, 2855
    and Potash Solution, 1082
    Concentrated, 1081, 2855
Glycerol, 1080
    Concentrated, 1081
Glyceryl Monostearate, 1082, 2883
Glycine, 1083, 2855
Glycyrrhiza, 2013
    Extract, 2015
    Extract, Crude, 2016
    Powdered, 2014
    Prepared, 2105, 2916
Gonadorelin Acetate, 1083
Goreisan Extract, 2017
Goshajinkigan Extract, 2018, 2911
Goshuyuto Extract, 2021, 2912
Granules
    Aciclovir, 408
    Aldioxa, 425
    Azelastine Hydrochloride, 501
    Calcium Paraaminosalicylate, 604
    Cefaclor Combination, 642
    Cefalexin Combination, 650
    Colestimide, 809
    Ecabet Sodium, 913
    L-Isoleucine, L-Leucine and L-Valine,
        1197
    Minocycline Hydrochloride, 1365
    Montelukast Sodium, 1379
    Pas-calcium, 604
    Polaprezinc, 1548

2962　*Index*　　　　　　　　　　　　　　　　　　　　　　　　　　　　　*Supplement I, JP XVIII*

Granules (*continued*)
　Ursodeoxycholic Acid,　1892
Guaifenesin,　1088, 2855
Guanabenz Acetate,　1089, 2855
Guanethidine Sulfate,　1090, 2856
Gypsum,　2023

H

Hachimijiogan Extract,　2024, 2912
Haloperidol,　1090, 2856
　Fine Granules,　1091
　Injection,　1092
　Tablets,　1093
Halothane,　1094
Haloxazolam,　1095, 2856
Hangekobokuto Extract,　2027, 2913
Hangeshashinto Extract,　2028
Hedysarum Root,　2031
Hemp Fruit,　2031
Heparin
　Calcium,　1096, 2856
　Sodium,　1100, 2856
　Sodium Injection,　1104, 2856
　Sodium Lock Solution,　1104
　Sodium Solution for Dialysis,　1105
L-Histidine,　1106, 2856
　Hydrochloride Hydrate,　1107, 2856
Hochuekkito Extract,　2032
Homatropine Hydrobromide,　1107
Homochlorcyclizine Hydrochloride,
　1108, 2856
Honey,　2035
Houttuynia Herb,　2035
Human
　Chorionic Gonadotrophin,　1085
　Chorionic Gonadotrophin for Injec-
　　tion,　1086
　Menopausal Gonadotrophin,　1087
　Normal Immunoglobulin,　1109
Hydralazine Hydrochloride,　1109,
　2856
　for Injection,　1109
　Powder,　1110
　Tablets,　1110
Hydrochloric Acid,　1111, 2856
　Dilute,　1111, 2856
　Lemonade,　1112
Hydrochlorothiazide,　1112, 2856
Hydrocortisone,　1113
　Acetate,　1114
　and Diphenhydramine Ointment,
　　1115
　Butyrate,　1115, 2856
　Sodium Phosphate,　1116, 2856
　Sodium Succinate,　1117
　Succinate,　1118
Hydrocotarnine Hydrochloride Hy-
　drate,　1119, 2856
Hydrogenated Oil,　1120, 2856
Hydrophilic
　Cream,　815
　Petrolatum,　1502

Hydrous Lanolin,　2061
Hydroxocobalamin Acetate,　1120
Hydroxyethylcellulose,　1121, 2856
Hydroxypropylcellulose,　1123, 2856
Hydroxyzine
　Hydrochloride,　1125, 2856
　Pamoate,　1126, 2856
Hymecromone,　1127, 2856
Hypromellose,　1127, 2856
　Acetate Succinate,　1129, 2856
　Capsules,　622
　Phthalate,　1131, 2856, 2883

I

Ibudilast,　1132, 2856
Ibuprofen,　1133, 2856
　Piconol,　1133, 2856
　Piconol Cream,　1134
　Piconol Ointment,　1135
Ichthammol,　1135
Idarubicin Hydrochloride,　1136, 2856
　for Injection,　1137
Idoxuridine,　1138, 2856
　Ophthalmic Solution,　1139
Ifenprodil Tartrate,　1140, 2856
　Fine Granules,　1140
　Tablets,　1141
Imidapril Hydrochloride,　1142, 2856
　Tablets,　1143
Imipenem
　and Cilastatin Sodium for Injection,
　　1145, 2884
　Hydrate,　1144, 2856
Imipramine Hydrochloride,　1146
　Tablets,　1147
Immature Orange,　2036
Imperata Rhizome,　2036
Indapamide,　1148, 2856
　Tablets,　1149
Indenolol Hydrochloride,　1150, 2856
Indigocarmine,　1151, 2856
　Injection,　1152
Indium (^{111}In) Chloride Injection,
　1152
Indometacin,　1152, 2857
　Capsules,　1153
　Suppositories,　1154
Influenza HA Vaccine,　1155
Injection
　Acetylcholine Chloride for,　406,
　　2845
　Aciclovir,　409
　Aciclovir for,　410
　Adrenaline,　418
　Alendronate Sodium,　428
　Alprostadil,　436, 2845
　Amikacin Sulfate,　447
　Amikacin Sulfate for,　448
　Aminophylline,　449
　Amphotericin B for,　466, 2868
　Ampicillin Sodium and Sulbactam
　　Sodium for,　471, 2868

Ampicillin Sodium for,　471
Arbekacin Sulfate,　479
L-Arginine Hydrochloride,　482
Ascorbic Acid,　484
Atropine Sulfate,　495
Aztreonam for,　507
Benzylpenicillin Potassium for,　528
Calcium Chloride,　596
Carboplatin,　629
Cefalotin Sodium for,　653
Cefazolin Sodium for,　657
Cefepime Dihydrochloride for,　671
Cefmetazole Sodium for,　678
Cefoperazone Sodium and Sulbac-
　tam Sodium for,　683, 2878
Cefoperazone Sodium for,　682
Cefotiam Hydrochloride for,　690
Cefozopran Hydrochloride for,　692
Ceftazidime for,　704
Chlorpheniramine Maleate,　741
Chlorpromazine Hydrochloride,
　745
Chorionic Gonadotrophin for,
　1086
Clindamycin Phosphate,　778
Compound Oxycodone,　1460
Compound Oxycodone and Atro-
　pine,　1460
Cyanocobalamin,　821
Dehydrocholic Acid,　833, 2852
Deslanoside,　836
Dextran 40,　838
Digoxin,　854
Dimercaprol,　868
Dimorpholamine,　869
Docetaxel,　879
Docetaxel for,　880
Dopamine Hydrochloride,　886
Doripenem for,　889
Doxorubicin Hydrochloride for,
　900
Edaravone,　915
Edrophonium Chloride,　918
Ephedrine Hydrochloride,　935
Epinephrine,　418
Ergometrine Maleate,　949
Estradiol Benzoate (Aqueous Suspen-
　sion),　960
Estriol (Aqueous Suspension),　961
Famotidine,　989
Famotidine for,　990
Filgrastim (Genetical Recombina-
　tion),　1009
Flomoxef Sodium for,　1016
Fluconazole,　1020
Folic Acid,　1037
Fosfomycin Sodium for,　1044
Fructose,　1046, 2855
Furosemide,　1050
Gallium (^{67}Ga) Citrate,　1055
Gentamicin Sulfate,　1066
Glucose,　1076
Haloperidol,　1092

Heparin Sodium, 1104, 2856
Human Chorionic Gonadotrophin for, 1086
Hydralazine Hydrochloride for, 1109
Idarubicin Hydrochloride for, 1137
Imipenem and Cilastatin Sodium for, 1145, 2884
Indigocarmine, 1152
Indium (^{111}In) Chloride, 1152
Insulin Human (Genetical Recombination), 1157, 2885
Insulin Glargine (Genetical Recombination), 1164
Interferon Alfa (NAMALWA), 1168
Iodinated (^{131}I) Human Serum Albumin, 1169
Iohexol, 1177
Iopamidol, 1178
Irinotecan Hydrochloride, 1189
Isepamicin Sulfate, 1194
Isoniazid, 1201
Levallorphan Tartrate, 1254
Levofloxacin, 1258
Lidocaine, 1264
Lincomycin Hydrochloride, 1267
Magnesium Sulfate, 1294
D-Mannitol, 1300
Meglumine Iotalamate, 1311
Meglumine Sodium Amidotrizoate, 1312
Mepivacaine Hydrochloride, 1318
Meropenem for, 1322
Metenolone Enanthate, 1328
Methotrexate for, 1333
Minocycline Hydrochloride for, 1366
Mitomycin C for, 1372
Morphine and Atropine, 1385
Morphine Hydrochloride, 1383
Nartograstim for (Genetical Recombination), 1405, 2891
Neostigmine Methylsulfate, 1409
Nicardipine Hydrochloride, 1410
Nicotinic Acid, 1419
Noradrenaline, 1433
Norepinephrine, 1433
Opial, 1449
Opium Alkaloids and Atropine, 1450
Opium Alkaloids and Scopolamine, 1451
Opium Alkaloids Hydrochlorides, 1449
Oxytocin, 1467
Ozagrel Sodium, 1469
Ozagrel Sodium for, 1470
Panipenem and Betamipron for, 1473
Papaverine Hydrochloride, 1476
Pazufloxacin Mesilate, 1486
Penicillin G Potassium for, 528

Peplomycin Sulfate for, 1496
Pethidine Hydrochloride, 1501
Phenolsulfonphthalein, 1510
Phenytoin Sodium for, 1514
Piperacillin Sodium for, 1534
Prednisolone Sodium Succinate for, 1576
Procainamide Hydrochloride, 1543
Procaine Hydrochloride, 1585
Progesterone, 1590
Protamine Sulfate, 1604
Purified Sodium Hyaluronate, 1710
Pyridoxine Hydrochloride, 1611
Reserpine, 1629
Riboflavin Sodium Phosphate, 1638
Ritodrine Hydrochloride, 1650
Roxatidine Acetate Hydrochloride for, 1659
Sivelestat Sodium for, 1695
Sodium Bicarbonate, 1699
Sodium Chloride, 0.9%, 1703
Sodium Chloride, 10%, 1703
Sodium Chromate (^{51}Cr), 1704
Sodium Citrate for Transfusion, 1704
Sodium Iodohippurate (^{131}I), 1714
Sodium Iotalamate, 1714
Sodium Pertechnetate (^{99m}Tc), 1719
Sodium Thiosulfate, 1727
Spectinomycin Hydrochloride for, 1735, 2899
Sterile Water for, in Containers, 1920
Streptomycin Sulfate for, 1746
Sulfobromophthalein Sodium, 1756
Sulpyrine, 1760
Suxamethonium Chloride, 1765
Suxamethonium Chloride for, 1766
Tazobactam and Piperacillin for, 1782
Teceleukin for (Genetical Recombination), 1789
Temozolomide for, 2902
Testosterone Enanthate, 1810
Testosterone Propionate, 1811
Thallium (^{201}Tl) Chloride, 1813
Thiamine Chloride Hydrochloride, 1816
Thiamylal Sodium for, 1819
Thiopental Sodium for, 1822, 2866
Tobramycin, 1838
Tranexamic Acid, 1852
Vancomycin Hydrochloride for, 1904
Vasopressin, 1904
Verapamil Hydrochloride, 1906
Vinblastine Sulfate for, 1908
Vitamin B$_1$ Hydrochloride, 1816
Vitamin B$_2$ Phosphate Ester, 1638
Vitamin B$_6$, 1611
Vitamin B$_{12}$, 821

Vitamin C, 484
Voriconazole for, 1915
Water for, 1920
Weak Opium Alkaloids and Scopolamine, 1452
Xylite, 1924
Xylitol, 1924
Insulin
    Human (Genetical Recombination), 1155, 2884
    Human (Genetical Recombination) Injection, 1157, 2885
    Aspart (GeneticalRecombination), 1160
    Glargine (Genetical Recombination), 1162
    Glargine (Genetical Recombination) Injection, 1164
Interferon Alfa (NAMALWA), 1165
Interferon Alfa (NAMALWA) Injection, 1168
Iodinated (^{131}I) Human Serum Albumin Injection, 1169
Iodine, 1170
    Glycerin, Compound, 1171
    Glycerin, Dental, 1172
    , Salicylic Acid and Phenol Spirit, 1173
    Tincture, 1170
    Tincture, Dilute, 1171
Iodoform, 1174
Iohexol, 1175, 2857
    Injection, 1177
Iopamidol, 1177, 2857
    Injection, 1178
Iotalamic Acid, 1179, 2857
Iotroxic Acid, 1180, 2857
Ipecac, 2036
    Powdered, 2037
    Syrup, 2038
Ipratropium Bromide Hydrate, 1181, 2857
Ipriflavone, 1182, 2857
    Tablets, 1183
Irbesartan, 1183, 2857
    and Amlodipine Besilate Tablets, 1185
    Tablets, 1184
Irinotecan Hydrochloride
    Hydrate, 1187, 2857
    Injection, 1189
Irsogladine Maleate, 1190, 2857
    Fine Granules, 1191
    Tablets, 1192
Isepamicin Sulfate, 1193, 2857
    Injection, 1194
Isoflurane, 1195
L-Isoleucine, 1196, 2857
    , L-Leucine and L-Valine Granules, 1197
Isomalt, 1198
    Hydrate, 1198, 2857
Isoniazid, 1200, 2857

Injection, 1201
Tablets, 1201
Isophane Insulin Human (Genetical Recombination) Injectable Aqueous Suspension, 1158, 2885
l-Isoprenaline Hydrochloride, 1202, 2857
Isopropanol, 1203
Isopropyl Alcohol, 1203
Isopropylantipyrine, 1203, 2857
Isosorbide, 1204, 2857
Dinitrate, 1205, 2857
Dinitrate Tablets, 1205
Mononitrate 70%/Lactose 30%, 1206, 2857
Mononitrate Tablets, 1208
Isotonic Sodium Chloride Solution, 1703, 2864
Isoxsuprine Hydrochloride, 1209, 2857
Tablets, 1210
Itraconazole, 1211, 2857

J

Japanese
Angelica Root, 2039
Angelica Root, Powdered, 2039
Gentian, 2040
Gentian, Powdered, 2040
Valerian, 2040
Valerian, Powdered, 2041
Zanthoxylum Peel, 2041
Zanthoxylum Peel, Powdered, 2042
Josamycin, 1212, 2857
Propionate, 1214, 2857
Tablets, 1213
Jujube, 2042
Seed, 2042
Juzentaihoto Extract, 2043

K

Kainic Acid
and Santonin Powder, 1215
Hydrate, 1215, 2857
Kakkonto Extract, 2046
Kakkontokasenkyushin'i Extract, 2049
Kallidinogenase, 1216
Kamikihito Extract, 2052
Kamishoyosan Extract, 2055
Kanamycin
Monosulfate, 1218, 2857
Sulfate, 1219, 2857
Kaolin, 1220
Keishibukuryogan Extract, 2058, 2913
Ketamine Hydrochloride, 1221, 2857
Ketoconazole, 1221, 2857
Cream, 1222
Lotion, 1223
Solution, 1223

Ketoprofen, 1224, 2857
Ketotifen Fumarate, 1225, 2857
Kitasamycin, 1226
Acetate, 1227
Tartrate, 1228, 2857
Koi, 2060

L

Labetalol Hydrochloride, 1230, 2857
Tablets, 1231
Lactic Acid, 1232, 2857
L-Lactic Acid, 1232, 2857
Lactose
Anhydrous, 1233, 2857
Hydrate, 1234, 2857
Lactulose, 1235, 2857
Lafutidine, 1236, 2858
Tablets, 1237
Lanoconazole, 1238, 2858
Cream, 1239
Cutaneous Solution, 1240
Ointment, 1240
Lanolin
Hydrous, 2061
Purified, 2061
Lansoprazole, 1241, 2858
Delayed-release Capsules, 1242
Delayed-release Orally Disintegrating Tablets, 1243
Lard, 2062
Latamoxef Sodium, 1245, 2858
Lauromacrogol, 1246
Lemonades
Hydrochloric Acid, 1112
Lenampicillin Hydrochloride, 1246, 2858
Lenograstim (Genetical Recombination), 1248
Leonurus Herb, 2063, 2913
L-Leucine, 1251, 2858
Leuprorelin Acetate, 1252
Levallorphan Tartrate, 1254, 2858
Injection, 1254
Levodopa, 1255, 2858
Levofloxacin
Fine Granules, 1257
Hydrate, 1256, 2858
Injection, 1258
Ophthalmic Solution, 1258
Tablets, 1259
Levomepromazine Maleate, 1261, 2858
Levothyroxine Sodium
Hydrate, 1261
Tablets, 1262
Lidocaine, 1263, 2858
Injection, 1264
Light
Anhydrous Silicic Acid, 1680, 2864
Liquid Paraffin, 1478, 2861
Lilium Bulb, 2063
Limaprost Alfadex, 1264

Lincomycin Hydrochloride
Hydrate, 1266, 2858
Injection, 1267
Lindera Root, 2064
Liniments
Diphenhydramine, Phenol and Zinc Oxide, 872
Phenol and Zinc Oxide, 1509
Liothyronine Sodium, 1267
Tablets, 1268
Liquefied Phenol, 1507
Liquid Paraffin, 1477, 2861
Lisinopril
Hydrate, 1269, 2858
Tablets, 1270
Lithium Carbonate, 1271, 2858
Lithospermum Root, 2064
Lobenzarit Sodium, 1273, 2858
Longan Aril, 2065
Longgu, 2065
Powdered, 2065
Lonicera Leaf and Stem, 2066
Loquat Leaf, 2066
Lorazepam, 1273, 2858
Losartan Potassium, 1274, 2858
and Hydrochlorothiazide Tablets, 1276
Tablets, 1275
Lotions
Ketoconazole, 1223
Sulfur and Camphor, 1756
Tacalcitol, 1767
Low Substituted Hydroxypropylcellulose, 1124, 2856
Loxoprofen Sodium
Hydrate, 1279, 2858
Tablets, 1280
Lycium
Bark, 2067
Fruit, 2067
L-Lysine
Acetate, 1281, 2858
Hydrochloride, 1282, 2858
Lysozyme Hydrochloride, 1283, 2858

M

Macrogol
400, 1284
1500, 1284
4000, 1285
6000, 1285
20000, 1286
Ointment, 1286
Magnesium
Aluminometasilicate, 1288, 2858
Aluminosilicate, 1287, 2858
Carbonate, 1289, 2858
Oxide, 1290, 2858
Silicate, 1291
Stearate, 1292, 2858, 2886
Sulfate Hydrate, 1294, 2858
Sulfate Injection, 1294

Supplement I, JP XVIII
Index 2965

Sulfate Mixture, 1295
Magnolia
 Bark, 2067, 2914
 Bark, Powdered, 2068
 Flower, 2069
Mallotus Bark, 2069
Malt, 2069
Maltose Hydrate, 1295, 2858
Manidipine Hydrochloride, 1296, 2858
 Tablets, 1297
D-Mannitol, 1298, 2858, 2888
 Injection, 1300
Maoto Extract, 2070, 2914
Maprotiline Hydrochloride, 1300, 2858
Meclofenoxate Hydrochloride, 1301, 2858
Mecobalamin, 1302
 Tablets, 1303
Medazepam, 1304, 2858
Medicinal
 Carbon, 1305, 2858
 Soap, 1306, 2858
Medroxyprogesterone Acetate, 1306, 2858
Mefenamic Acid, 1307, 2858
Mefloquine Hydrochloride, 1308, 2859
Mefruside, 1309, 2859
 Tablets, 1310
Meglumine, 1310, 2859
 Iotalamate Injection, 1311
 Sodium Amidotrizoate Injection, 1312
Melphalan, 1313, 2859
Menatetrenone, 1314, 2859
Mentha
 Herb, 2072
 Oil, 2072
 Water, 2073
dl-Menthol, 1315, 2889
l-Menthol, 1315, 2890
Mepenzolate Bromide, 1316, 2859
Mepitiostane, 1316, 2859
Mepivacaine Hydrochloride, 1317, 2859
 Injection, 1318
Mequitazine, 1319, 2859
 Tablets, 1319
Mercaptopurine Hydrate, 1320, 2859
Meropenem
 for Injection, 1322
 Hydrate, 1321, 2859
Mesalazine, 1323, 2859
 Extended-release Tablets, 1325
Mestranol, 1326, 2859
Metenolone
 Acetate, 1327, 2859
 Enanthate, 1328, 2859
 Enanthate Injection, 1328
Metformin Hydrochloride, 1329, 2859

Tablets, 1329
Methamphetamine Hydrochloride, 1330
L-Methionine, 1331, 2859
Methotrexate, 1331
 Capsules, 1332
 for Injection, 1333
 Tablets, 1334
Methoxsalen, 1335, 2859
Methyl
 Parahydroxybenzoate, 1343, 2859, 2890
 Salicylate, 1346, 2859
 Salicylate Spirit, Compound, 1347
Methylbenactyzium Bromide, 1336
Methylcellulose, 1336, 2859
Methyldopa
 Hydrate, 1338, 2859
 Tablets, 1339
dl-Methylephedrine Hydrochloride, 1340, 2859
 Powder, 10%, 1341
Methylergometrine Maleate, 1342
 Tablets, 1342
Methylprednisolone, 1344
 Succinate, 1345, 2859
Methyltestosterone, 1347
 Tablets, 1348
Meticrane, 1349, 2859
Metildigoxin, 1350, 2859
Metoclopramide, 1351, 2859
 Tablets, 1351
Metoprolol Tartrate, 1352, 2859
 Tablets, 1353
Metronidazole, 1354, 2859
 Tablets, 1354
Metyrapone, 1355, 2859
Mexiletine Hydrochloride, 1356, 2859
Miconazole, 1357, 2859
 Nitrate, 1358, 2859
Microcrystalline Cellulose, 716, 2850
Micronomicin Sulfate, 1358, 2859
Midecamycin, 1359, 2859
 Acetate, 1360, 2859
Miglitol, 1361, 2859
 Tablets, 1362
Migrenin, 1363, 2860
Minocycline Hydrochloride, 1364, 2860
 for Injection, 1366
 Granules, 1365
 Tablets, 1367
Mitiglinide Calcium
 Hydrate, 1368, 2860
 Tablets, 1369
Mitomycin C, 1371
 for Injection, 1372
Mizoribine, 1372, 2860
 Tablets, 1373
Monobasic Calcium Phosphate Hydrate, 606, 2848
Montelukast Sodium, 1334, 2860
 Chewable Tablets, 1377

Granules, 1379
 Tablets, 1380
Morphine
 and Atropine Injection, 1385
 Hydrochloride Hydrate, 1382
 Hydrochloride Injection, 1383
 Hydrochloride Tablets, 1384
 Sulfate Hydrate, 1386
Mosapride Citrate
 Hydrate, 1387, 2860
 Powder, 1388
 Tablets, 1389
Moutan Bark, 2073
 Powdered, 2074
Mukoi-Daikenchuto Extract, 2075, 2914
Mulberry Bark, 2076
Mupirocin Calcium
 Hydrate, 1390, 2860
 Ointment, 1392

N

Nabumetone, 1392, 2860
 Tablets, 1393
Nadolol, 1394, 2860
Nafamostat Mesilate, 1395, 2860
Naftopidil, 1396, 2860
 Orally Disintegrating Tablets, 1397
 Tablets, 1398
Nalidixic Acid, 1399, 2860
Naloxone Hydrochloride, 1400
Naphazoline
 and Chlorpheniramine Solution, 1401
 Hydrochloride, 1400
 Nitrate, 1401, 2860
Naproxen, 1402, 2860
Nartograstim (Genetical Recombination), 1403, 2891
 for Injection, 1405, 2891
Natamycin, 1520
Nateglinide, 1406, 2860
 Tablets, 1407
Natural Aluminum Silicate, 442, 2845
Nelumbo Seed, 2077
Neomycin Sulfate, 1045
Neostigmine Methylsulfate, 1408
 Injection, 1409
Nicardipine Hydrochloride, 1410, 2860
 Injection, 1410
Nicergoline, 1411, 2860
 Powder, 1412
 Tablets, 1413
Niceritrol, 1414, 2860
Nicomol, 1415, 2860
 Tablets, 1416
Nicorandil, 1417, 2860
Nicotinamide, 1417, 2860
Nicotinic Acid, 1418, 2860
 Injection, 1419
Nifedipine, 1420, 2860

Delayed-release Fine Granules, 1420
Extended-release Capsules, 1422
Fine Granules, 1422
Nilvadipine, 1423, 2860
Tablets, 1424
Nitrazepam, 1426, 2860
Nitrendipine, 1426, 2860
Tablets, 1427
Nitrogen, 1428
Nitroglycerin Tablets, 1429
Nitrous Oxide, 1430
Nizatidine, 1431, 2860
Capsules, 1432
Noradrenaline, 1433
Injection, 1433
Norepinephrine, 1433
Injection, 1433
Norethisterone, 1434
Norfloxacin, 1434, 2860
Norgestrel, 1435, 2860
and Ethinylestradiol Tablets, 1436
Nortriptyline Hydrochloride, 1437, 2860
Tablets, 1438
Noscapine, 1439, 2860
Hydrochloride Hydrate, 1439
Notopterygium, 2077
Nuphar Rhizome, 2077
Nutmeg, 2078, 2915
Nux Vomica, 2078
Extract, 2079
Extract Powder, 2080
Tincture, 2080
Nystatin, 1440, 2860

O

Ofloxacin, 1441, 2860
Ointments
Aciclovir, 410
Aciclovir Ophthalmic, 411
Acrinol and Zinc Oxide, 416
Betamethasone Valerate and Gentamicin Sulfate, 544
Gentamicin Sulfate, 1066
Hydrocortisone and Diphenhydramine, 1115
Ibuprofen Piconol, 1135
Lanoconazole, 1240
Macrogol, 1286
Mupirocin Calcium, 1392
Polyethylene Glycol, 1286
Simple, 2153
Sulfur, Salicylic Acid and Thianthol, 1757
Tacalcitol, 1768
White, 1921
Zinc Oxide, 1929
Olive Oil, 2081
Olmesartan Medoxomil, 1442, 2860
Tablets, 1443
Olopatadine Hydrochloride, 1444,

2860
Tablets, 1445
Omeprazole, 1446, 2860
Delayed-release Tablets, 1447
Ophiopogon Root, 2081
Ophthalmic Solution
Bromfenac Sodium, 565
Chloramphenicol and Colistin Sodium Methanesulfonate, 731
Dibekacin Sulfate, 845
Dorzolamide Hydrochloride, 892
Dorzolamide Hydrochloride and Timolol Maleate, 893
Gatifloxacin, 1057
Gentamicin Sulfate, 1067
Idoxuridine, 1139
Levofloxacin, 1258
Pemirolast Potassium, 1487
Purified Sodium Hyaluronate, 1711
Silver Nitrate, 1687
Tranilast, 1856
Zinc Sulfate, 1931
Ophthalmic Ointment
Aciclovir, 411
Opium
Ipecac Powder, 2083
Powder, Diluted, 2082
Powdered, 2082
Tincture, 2083
Opium Alkaloids
and Atropine Injection, 1450
and Scopolamine Injection, 1451
Hydrochlorides, 1448
Hydrochlorides Injection, 1449
Orange
Oil, 2083
Peel Syrup, 2084
Peel Tincture, 2084
Orciprenaline Sulfate, 1454, 2860
Orengedokuto Extract, 2084
Oriental Bezoar, 2086
Otsujito Extract, 2087
Oxapium Iodide, 1454, 2861
Oxaprozin, 1455, 2861
Oxazolam, 1456, 2861
Oxetacaine, 1457
Oxethazaine, 1457, 2861
Oxprenolol Hydrochloride, 1457, 2861
Oxybuprocaine Hydrochloride, 1458, 2861
Oxybutynin Hydrochloride, 2891
Oxycodone Hydrochloride Hydrate, 1459
Oxydol, 1462, 2861
Oxygen, 1462
Oxymetholone, 1463
Oxytetracycline Hydrochloride, 1464, 2861
Oxytocin, 1465
Injection, 1467
Oyster Shell, 2090
Powdered, 2090

Ozagrel Sodium, 1468, 2861
for Injection, 1470
Injection, 1469

P

Panax Japonicus Rhizome, 2090
Powdered, 2091
Pancreatin, 1470
Pancuronium Bromide, 1471
Panipenem, 1471, 2861
and Betamipron for Injection, 1473
Pantethine, 1475, 2861
Papaverine Hydrochloride, 1475
Injection, 1476
Paracetamol, 402
Paraffin, 1476, 2861
Light Liquid, 1478, 2861
Liquid, 1477, 2861
Paraformaldehyde, 1478
Paste, Dental, 1479
Parnaparin Sodium, 1480, 2861
Paroxetine Hydrochloride
Hydrate, 1482, 2861
Tablets, 1483
Pas-calcium
Granules, 604
Hydrate, 603
Paste
Arsenical, 483
Dental Paraformaldehyde, 1479
Dental Triozinc, 1877
Pazufloxacin Mesilate, 1485, 2861
Injection, 1486
Peach Kernel, 2091, 2915
Powdered, 2092, 2915
Peanut Oil, 2093
Pemirolast Potassium, 1486, 2861
for Syrup, 1489
Ophthalmic Solution, 1487
Tablets, 1489
Penbutolol Sulfate, 1490, 2861
Penicillin G Potassium, 527
for Injection, 528
Pentazocine, 1491, 2861
Pentobarbital Calcium, 1491, 2861
Tablets, 1492
Pentoxyverine Citrate, 1493, 2861
Peony Root, 2093
Powdered, 2094
Peplomycin Sulfate, 1494, 2861
for Injection, 1496
Perilla Herb, 2095
Perphenazine, 1497, 2861
Maleate, 1498, 2861
Maleate Tablets, 1499
Tablets, 1497
Pethidine Hydrochloride, 1500
Injection, 1501
Petrolatum, 2893
White, 1501, 2861, 2892
Yellow, 1502, 2861, 2893
Petroleum Benzin, 1503

Supplement I, JP XVIII   Index   2967

Peucedanum Root, 2095
Pharbitis Seed, 2096
Phellodendron
    , Albumin Tannate and Bismuth Sub-
        nitrate Powder, 2098
    Bark, 2096
    Bark, Powdered, 2097
    Powder for Cataplasm, Compound,
        2098
Phenazone, 475
Phenethicillin Potassium, 1503, 2861
Phenobarbital, 1504, 2861
    Powder, 10%, 1505
    Tablets, 1506
Phenol, 1507
    and Zinc Oxide Liniment, 1509
    for Disinfection, 1507
    Liquefied, 1507
    with Camphor, Dental, 1508
Phenolated Water, 1508
    for Disinfection, 1508
Phenolsulfonphthalein, 1509
    Injection, 1510
L-Phenylalanine, 1510, 2861
Phenylbutazone, 1511, 2861
Phenylephrine Hydrochloride, 1512
Phenytoin, 1512, 2861
    Powder, 1513
    Sodium for Injection, 1514, 2861
    Tablets, 1513
Phytonadione, 1515, 2861
Picrasma Wood, 2099, 2915
    Powdered, 2099, 2916
Pilocarpine Hydrochloride, 1516
    Tablets, 1516
Pilsicainide Hydrochloride
    Capsules, 1519
    Hydrate, 1518, 2861
Pimaricin, 1520, 2861
Pimozide, 1521, 2861
Pindolol, 1522, 2862
Pinellia Tuber, 2100
Pioglitazone Hydrochloride, 1522,
    2862
    and Glimepiride Tablets, 1524
    and Metformin Hydrochloride
        Tablets, 1527
    Tablets, 1523
Pipemidic Acid Hydrate, 1530, 2862
Piperacillin
    Hydrate, 1530, 2862
    Sodium, 1532, 2862
    Sodiumfor Injection, 1534
Piperazine
    Adipate, 1534, 2862
    Phosphate Hydrate, 1535, 2862
    Phosphate Tablets, 1535
Pirarubicin, 1536, 2862
Pirenoxine, 1537, 2862
Pirenzepine Hydrochloride Hydrate,
    1538, 2862
Piroxicam, 1539, 2862
Pitavastatin Calcium

Hydrate, 1540, 2862
Orally Disintegrating Tablets, 1541
Tablets, 1543
Pivmecillinam Hydrochloride, 1545,
    2862
    Tablets, 1546
Plantago
    Herb, 2100, 2916
    Seed, 2100
Platycodon
    Fluidextract, 2102
    Root, 2101
    Root, Powdered, 2101
Pogostemon Herb, 2102
Polaprezinc, 1546, 2862
    Granules, 1548
Polyethylene Glycol
    400, 1284
    1500, 1284
    4000, 1285
    6000, 1285
    20000, 1286
    Ointment, 1286
Polygala Root, 2102
    Powdered, 2103
Polygonatum Rhizome, 2103
Polygonum Root, 2104
Polymixin B Sulfate, 1543, 2862
Polyoxyl 40 Stearate, 1550, 2862
Polyporus Sclerotium, 2104
    Powdered, 2104
Polysorbate 80, 1550, 2862, 2894
Poria Sclerotium, 2105
    Powdered, 2105
Potash Soap, 1552
Potassium
    Bromide, 1552, 2862
    Canrenoate, 1553, 2862
    Carbonate, 1553, 2862
    Chloride, 1554, 2862
    Clavulanate, 1554, 2862
    Guaiacolsulfonate, 1556
    Hydroxide, 1556, 2862
    Iodide, 1557, 2862
    Permanganate, 1558, 2862
    Sulfate, 1558, 2862
Potato Starch, 1739
Povidone, 1559, 2862
    -Iodine, 1561, 2862
Powder
    Ascorbic Acid, 485
    Chlordiazepoxide, 733
    Chlorpheniramine Maleate, 741
    Codeine Phosphate, 1%, 804
    Codeine Phosphate, 10%, 805
    Compound Diastase and Sodium Bi-
        carbonate, 843
    Compound Phellodendron, for
        Cataplasm, 2098
    Compound Rhubarb and Senna,
        2115
    Compound ScopoliaExtract and Di-
        astase, 2136

Diastase and Sodium Bicarbonate,
    843
Dihydrocodeine Phosphate, 1%,
    857
Dihydrocodeine Phosphate, 10%,
    858
Diluted Opium, 2082
Diphenhydramine and
    Bromovalerylurea, 871
Ephedrine Hydrochloride, 10%,
    936
Famotidine, 991
Gentian and Sodium Bicarbonate,
    2008
Hydralazine Hydrochloride, 1110
Kainic Acid and Santonin, 1215
dl-Methylephedrine Hydrochloride,
    10%, 1341
Mosapride Citrate, 1388
Nicergoline, 1412
Nux Vomica Extract, 2080
Opium Ipecac, 2083
Phellodendron, Albumin Tannate
    and Bismuth Subnitrate, 2098
Phenobarbital, 10%, 1505
Phenytoin, 1513
Reserpine, 0.1%, 1630
Riboflavin, 1635
Scopolia Extract and Carbon, 2136
Scopolia Extract and Ethyl
    Aminobenzoate, 2137
Salicylated Alum, 1670
Scopolia Extract, 2135
Swertia and Sodium Bicarbonate,
    2158
Thiamine Chloride Hydrochloride,
    1817
Vitamin B₁ Hydrochloride, 1817
Vitamin B₂, 1635
Vitamin C, 485
Zinc Oxide Starch, 1930
Powdered
    Acacia, 1939
    Agar, 1941
    Alisma Tuber, 1942
    Aloe, 1943
    Amomum Seed, 1945
    Atractylodes Lancea Rhizome,
        1951
    Atractylodes Rhizome, 1952
    Calumba, 1972
    Capsicum, 1973
    Cellulose, 719, 2850, 2878
    Cinnamon Bark, 1981
    Clove, 1984
    Cnidium Rhizome, 1986
    Coix Seed, 1987
    Coptis Rhizome, 1989
    Corydalis Tuber, 1992, 2910
    Cyperus Rhizome, 1994
    Dioscorea Rhizome, 1999
    Fennel, 2003
    Gambir, 2005

Gardenia Fruit, 2006
Gentian, 2008
Geranium Herb, 2009
Ginger, 2010, 2911
Ginseng, 2012
Glycyrrhiza, 2014
Ipecac, 2037
Japanese Angelica Root, 2039
Japanese Gentian, 2040
Japanese Valerian, 2041
Japanese Zanthoxylum Peel, 2042
Longgu, 2065
Magnolia Bark, 2068
Moutan Bark, 2074
Opium, 2082
Oyster Shell, 2090
Panax Japonicus Rhizome, 2091
Peach Kernel, 2092, 2915
Peony Root, 2094
Phellodendron Bark, 2097
Picrasma Wood, 2099, 2916
Platycodon Root, 2101
Polygala Root, 2103
Polyporus Sclerotium, 2104
Poria Sclerotium, 2105
Processed Aconite Root, 2108
Rhubarb, 2114
Rose Fruit, 2118
Scutellaria Root, 2139
Senega, 2140
Senna Leaf, 2142, 2920
Smilax Rhizome, 2154
Sophora Root, 2155
Sweet Hydrangea Leaf, 2156
Swertia Herb, 2158
Tragacanth, 2165
Turmeric, 2167
Pranlukast Hydrate, 1562, 2862
Pranoprofen, 1563, 2862
Prasterone Sodium Sulfate Hydrate, 1564, 2862
Pravastatin Sodium, 1564, 2862
Fine Granules, 1566
Solution, 1567
Tablets, 1568
Prazepam, 1570, 2862
Tablets, 1570
Prazosin Hydrochloride, 1571, 2862
Precipitated Calcium Carbonate, 594, 2848
Fine Granules, 594
Tablets, 595
Prednisolone, 1572, 2862
Acetate, 1574
Sodium Phosphate, 1575, 2862
Sodium Succinate for Injection, 1576
Succinate, 1576
Tablets, 1573
Prepared Glycyrrhiza, 2105, 2916
Primidone, 1578, 2862
Probenecid, 1578, 2863
Tablets, 1579

Probucol, 1580, 2863
Fine Granules, 1581
Tablets, 1582
Procainamide Hydrochloride, 1582, 2863
Injection, 1543
Tablets, 1584
Procaine Hydrochloride, 1585, 2863
Injection, 1585
Procarbazine Hydrochloride, 1586, 2863
Procaterol Hydrochloride Hydrate, 1587, 2863
Processed
Aconite Root, 2106
Aconite Root, Powdered, 2108
Ginger, 2109, 2916
Prochlorperazine Maleate, 1588, 2863
Tablets, 1588
Progesterone, 1589
Injection, 1590
Proglumide, 1591, 2863
L-Proline, 1591, 2863
Promethazine Hydrochloride, 1593, 2863
Propafenone Hydrochloride, 1593, 2863
Tablets, 1594
Propantheline Bromide, 1595
Propiverine Hydrochloride, 1596, 2863
Tablets, 1597
Propranolol Hydrochloride, 1598, 2863
Tablets, 1599
Propylene Glycol, 1600, 2863
Propyl Parahydroxybenzoate, 1601, 2863, 2896
Propylthiouracil, 1602
Tablets, 1603
Propyphenazone, 1203
Protamine Sulfate, 1603
Injection, 1604
Prothionamide, 1605, 2863
Protirelin, 1605, 2863
Tartrate Hydrate, 1606, 2863
Prunella Spike, 2110
Pueraria Root, 2110
Pullulan, 1607, 2863
Capsules, 622
Purified
Dehydrocholic Acid, 832, 2852
Gelatin, 1062, 2855
Glucose, 1075, 2855
Lanolin, 2061
Shellac, 1679, 2864
Sodium Hyaluronate, 1709, 2865
Sodium Hyaluronate Injection, 1710
Sodium Hyaluronate Ophthalmic Solution, 1711
Water, 1919
Water in Containers, 1919

Pyrantel Pamoate, 1607, 2863
Pyrazinamide, 1608, 2863
Pyridostigmine Bromide, 1609, 2863
Pyridoxal Phosphate Hydrate, 1609, 2863
Pyridoxine Hydrochloride, 1611, 2863
Injection, 1611
Pyroxylin, 1612
Pyrrolnitrin, 1612

Q

Quercus Bark, 2111
Quetiapine Fumarate, 1613, 2863
Fine Granules, 1615
Tablets, 1615
Quinapril Hydrochloride, 1617, 2863
Tablets, 1618
Quinidine Sulfate Hydrate, 1620
Quinine
Ethyl Carbonate, 1621, 2863
Hydrochloride Hydrate, 1622
Sulfate Hydrate, 1623, 2863

R

Rabeprazole Sodium, 1624, 2863
Ranitidine Hydrochloride, 1625, 2863
Rape Seed Oil, 2111
Rebamipide, 1626, 2863
Tablets, 1627
Red Ginseng, 2112
Rehmannia Root, 2113
Reserpine, 1628
Injection, 1629
Tablets, 1630
Powder, 0.1%, 1630
Retinol
Acetate, 1631
Palmitate, 1632
Rhubarb, 2113
and Senna Powder, Compound, 2115
Powdered, 2114
Ribavirin, 1632, 2863
Capsules, 1633
Riboflavin, 1635
Butyrate, 1636, 2863
Powder, 1635
Sodium Phosphate, 1637
Sodium Phosphate Injection, 1638
Ribostamycin Sulfate, 1638, 2863
Rice Starch, 1740
Rifampicin, 1639, 2863
Capsules, 1640
Rikkunshito Extract, 2116
Rilmazafone Hydrochloride
Hydrate, 1642, 2863
Tablets, 1643
Ringer's Solution, 1644, 2863
Risperidone, 1645, 2864
Fine Granules, 1645

Oral Solution, 1647
Tablets, 1648
Ritodrine Hydrochloride, 1649, 2864
Injection, 1650
Tablets, 1651
Rose Fruit, 2118
Powdered, 2118
Rosin, 2118
Rosuvastatin Calcium, 1652, 2864
Tablets, 1654
Roxatidine Acetate Hydrochloride, 1656, 2864
Extended-release Capsules, 1657
Extended-release Tablets, 1658
for Injection, 1659
Roxithromycin, 1660, 2864
Tablets, 1661
Royal Jelly, 2119
Ryokeijutsukanto Extract, 2119

S

Saccharated Pepsin, 1662
Saccharin, 1663, 2864
Sodium Hydrate, 1664, 2864
Safflower, 2121
Saffron, 2122
Saibokuto Extract, 2122
Saikokeishikankyoto Extract, 2916
Saikokeishito Extract, 2125
Saireito Extract, 2128
Salazosulfapyridine, 1666, 2864
Salbutamol Sulfate, 1667, 2864
Salicylated Alum Powder, 1670
Salicylic Acid, 1667, 2864
Adhesive Plaster, 1668
Spirit, 1669
Spirit, Compound, 1669
Salvia Miltiorrhiza Root, 2131
Santonin, 1671
Saponated Cresol Solution, 816
Saposhnikovia Root and Rhizome, 2132
Sappan Wood, 2132
Sarpogrelate Hydrochloride, 1671, 2864
Fine Granules, 1672, 2898
Tablets, 1674
Saussurea Root, 2132
Schisandra Fruit, 2133
Schizonepeta Spike, 2133
Scopolamine
Butylbromide, 1675, 2864
Hydrobromide Hydrate, 1676
Scopolia
Extract, 2135
Extract and Carbon Powder, 2136
Extract and Ethyl Aminobenzoate Powder, 2137
Extract and Tannic Acid Suppositories, 2138
Extract Powder, 2135
Rhizome, 2133

Scutellaria Root, 2138
Powdered, 2139
Senega, 2140
Powdered, 2140
Syrup, 2140
Senna Leaf, 2141, 2920
Powdered, 2142, 2920
L-Serine, 1677, 2864
Sesame, 2143
Oil, 2143
Sevoflurane, 1677
Shakuyakukanzoto Extract, 2143
Shellac
Purified, 1679, 2864
White, 1679, 2864
Shimbuto Extract, 2145, 2920
Shosaikoto Extract, 2147
Shoseiryuto Extract, 2150
Silodosin, 1681, 2864
Orally Disintegrating Tablets, 1683
Tablets, 1684
Silver
Nitrate, 1686, 2864
Nitrate Ophthalmic Solution, 1687
Protein, 1687
Protein Solution, 1687
Simple
Ointment, 2153
Syrup, 1688
Simvastatin, 1688, 2864
Tablets, 1689
Sinomenium Stem and Rhizome, 2153, 2920
Sitagliptin Phosphate
Hydrate, 1691, 2864
Tablets, 1692
Sivelestat Sodium
for Injection, 1695
Hydrate, 1694, 2864
Smilax Rhizome, 2153
Powdered, 2154
Sodium
Acetate Hydrate, 1696, 2864
Aurothiomalate, 1697, 2864
Benzoate, 1698, 2864
Bicarbonate and Bitter Tincture Mixture, 2154
Bicarbonate, 1698, 2864
Bicarbonate Injection, 1699
Bisulfite, 1699, 2864
Borate, 1700, 2864
Bromide, 1700, 2864
Carbonate Hydrate, 1701, 2864
Chloride, 1702, 2864, 2898
Chloride Injection, 0.9%, 1703
Chloride Injection, 10%, 1703
Chromate (^{51}Cr) Injection, 1704
Citrate Hydrate, 1704, 2864
Citrate Injection for Transfusion, 1704
Cromoglicate, 1705, 2864
Fusidate, 1707, 2864
Hyaluronate, Purified, 1709, 2865

Hyaluronate Injection, Purified, 1710
Hyaluronate Ophthalmic Solution, Purified, 1711
Hydrogen Carbonate, 1698
Hydroxide, 1712, 2865
Iodide, 1713, 2865
Iodide (^{123}I) Capsules, 1714
Iodide (^{131}I) Capsules, 1714
Iodide (^{131}I) Solution, 1714
Iodohippurate (^{131}I) Injection, 1714
Iotalamate Injection, 1714
L-Lactate Ringer's Solution, 1716, 2865
L-Lactate Solution, 1715, 2865
Lauryl Sulfate, 1718
Metabisulfite, 1722
Pertechnetate (^{99m}Tc) Injection, 1719
Picosulfate Hydrate, 1720, 2865
Polystyrene Sulfonate, 1721, 2865
Pyrosulfite, 1722, 2865
Risedronate Hydrate, 1722, 2865
Risedronate Tablets, 1724
Salicylate, 1725, 2865
Starch Glycolate, 1725, 2865
Sulfate, Anhydrous, 2154
Sulfate Hydrate, 2155
Thiosulfate Hydrate, 1727, 2865
Thiosulfate Injection, 1727
Valproate, 1728, 2865
Valproate Extended-release Tablets A, 1729
Valproate Extended-release Tablets B, 1730
Valproate Syrup, 1731
Valproate Tablets, 1731
Solution
Adrenaline, 418
Alum, 439
Benzalkonium Chloride, 520
Benzethonium Chloride, 522
Butenafine Hydrochloride, 582
Chlorhexidine Gluconate, 735
Compound Thianthol and Salicylic Acid, 1820
Cresol, 816
Dental Sodium Hypochlorite, 475
Diagnostic Sodium Citrate, 1705
Epinephrine, 418
Glycerin and Potash, 1082
Heparin Sodium Lock, 1104
Heparin Sodium, for Dialysis, 1105
Isotonic Sodium Chloride, 1703
Ketoconazole, 1223
Lanoconazole Cutaneous, 1240
Naphazoline and Chlorpheniramine, 1401
Pravastatin Sodium, 1567
Ringer's, 1644
Risperidone Oral, 1647
Saponated Cresol, 816
Silver Protein, 1687

2970 *Index*

Solution (*continued*)
Sodium Iodide (^{131}I), 1714
Sodium L-Lactate, 1715, 2865
Sodium L-Lactate Ringer's, 1716, 2865
D-Sorbitol, 1733, 2865
Terbinafine Hydrochloride, 1806
Tolnaftate, 1845
Sophora Root, 2155
Powdered, 2155
Sorbitan Sesquioleate, 1732, 2865
D-Sorbitol, 1733, 2865
Solution, 1733, 2865
Soybean Oil, 2156
Spectinomycin Hydrochloride
for Injection, 1735, 2899
Hydrate, 1734
Spiramycin Acetate, 1736, 2865
Spirit
Capsicum and Salicylic Acid, 1975
Compound Methyl Salicylate, 1347
Compound Salicylic Acid, 1669
Foeniculated Ammonia, 2004
Iodine, Salicylic Acid and Phenol, 1173
Salicylic Acid, 1669
Spironolactone, 1737
Tablets, 1737
Spray
Butenafine Hydrochloride, 583
Terbinafine Hydrochloride, 1807
Starch
Corn, 1738
Potato, 1739
Rice, 1740
Wheat, 1741, 2899
Stearic Acid, 1743, 2865, 2899
Stearyl Alcohol, 1744
Sterile
Purified Water in Containers, 1920
Water for Injection in Containers, 1920
Streptomycin Sulfate, 1745, 2865
for Injection, 1746
Sucralfate Hydrate, 1746, 2865
Sucrose, 1748
Sulbactam Sodium, 1749, 2865
Sulbenicillin Sodium, 1750, 2865
Sulfadiazine Silver, 1751
Sulfafurazole, 1754
Sulfamethizole, 1752, 2865
Sulfamethoxazole, 1753, 2865
Sulfamonomethoxine Hydrate, 1713, 2865
Sulfasalazine, 1666
Sulfisoxazole, 1754, 2865
Sulfobromophthalein Sodium, 1755, 2865
Injection, 1756
Sulfur, 1756, 2865
and Camphor Lotion, 1756
, Salicylic Acid and Thianthol Ointment, 1757

Sulindac, 1757, 2865
Sulpiride, 1758, 2865
Capsules, 1758
Tablets, 1759
Sulpyrine
Hydrate, 1760, 2865
Injection, 1760
Sultamicillin Tosilate
Hydrate, 1761, 2865
Tablets, 1762
Sultiame, 1764, 2865
Suppositories
Bisacodyl, 554
Diclofenac Sodium, 847
Indometacin, 1154
ScopoliaExtract and Tannic Acid, 2138
Suxamethonium Chloride
for Injection, 1766
Hydrate, 1764
Injection, 1765
Sweet Hydrangea Leaf, 2156
Powdered, 2156
Swertia
and Sodium Bicarbonate Powder, 2158
Herb, 2157
Herb, Powdered, 2158
Synthetic Aluminum Silicate, 443, 2845
Syrup
Aciclovir, 411
Aciclovir for, 412
Amphotericin B, 466
Cefadroxil for, 647
Cefalexin for, 651
Cefatrizine Propylene Glycolate for, 655
Cefpodoxime Proxetil for, 696
Cefroxadine for, 700
Clarithromycin for, 771
Faropenem Sodium for, 994
Fosfomycin Calcium for, 1042
Ipecac, 2038
Orange Peel, 2084
Pemirolast Potassium for, 1489
Senega, 2140
Simple, 1688
Sodium Valproate, 1731
Tranilast for, 1856
Triclofos Sodium, 1869

T

Tablets
Acemetacin, 401
Acetylsalicylic Acid, 488
Aciclovir, 413
Ajmaline, 420
Alacepril, 422
Aldioxa, 426
Alendronate Sodium, 429
Allopurinol, 431

Alminoprofen, 433
Amiodarone Hydrochloride, 451
Amitriptyline Hydrochloride, 453
Amlexanox, 455
Amlodipine Besilate, 458
Amlodipine Besilate Orally Disintegrating, 457
Amosulalol Hydrochloride, 461
Amphotericin B, 467, 2868
Anastrozole, 2870
Ascorbic Acid and Calcium Pantothenate, 485
Aspirin, 488
Atorvastatin Calcium, 493
Auranofin, 497
Azathioprine, 499
Azelnidipine, 502
Azosemide, 505
Baclofen, 511
Benidipine Hydrochloride, 516
Bepotastine Besilate, 530
Beraprost Sodium, 532
Betahistine Mesilate, 536
Betamethasone, 539
Bezafibrate Extended-release, 549
Bicalutamide, 2872
Bisoprolol Fumarate, 557
Brotizolam, 568
Bucillamine, 570
Buformin Hydrochloride Delayed-release, 574
Buformin Hydrochloride, 575
Cadralazine, 587
Candesartan Cilexetil, 613
Candesartan Cilexetil and Amlodipine Besylate, 615
Candesartan Cilexetil and Hydrochlorothiazide, 618
L-Carbocisteine, 626
Carvedilol, 638
Cefcapene Pivoxil Hydrochloride, 663
Cefditoren Pivoxil, 668
Cefpodoxime Proxetil, 697
Cefteram Pivoxil, 706
Cetirizine Hydrochloride, 724
Chlordiazepoxide, 734
Chlorpheniramine Maleate, 742
Chlorpromazine Hydrochloride, 745
Chlorpropamide, 747
Chlorphenesin Carbamate, 739
Cibenzoline Succinate, 750
Cilazapril, 755
Cilnidipine, 758
Cilostazol, 760
Clarithromycin, 772
Clomifene Citrate, 784
Clomipramine Hydrochloride, 786
Clonazepam, 788
Cloperastine Fendizoate, 791
Clopidogrel Sulfate, 794
Clotiazepam, 798

Codeine Phosphate, 805
Colestimide, 809
Cyclophosphamide, 822
Diazepam, 844
Diethylcarbamazine Citrate, 849
Digoxin, 855
Dimenhydrinate, 866
Distigmine Bromide, 876
Donepezil Hydrochloride, 884
Doxazosin Mesilate, 897
Doxycycline Hydrochloride, 903
Dydrogesterone, 908
Ebastine, 911
Ebastine Orally Disintegrating, 909
Emorfazone, 924
Enalapril Maleate, 926
Entacapone, 930
Epalrestat, 933
Ephedrine Hydrochloride, 937
Eplerenone, 941
Ergometrine Maleate, 950
Erythromycin Delayed-release, 956
Estriol, 961
Etacrynic Acid, 963
Ethinylestradiol, 969
Ethyl Loflazepate, 978
Etidronate Disodium, 981
Etilefrine Hydrochloride, 983
Etizolam, 985
Famotidine, 992
Faropenem Sodium, 995
Felodipine, 999
Fenofibrate, 1002
Fexofenadine Hydrochloride, 1005
Flecainide Acetate, 1013
Fludiazepam, 1022
Flutoprazepam, 1033
Fluvoxamine Maleate, 1036
Folic Acid, 1038
Fudosteine, 1048
Furosemide, 1050
Glimepiride, 1070
Haloperidol, 1093
Hydralazine Hydrochloride, 1110
Ifenprodil Tartrate, 1141
Imidapril Hydrochloride, 1143
Imipramine Hydrochloride, 1147
Indapamide, 1149
Ipriflavone, 1183
Irbesartan, 1184
Irbesartan and Amlodipine Besilate, 1185
Irsogladine Maleate, 1192
Isoniazid, 1201
Isosorbide Dinitrate, 1205
Isosorbide Mononitrate, 1208
Isoxsuprine Hydrochloride, 1210
Josamycin, 1213
Labetalol Hydrochloride, 1231
Lafutidine, 1237
Lansoprazole Delayed-release Orally Disintegrating, 1243
Levofloxacin, 1259

Levothyroxine Sodium, 1262
Liothyronine Sodium, 1268
Lisinopril, 1270
Losartan Potassium, 1275
Losartan Potassium and Hydrochlorothiazide, 1276
Loxoprofen Sodium, 1280
Manidipine Hydrochloride, 1297
Mecobalamin, 1303
Mefruside, 1310
Mequitazine, 1319
Mesalazine Extended-release, 1325
Metformin Hydrochloride, 1329
Methotrexate, 1334
Methyldopa, 1339
Methylergometrine Maleate, 1342
Methyltestosterone, 1348
Metoclopramide, 1351
Metoprolol Tartrate, 1353
Metronidazole, 1354
Miglitol, 1362
Minocycline Hydrochloride, 1367
Mitiglinide Calcium, 1369
Mizoribine, 1373
Montelukast Sodium Chewable, 1377
Montelukast Sodium, 1380
Morphine Hydrochloride, 1384
Mosapride Citrate, 1389
Nabumetone, 1393
Naftopidil Orally Disintegrating, 1397
Naftopidil, 1398
Nateglinide, 1407
Nicergoline, 1413
Nicomol, 1416
Nilvadipine, 1424
Nitrendipine, 1427
Nitroglycerin, 1429
Norgestrel and Ethinylestradiol, 1436
Nortriptyline Hydrochloride, 1438
Olmesartan Medoxomil, 1443
Olopatadine Hydrochloride, 1445
Omeprazole Delayed-release, 1447
Paroxetine Hydrochloride, 1483
Pemirolast Potassium, 1489
Pentobarbital Calcium, 1492
Perphenazine Maleate, 1499
Perphenazine, 1497
Phenobarbital, 1506
Phenytoin, 1513
Pilocarpine Hydrochloride, 1516
Pioglitazone Hydrochloride, 1523
Pioglitazone Hydrochloride and Glimepiride, 1524
Pioglitazone Hydrochloride and Metformin Hydrochloride, 1527
Piperazine Phosphate, 1535
Pitavastatin Calcium, 1543
Pitavastatin Calcium Orally Disintegrating, 1541
Pivmecillinam Hydrochloride, 1546

Pravastatin Sodium, 1568
Prazepam, 1570
Precipitated Calcium Carbonate, 595
Prednisolone, 1573
Probenecid, 1579
Probucol, 1582
Procainamide Hydrochloride, 1584
Prochlorperazine Maleate, 1588
Propafenone Hydrochloride, 1594
Propiverine Hydrochloride, 1597
Propranolol Hydrochloride, 1599
Propylthiouracil, 1603
Quetiapine Fumarate, 1615
Quinapril Hydrochloride, 1618
Rebamipide, 1627
Reserpine, 1630
Rilmazafone Hydrochloride, 1643
Risperidone, 1648
Ritodrine Hydrochloride, 1651
Rosuvastatin Calcium, 1654
Roxatidine Acetate Hydrochloride Extended-release, 1658
Roxithromycin, 1661
Sarpogrelate Hydrochloride, 1674
Silodosin, 1684
Silodosin Orally Disintegrating, 1683
Simvastatin, 1689
Sitagliptin Phosphate, 1692
Sodium Risedronate, 1724
Sodium Valproate, 1731
Sodium Valproate Extended-release, A, 1729
Sodium Valproate Extended-release, B, 1730
Spironolactone, 1737
Sulpiride, 1759
Sultamicillin Tosilate, 1762
Taltirelin, 1775
Taltirelin Orally Disintegrating, 1774
Tamsulosin Hydrochloride Extended-release, 1779
Telmisartan, 1797
Telmisartan and Amlodipine Besilate, 1795
Telmisartan and Hydrochlorothiazide, 1798
Temocapril Hydrochloride, 1801
Terbinafine Hydrochloride, 1807
Thiamazole, 1815
Tiapride Hydrochloride, 1826
Tiaramide Hydrochloride, 1828
Ticlopidine Hydrochloride, 1829
Tipepidine Hibenzate, 1834
Tolbutamide, 1844
Tosufloxacin Tosilate, 1848
Tranexamic Acid, 1852
Trichlormethiazide, 1865
Trihexyphenidyl Hydrochloride, 1871
Trimetazidine Hydrochloride, 1874

2972   *Index*   *Supplement I, JP XVIII*

Tablets (*continued*)
  Troxipide,   1879
  Ursodeoxycholic Acid,   1893
  Valaciclovir Hydrochloride,   1896
  Valsartan,   1899
  Valsartan and Hydrochlorothiazide,
    1900
  Verapamil Hydrochloride,   1907
  Voglibose,   1912, 2905
  Voglibose Orally Disintegrating,
    2903
  Voriconazole,   1916
  Warfarin Potassium,   1918
  Zaltoprofen,   1926
  Zolpidem Tartrate,   1932
  Zonisamide,   1934
  Zopiclone,   1936
Tacalcitol
  Hydrate,   1766
  Lotion,   1767
  Ointment,   1768
Tacrolimus
  Capsules,   1770
  Hydrate,   1769, 2865
Talampicillin Hydrochloride,   1771,
    2866
Talc,   1772
Taltirelin
  Hydrate,   1773, 2866
  Orally Disintegrating Tablets,   1774
  Tablets,   1775
Tamoxifen Citrate,   1777, 2866
Tamsulosin Hydrochloride,   1778,
    2866
  Extended-release Tablets,   1779
Tannic Acid,   1780
Tartaric Acid,   1780, 2866
Taurine,   1780, 2866
Tazobactam,   1781, 2866
  and Piperacillin for Injection,   1782
Teceleukin
  for Injection (Genetical Recombina-
    tion),   1789
  (Genetical Recombination),   1784
Tegafur,   1790, 2866
Teicoplanin,   1791, 2866
Telmisartan,   1794, 2866
  and Amlodipine Besilate Tablets,
    1795
  and Hydrochlorothiazide Tablets,
    1798
  Tablets,   1797
Temocapril Hydrochloride,   1800,
    2866
  Tablets,   1801
Temozolomide,   2900
  Capsules,   2901
  for Injection,   2902
Teprenone,   1802, 2866
  Capsules,   1804
Terbinafine Hydrochloride,   1805,
    2866
  Cream,   1806

Solution,   1806
Spray,   1807
Tablets,   1807
Terbutaline Sulfate,   1808, 2866
Testosterone
  Enanthate,   1809
  Enanthate Injection,   1810
  Propionate,   1810
  Propionate Injection,   1811
Tetracaine Hydrochloride,   1812, 2866
Tetracycline Hydrochloride,   1812,
    2866
Thallium (^{201}Tl) Chloride Injection,
    1813
Theophylline,   1813, 2866
Thiamazole,   1814, 2866
  Tablets,   1815
Thiamine Chloride Hydrochloride,
    1815, 2866
  Injection,   1816
  Powder,   1817
Thiamine Nitrate,   1817, 2866
Thiamylal Sodium,   1818, 2866
  for Injection,   1819
Thianthol,   1820
  and Salicylic Acid Solution, Com-
    pound,   1820
Thiopental Sodium,   1821, 2866
  for Injection,   1822, 2866
Thioridazine Hydrochloride,   1823,
    2866
L-Threonine,   1823, 2866
Thrombin,   1824
Thymol,   1825
Tiapride Hydrochloride,   1826, 2866
  Tablets,   1826
Tiaramide Hydrochloride,   1827, 2866
  Tablets,   1828
Ticlopidine Hydrochloride,   1829,
    2866
  Tablets,   1829
Timepidium Bromide Hydrate,   1830,
    2866
Timolol Maleate,   1831, 2866
Tincture
  Bitter,   1961
  Capsicum,   1974
  Iodine,   1170
  Iodine, Dilute,   1171
  Nux Vomica,   2080
  Opium,   2083
  Orange Peel,   2084
Tinidazole,   1832, 2866
Tipepidine Hibenzate,   1833, 2866
  Tablets,   1834
Titanium Oxide,   1835
Tizanidine Hydrochloride,   1836, 2866
Toad Cake,   2159
Tobramycin,   1837, 2866
  Injection,   1838
Tocopherol,   1838, 2866
  Acetate,   1839, 2866
  Calcium Succinate,   1840

Nicotinate,   1841, 2866
Todralazine Hydrochloride Hydrate,
    1842, 2867
Tofisopam,   1843, 2867
Tokakujokito Extract,   2160, 2921
Tokishakuyakusan Extract,   2162
Tolbutamide,   1843, 2867
  Tablets,   1844
Tolnaftate,   1844, 2867
  Solution,   1845
Tolperisone Hydrochloride,   1846,
    2867
Tosufloxacin Tosilate
  Hydrate,   1846, 2867
  Tablets,   1848
Tragacanth,   2165
  Powdered,   2165
Tramadol Hydrochloride,   1849, 2867
Tranexamic Acid,   1850, 2867
  Capsules,   1851
  Injection,   1852
  Tablets,   1852
Tranilast,   1853, 2867
  Capsules,   1854
  Fine Granules,   1855
  for Syrup,   1856
  Ophthalmic Solution,   1856
Trapidil,   1857, 2867
Trehalose Hydrate,   1858, 2867
Trepibutone,   1859, 2867
Triamcinolone,   1860, 2867
  Acetonide,   1861, 2867
Triamterene,   1862, 2867
Triazolam,   1862, 2867
Tribulus Fruit,   2165
Trichlormethiazide,   1864, 2867
  Tablets,   1865
Trichomycin,   1867
Trichosanthes Root,   2166
Triclofos Sodium,   1868, 2867
  Syrup,   1869
Trientine Hydrochloride,   1869, 2867
  Capsules,   1870
Trihexyphenidyl Hydrochloride,
    1870, 2867
  Tablets,   1871
Trimebutine Maleate,   1872, 2867
Trimetazidine Hydrochloride,   1873,
    2867
  Tablets,   1874
Trimethadione,   1875, 2867
Trimetoquinol Hydrochloride Hydrate,
    1876, 2867
Tropicamide,   1877, 2867
Troxipide,   1878, 2867
  Fine Granules,   1878
  Tablets,   1879
L-Tryptophan,   1880, 2867
Tulobuterol,   1881, 2867
  Hydrochloride,   1883, 2867
  Transdermal Tape,   1882
Turmeric,   2166, 2921
  Powdered,   2167

Supplement I, JP XVIII   *Index*   2973

Turpentine Oil,   2168
L-Tyrosine,   1883, 2867

U

Ubenimex,   1884, 2867
  Capsules,   1885
Ubidecarenone,   1886, 2867
Ulinastatin,   1887, 2867
Uncaria Hook,   2168, 2921
Unseiin Extract,   2169
Urapidil,   1889, 2867
Urea,   1890, 2867
Urokinase,   1890, 2867
Ursodeoxycholic Acid,   1891, 2867
  Granules,   1892
  Tablets,   1893
Uva Ursi Fluidextract,   2171

V

Vaccine
  BCG, Freeze-dried, (for Percutaneous Use),   514
  Diphtheria-Purified Pertussis-Tetanus Combined, Adsorbed,   873
  Hepatitis B, Adsorbed,   1106
  Influenza HA,   1155
  Inactivated Tissue Culture Rabies, Freeze-dried,   1625
  Live Attenuated Measles, Freeze-dried,   1301
  Live Attenuated Mumps, Freeze-dried,   1390
  Live Attenuated Rubella, Freeze-dried,   1662
  Purified Pertussis, Adsorbed,   1500
  Smallpox, Freeze-dried,   1696
  Smallpox, Freeze-dried, Prepared in Cell Culture,   1696
Valaciclovir Hydrochloride,   1894, 2868
  Tablets,   1896
L-Valine,   1897, 2868
Valsartan,   1898, 2868
  and Hydrochlorothiazide Tablets,   1900
  Tablets,   1899
Vancomycin Hydrochloride,   1902, 2868
  for Injection,   1904

Vasopressin Injection,   1904
Verapamil Hydrochloride,   1905, 2868
  Injection,   1906
  Tablets,   1907
Vinblastine Sulfate,   1907
  for Injection,   1908
Vincristine Sulfate,   1909
Vitamin A
  Acetate,   1631
  Oil,   1910
  Palmitate,   1632
Vitamin B_1
  Hydrochloride,   1815
  Hydrochloride Injection,   1816
  Hydrochloride Powder,   1817
  Nitrate,   1817
Vitamin B_2,   1635
  Butyrate,   1636
  Phosphate Ester,   1637
  Phosphate Ester Injection,   1638
  Powder,   1635
Vitamin B_6,   1611
  Injection,   1611
Vitamin B_{12},   820
  Injection,   821
Vitamin C,   484
  Injection,   484
  Powder,   485
Vitamin D_2,   948
Vitamin D_3,   748
Vitamin E,   1838
  Acetate,   1839
  Calcium Succinate,   1840
  Nicotinate,   1841
Vitamin K_1,   1515
Voglibose,   1911, 2868
  Orally Disintegrating Tablets,   2904
  Tablets,   1912, 2905
Voriconazole,   1913, 2868
  for Injection,   1915
  Tablets,   1916

W

Warfarin Potassium,   1917, 2868
  Tablets,   1918
Water,   1919
  for Injection,   1920
  for Injection in Containers, Sterile,   1920
  in Containers, Purified,   1919

  in Containers, Sterile, Purified,   1920
  Purified,   1919
Weak Opium Alkaloids and Scopolamine Injection,   1452
Wheat Starch,   1741, 2899
White
  Beeswax,   1956
  Ointment,   1921
  Petrolatum,   1501, 2861, 2892
  Shellac,   1679, 2864
  Soft Sugar,   1748, 2865
Whole Human Blood,   1921
Wine,   1921, 2868
Wood Creosote,   2171

X

Xylitol,   1923, 2868
  Injection,   1924

Y

Yellow
  Beeswax,   1956
  Petrolatum,   1502, 2861, 2893
Yokukansan Extract,   2173
Yokukansankachimpihange Extract,   2922

Z

Zaltoprofen,   1925, 2868
  Tablets,   1926
Zidovudine,   1927, 2868
Zinc
  Chloride,   1928, 2868
  Oxide,   1928, 2868
  Oxide Oil,   1929
  Oxide Ointment,   1929
  Oxide Starch Powder,   1930
  Sulfate Hydrate,   1930, 2868
  Sulfate Ophthalmic Solution,   1931
Zolpidem Tartrate,   1931, 2868
  Tablets,   1932
Zonisamide,   1933, 2868
  Tablets,   1934
Zopiclone,   1935, 2868
  Tablets,   1936

INDEX IN LATIN NAME

A

Achyranthis Radix, 1940
Aconiti Radix Processa, 2106
  Radix Processa et Pulverata, 2108
Adeps Lanae Purificatus, 2061
  Suillus, 2062
Agar, 1940
  Pulveratum, 1941
Akebiae Caulis, 1941
Alismatis Tuber, 1941
  Tuber Pulveratum, 1942
Aloe, 1942
  Pulverata, 1943
Alpiniae Fructus, 1960
  Officinarum Rhizoma, 1944
Amomi Semen, 1945
  Semen Pulveratum, 1945
Anemarrhenae Rhizoma, 1945
Angelicae Acutilobae Radix, 2039
  Acutilobae Radix Pulverata, 2039
  Dahuricae Radix, 1946
Apilac, 2119
Araliae Cordatae Rhizoma, 1947
Arctii Fructus, 1969
Arecae Semen, 1948
Armeniacae Semen, 1946
Artemisiae Capillaris Flos, 1948
  Folium, 1949
Asiasari Radix, 1949
Asparagi Radix, 1950
Astragali Radix, 1950
Atractylodis Lanceae Rhizoma, 1951
  Lanceae Rhizoma Pulveratum,
  1951
  Rhizoma, 1952
  Rhizoma Pulveratum, 1952
Aurantii Fructus Immaturus, 2036
  Pericarpium, 1960

B

Belladonnae Radix, 1957
Benincasae Semen, 1959
Benzoinum, 1960
Bezoar Bovis, 2086
Bufonis Crustum, 2159
Bupleuri Radix, 1968

C

Calumbae Radix, 1972
  Radix Pulverata, 1972
Cannabis Fructus, 2031
Capsici Fructus, 1973

Fructus Pulveratus, 1973
Cardamomi Fructus, 1975
Carthami Flos, 2121
Caryophylli Flos, 1984
  Flos Pulveratus, 1984
Cassiae Semen, 1976
Catalpae Fructus, 1976
Cera Alba, 1956
  Carnauba, 1975
  Flava, 1956
Chrysanthemi Flos, 1980
Cimicifugae Rhizoma, 1980
Cinnamomi Cortex, 1981
  Cortex Pulveratus, 1981
Cistanchis Herba, 1982
Citri Unshiu Pericarpium, 1983
Clematidis Radix, 1983
Cnidii Monnieri Fructus, 2909
Cnidii Monnieris Fructus, 1985
  Rhizoma, 1985
  Rhizoma Pulveratum, 1986
Codonopsis Radix, 1986
Coicis Semen, 1987
  Semen Pulveratum, 1987
Condurango Cortex, 1987
Coptidis Rhizoma, 1988
  Rhizoma Pulveratum, 1989
Corni Fructus, 1990
Corydalis Tuber, 1991
  Tuber Pulveratum, 1992
Crataegi Fructus, 1993
Creosotum Ligni, 2171
Crocus, 2122
Curcumae Longae Rhizoma, 2166
  Longae Rhizoma Pulveratum, 2167
  Rhizoma, 1993
Cyperi Rhizoma, 1994
  Rhizoma Pulveratum, 1994

D

Digenea, 1998
Dioscoreae Rhizoma, 1999
  Rhizoma Pulveratum, 1999
Dolichi Semen, 2000

E

Eleutherococci senticosi Rhizoma,
  2000
Ephedrae Herba, 2001
Epimedii Herba, 2001
Eriobotryae Folium, 2066
Eucommiae Cortex, 2002
Euodiae Fructus, 2003

F

Fel Ursi, 1955
Foeniculi Fructus, 2003
  Fructus Pulveratus, 2003
Forsythiae Fructus, 2004
Fossilia Ossis Mastodi, 2065
  Ossis Mastodi Pulveratum, 2065
Fritillariae Bulbus, 2005
Fructus Hordei Germinatus, 2069

G

Gambir, 2005
  Pulveratum, 2005
Gardeniae Fructus, 2006
  Fructus Pulveratus, 2006
Gastrodiae Tuber, 2007
Gentianae Radix, 2007
  Radix Pulverata, 2008
  Scabrae Radix, 2040
  Scabrae Radix Pulverata, 2040
Geranii Herba, 2009
  Herba Pulverata, 2009
Ginseng Radix, 2011
  Radix Pulverata, 2012
  Radix Rubra, 2112
Glehniae Radix cum Rhizoma, 2013
Glycyrrhizae Radix, 2013
  Radix Praeparata, 2105
  Radix Pulverata, 2014
Gummi Arabicum, 1939
  Arabicum Pulveratum, 1939
Gypsum Exsiccatum, 2023
  Fibrosum, 2023

H

Hedysari Radix, 2031
Houttuyniae Herba, 2035
Hydrangeae Dulcis Folium, 2156
  Dulcis Folium Pulveratum, 2156

I

Imperatae Rhizoma, 2036
Ipecacuanhae Radix, 2036
  Radix Pulverata, 2037

K

Kasseki, 1944
Koi, 2060

L

Leonuri Herba, 2063
Lilii Bulbus, 2063
Linderae Radix, 2064
Lithospermi Radix, 2064
Longan Arillus, 2065
Lonicerae Folium Cum Caulis, 2066
Lycii Cortex, 2067
   Fructus, 2067

M

Magnoliae Cortex, 2067
   Cortex Pulveratus, 2068
   Flos, 2069
Malloti Cortex, 2069
Mel, 2035
Menthae Herba, 2072
Mori Cortex, 2076
Moutan Cortex, 2073
   Cortex Pulveratus, 2074
Myristicae Semen, 2078

N

Nelumbinis Semen, 2077
Notopterygii Rhizoma, 2077
Nupharis Rhizoma, 2077

O

Oleum Arachidis, 2093
   Aurantii, 2083
   Cacao, 1972
   Camelliae, 1972
   Caryophylli, 1984
   Cinnamomi, 1982
   Cocois, 1986
   Eucalypti, 2002
   Foeniculi, 2004
   Maydis, 1990
   Menthae Japonicae, 2072
   Olivae, 2081
   Rapae, 2111
   Ricini, 1976
   Sesami, 2143
   Sojae, 2156
   Terebinthinae, 2168
Ophiopogonis Radix, 2081
Opium Pulveratum, 2082
Oryzae Fructus, 1968

Ostreae Testa, 2090
   Testa Pulverata, 2090

P

Paeoniae Radix, 2093
   Radix Pulverata, 2094
Panacis Japonici Rhizoma, 2090
   Japonici Rhizoma Pulveratum, 2091
Perillae Herba, 2095
Persicae Semen, 2091
   Semen Pulveratum, 2092
Peucedani Radix, 2095
Pharbitidis Semen, 2096
Phellodendri Cortex, 2096
   Cortex Pulveratus, 2097
Picrasmae Lignum, 2099
   Lignum Pulveratum, 2099
Pinelliae Tuber, 2100
Plantaginis Herba, 2100
   Semen, 2100
Platycodi Radix, 2101
   Radix Pulverata, 2101
Pogostemi Herba, 2102
Polygalae Radix, 2102
   Radix Pulverata, 2103
Polygonati Rhizoma, 2103
Polygoni Multiflori Radix, 2104
Polyporus, 2104
   Pulveratus, 2104
Poria, 2105
   Pulveratum, 2105
Prunellae Spica, 2110
Pruni Cortex, 1977
Puerariae Radix, 2110

Q

Quercus Cortex, 2111

R

Rehmanniae Radix, 2113
Resina Pini, 2118
Rhei Rhizoma, 2113
   Rhizoma Pulveratum, 2114
Rosae Fructus, 2118
   Fructus Pulveratus, 2118

S

Sal Mirabilis, 2155

Mirabilis Anhydricus, 2154
Salviae Miltiorrhizae Radix, 2131
Saposhnikoviae Radix, 2132
Sappan Lignum, 2132
Saussureae Radix, 2132
Schisandrae Fructus, 2133
Schizonepetae Spica, 2133
Scopoliae Rhizoma, 2133
Scutellariae Radix, 2138
   Radix Pulverata, 2139
Senegae Radix, 2140
   Radix Pulverata, 2140
Sennae Folium, 2141
   Folium Pulveratum, 2142
Sesami Semen, 2143
Sevum Bovinum, 1956
Sinomeni Caulis et Rhizoma, 2153
Smilacis Rhizoma, 2153
   Rhizoma Pulveratum, 2154
Sophorae Radix, 2155
   Radix Pulverata, 2155
Strychni Semen, 2078
Swertiae Herba, 2157
   Herba Pulverata, 2158

T

Tinctura Amara, 1961
Tragacantha, 2165
   Pulverata, 2165
Tribuli Fructus, 2165
Trichosanthis Radix, 2166

U

Uncariae Uncis Cum Ramulus, 2168
Uvae Ursi Folium, 1955

V

Valerianae Fauriei Radix, 2040
   Fauriei Radix Pulverata, 2041

Z

Zanthoxyli Piperiti Pericarpium, 2041
   Piperiti Pericarpium Pulveratum, 2042
Zingiberis Rhizoma, 2009
   Rhizoma Processum, 2109
   Rhizoma Pulveratum, 2010
Ziziphi Fructus, 2042
   Semen, 2042

INDEX IN JAPANESE

ア

亜鉛華デンプン　1930
亜鉛華軟膏　1929
アカメガシワ　2069
アクチノマイシンD　417
アクラルビシン塩酸塩　413
アクリノール・亜鉛華軟膏　416
アクリノール水和物　414
アクリノール・チンク油　415
アザチオプリン　498
アザチオプリン錠　499
亜酸化窒素　1430
アシクロビル　407
アシクロビル顆粒　408
アシクロビル眼軟膏　411
アシクロビル錠　413
アシクロビルシロップ　411
アシクロビル注射液　409
アシクロビル軟膏　410
アジスロマイシン水和物　504
アジマリン　420
アジマリン錠　420
亜硝酸アミル　474
アスコルビン酸　484
アスコルビン酸散　485
アスコルビン酸注射液　484
アスコルビン酸・パントテン酸カルシウム錠　485
アズトレオナム　506
L-アスパラギン酸　487
アスピリン　488
アスピリンアルミニウム　489
アスピリン錠　488
アスポキシシリン水和物　490
アセタゾラミド　403
アセチルシステイン　406
アセトアミノフェン　402
アセトヘキサミド　404
アセブトロール塩酸塩　399
アセメタシン　399
アセメタシンカプセル　400
アセメタシン錠　401
アゼラスチン塩酸塩　500
アゼラスチン塩酸塩顆粒　501
アゼルニジピン　502
アゼルニジピン錠　502
アセンヤク　2005
アセンヤク末　2005
アゾセミド　505
アゾセミド錠　505
アテノロール　491
アトルバスタチンカルシウム錠　493
アトルバスタチンカルシウム水和物　492

アドレナリン　417
アドレナリン液　418
アドレナリン注射液　418
アトロピン硫酸塩水和物　494
アトロピン硫酸塩注射液　495
アナストロゾール　2869
アナストロゾール錠　2870
亜ヒ酸パスタ　483
アプリンジン塩酸塩　476
アプリンジン塩酸塩カプセル　476
アフロクアロン　419
アヘンアルカロイド・アトロピン注射液　1450
アヘンアルカロイド・スコポラミン注射液　1451
アヘンアルカロイド塩酸塩　1448
アヘンアルカロイド塩酸塩注射液　1449
アヘン散　2082
アヘンチンキ　2083
アヘン・トコン散　2083
アヘン末　2082
アマチャ　2156
アマチャ末　2156
アマンタジン塩酸塩　444
アミオダロン塩酸塩　450
アミオダロン塩酸塩錠　451
アミカシン硫酸塩　446
アミカシン硫酸塩注射液　447
アミドトリゾ酸　445
アミドトリゾ酸ナトリウムメグルミン注射液　1312
アミトリプチリン塩酸塩　452
アミトリプチリン塩酸塩錠　453
アミノ安息香酸エチル　971
アミノフィリン水和物　448
アミノフィリン注射液　449
アムホテリシンB　465
アムホテリシンB錠　467, 2868
アムホテリシンBシロップ　466
アムロジピンベシル酸塩　456
アムロジピンベシル酸塩口腔内崩壊錠　457
アムロジピンベシル酸塩錠　458
アモキサピン　462
アモキシシリンカプセル　464
アモキシシリン水和物　463
アモスラロール塩酸塩　460
アモスラロール塩酸塩錠　461
アモバルビタール　459
アラセプリル　421
アラセプリル錠　422
L-アラニン　423
アラビアゴム　1939
アラビアゴム末　1939
アリメマジン酒石酸塩　430

亜硫酸水素ナトリウム　1699
アルガトロバン水和物　479
L-アルギニン　481
L-アルギニン塩酸塩　481
L-アルギニン塩酸塩注射液　482
アルジオキサ　424
アルジオキサ顆粒　425
アルジオキサ錠　426
アルプラゾラム　434
アルプレノロール塩酸塩　434
アルプロスタジル　435
アルプロスタジル　アルファデクス　438
アルプロスタジル注射液　436
アルベカシン硫酸塩　477
アルベカシン硫酸塩注射液　479
アルミノプロフェン　432
アルミノプロフェン錠　433
アレンドロン酸ナトリウム錠　429
アレンドロン酸ナトリウム水和物　426
アレンドロン酸ナトリウム注射液　428
アロエ　1942
アロエ末　1943
アロチノロール塩酸塩　482
アロプリノール　430
アロプリノール錠　431
安息香酸　523
安息香酸ナトリウム　1698
安息香酸ナトリウムカフェイン　590
安息香酸ベンジル　525
アンソッコウ　1960
アンチピリン　475
アンピシリン水和物　468
アンピシリンナトリウム　470
アンピロキシカム　473
アンピロキシカムカプセル　473
アンベノニウム塩化物　445
アンモニア・ウイキョウ精　2004
アンモニア水　459
アンレキサノクス　453
アンレキサノクス錠　455

イ

イオウ　1756
イオウ・カンフルローション　1756
イオウ・サリチル酸・チアントール軟膏　1757
イオタラム酸　1179
イオタラム酸ナトリウム注射液　1714
イオタラム酸メグルミン注射液　1311
イオトロクス酸　1180
イオパミドール　1177
イオパミドール注射液　1178

イオヘキソール　1175
イオヘキソール注射液　1177
イクタモール　1135
イコサペント酸エチル　974
イコサペント酸エチルカプセル　975
イセパマイシン硫酸塩　1193
イセパマイシン硫酸塩注射液　1194
イソクスプリン塩酸塩　1209
イソクスプリン塩酸塩錠　1210
イソソルビド　1204
イソニアジド　1200
イソニアジド錠　1201
イソニアジド注射液　1201
イソフェンインスリン　ヒト(遺伝子
　組換え)水性懸濁注射液　1158,
　2885
イソフルラン　1195
l-イソプレナリン塩酸塩　1202
イソプロパノール　1203
イソプロピルアンチピリン　1203
イソマル水和物　1198
L-イソロイシン　1196
イソロイシン・ロイシン・バリン顆粒
　1197
イダルビシン塩酸塩　1136
一硝酸イソソルビド錠　1208
70%一硝酸イソソルビド乳糖末　1206
イドクスウリジン　1138
イドクスウリジン点眼液　1139
イトラコナゾール　1211
イフェンプロジル酒石酸塩　1140
イフェンプロジル酒石酸塩細粒　1140
イフェンプロジル酒石酸塩錠　1141
イブジラスト　1132
イブプロフェン　1133
イブプロフェンピコノール　1133
イブプロフェンピコノールクリーム
　1134
イブプロフェンピコノール軟膏　1135
イプラトロピウム臭化物水和物　1181
イプリフラボン　1182
イプリフラボン錠　1183
イミダプリル塩酸塩　1142
イミダプリル塩酸塩錠　1143
イミプラミン塩酸塩　1146
イミプラミン塩酸塩錠　1147
イミペネム水和物　1144
イリノテカン塩酸塩水和物　1187
イリノテカン塩酸塩注射液　1189
イルソグラジンマレイン酸塩　1190
イルソグラジンマレイン酸塩細粒
　1191
イルソグラジンマレイン酸塩錠　1192
イルベサルタン　1183
イルベサルタン・アムロジピンベシル
　酸塩錠　1185
イルベサルタン錠　1184
イレイセン　1983
インジゴカルミン　1151
インジゴカルミン注射液　1152
インスリン　ヒト(遺伝子組換え)
　1155, 2884
インスリン　ヒト(遺伝子組換え)注射

液　1157, 2885
インスリン　アスパルト(遺伝子組換
　え)　1160
インスリン　グラルギン(遺伝子組換
　え)　1162
インスリン　グラルギン(遺伝子組換
　え)注射液　1164
インダパミド　1148
インダパミド錠　1149
インターフェロン　アルファ
　(NAMALWA)　1165
インターフェロン　アルファ
　(NAMALWA)注射液　1168
インチンコウ　1948, 2907
インデノロール塩酸塩　1150
インドメタシン　1152
インドメタシンカプセル　1153
インドメタシン坐剤　1154
インフルエンザ HA ワクチン　1155
インヨウカク　2001

ウ

ウイキョウ　2003
ウイキョウ末　2003
ウイキョウ油　2004
ウコン　2166, 2921
ウコン末　2167
ウベニメクス　1884
ウベニメクスカプセル　1885
ウヤク　2064
ウラピジル　1889
ウリナスタチン　1887
ウルソデオキシコール酸　1891
ウルソデオキシコール酸顆粒　1892
ウルソデオキシコール酸錠　1893
ウロキナーゼ　1890
ウワウルシ　1955, 2908
ウワウルシ流エキス　2171
温清飲エキス　2169

エ

エイジツ　2118
エイジツ末　2118
エカベトナトリウム顆粒　913
エカベトナトリウム水和物　912
液状フェノール　1507
エコチオパートヨウ化物　914
エスタゾラム　958
エストラジオール安息香酸エステル
　959
エストラジオール安息香酸エステル水
　性懸濁注射液　960
エストリオール　960
エストリオール錠　961
エストリオール水性懸濁注射液　961
エタクリン酸　962
エタクリン酸錠　963
エタノール　964, 2880
エダラボン　915
エダラボン注射液　915
エタンブトール塩酸塩　964

エチオナミド　970
エチゾラム　984
エチゾラム細粒　984
エチゾラム錠　985
エチドロン酸二ナトリウム　980
エチドロン酸二ナトリウム錠　981
エチニルエストラジオール　968
エチニルエストラジオール錠　969
L-エチルシステイン塩酸塩　973
エチルセルロース　971
エチルモルヒネ塩酸塩水和物　979
エチレフリン塩酸塩　982
エチレフリン塩酸塩錠　983
エチレンジアミン　974
エデト酸カルシウムナトリウム水和物
　608
エデト酸ナトリウム水和物　1706
エーテル　967
エテンザミド　967
エトスクシミド　970
エトドラク　987
エトポシド　987
エドロホニウム塩化物　917
エドロホニウム塩化物注射液　918
エナラプリルマレイン酸塩　924
エナラプリルマレイン酸塩錠　926
エノキサシン水和物　928
エバスチン　909
エバスチン口腔内崩壊錠　909
エバスチン錠　911
エパルレスタット　932
エパルレスタット錠　933
エピリゾール　938
エピルビシン塩酸塩　939
エフェドリン塩酸塩　935
エフェドリン塩酸塩散10%　936
エフェドリン塩酸塩錠　937
エフェドリン塩酸塩注射液　935
エペリゾン塩酸塩　934
エプレレノン　940
エプレレノン錠　941
エポエチン　アルファ(遺伝子組換え)
　942
エポエチン　ベータ(遺伝子組換え)
　945, 2879
エメダスチンフマル酸塩　921
エメダスチンフマル酸塩徐放カプセル
　922
エモルファゾン　923
エモルファゾン錠　924
エリスロマイシン　955
エリスロマイシンエチルコハク酸エス
　テル　956
エリスロマイシンステアリン酸塩
　958
エリスロマイシン腸溶錠　956
エリスロマイシンラクトビオン酸塩
　957
エリブリンメシル酸塩　951
エルカトニン　919
エルゴカルシフェロール　948
エルゴタミン酒石酸塩　950
エルゴメトリンマレイン酸塩　949

エルゴメトリンマレイン酸塩錠 950
エルゴメトリンマレイン酸塩注射液 949
塩化亜鉛 1928
塩化インジウム(^{111}In)注射液 1152
塩化カリウム 1554
塩化カルシウム水和物 596
塩化カルシウム注射液 596
塩化タリウム(^{201}Tl)注射液 1813
塩化ナトリウム 1702, 2898
10％塩化ナトリウム注射液 1703
エンゴサク 1991, 2909
エンゴサク末 1992, 2910
塩酸 1111
塩酸リモナーデ 1112
エンタカポン 928
エンタカポン錠 930
エンビオマイシン硫酸塩 931, 2879
エンフルラン 927

オ

オウギ 1950
オウゴン 2138
オウゴン末 2139
黄色ワセリン 1502, 2893
オウセイ 2103
オウバク 2096
オウバク・タンナルビン・ビスマス散 2098
オウバク末 2097
オウヒ 1977
オウレン 1988
黄連解毒湯エキス 2084
オウレン末 1989
オキサゾラム 1456
オキサピウムヨウ化物 1454
オキサプロジン 1455
オキシコドン塩酸塩水和物 1459
オキシテトラサイクリン塩酸塩 1464
オキシトシン 1465
オキシトシン注射液 1467
オキシドール 1462
オキシブチニン塩酸塩 2891
オキシブプロカイン塩酸塩 1458
オキシメトロン 1463
オキセサゼイン 1457
オクスプレノロール塩酸塩 1457
オザグレルナトリウム 1468
オザグレルナトリウム注射液 1469
乙字湯エキス 2087
オフロキサシン 1441
オメプラゾール 1446
オメプラゾール腸溶錠 1447
オーラノフィン 496
オーラノフィン錠 497
オリブ油 2081
オルシプレナリン硫酸塩 1454
オルメサルタン メドキソミル 1442
オルメサルタン メドキソミル錠 1443
オレンジ油 2083
オロパタジン塩酸塩 1444

オロパタジン塩酸塩錠 1445
オンジ 2102
オンジ末 2103

カ

カイニン酸・サントニン散 1215
カイニン酸水和物 1215
ガイヨウ 1949, 2907
カオリン 1220
カカオ脂 1972
加香ヒマシ油 1976
カゴソウ 2110
カシュウ 2104
ガジュツ 1993
加水ラノリン 2061
ガチフロキサシン水和物 1055
ガチフロキサシン点眼液 1057
カッコウ 2102
カッコン 2110
葛根湯エキス 2046
葛根湯加川芎辛夷エキス 2049
カッセキ 1944
過テクネチウム酸ナトリウム(^{99m}Tc)注射液 1719
果糖 1046
果糖注射液 1046
カドララジン 587
カドララジン錠 587
カナマイシン一硫酸塩 1218
カナマイシン硫酸塩 1219
カノコソウ 2040
カノコソウ末 2041
カフェイン水和物 589
カプセル 622
カプトプリル 622
ガベキサートメシル酸塩 1052
カベルゴリン 585
過マンガン酸カリウム 1558
加味帰脾湯エキス 2052
加味逍遙散エキス 2055
カモスタットメシル酸塩 610
β-ガラクトシダーゼ（アスペルギルス） 1053
β-ガラクトシダーゼ（ペニシリウム） 1054
カリジノゲナーゼ 1216
カリ石ケン 1552
カルシトニン サケ 591
カルテオロール塩酸塩 635
カルナウバロウ 1975
カルバゾクロムスルホン酸ナトリウム水和物 624
カルバマゼピン 623
カルビドパ水和物 625
カルベジロール 637
カルベジロール錠 638
L-カルボシステイン 626
L-カルボシステイン錠 626
カルボプラチン 628
カルボプラチン注射液 629
カルメロース 630
カルメロースカルシウム 631

カルメロースナトリウム 632
カルモナムナトリウム 635
カルモフール 634
カロコン 2166
カンキョウ 2109, 2916
カンゾウ 2013
乾燥亜硫酸ナトリウム 1727
カンゾウエキス 2015
乾燥甲状腺 1825
乾燥酵母 1924
乾燥細胞培養痘そうワクチン 1696
乾燥ジフテリアウマ抗毒素 873
乾燥弱毒生おたふくかぜワクチン 1390
乾燥弱毒生風しんワクチン 1662
乾燥弱毒生麻しんワクチン 1301
乾燥水酸化アルミニウムゲル 440
乾燥水酸化アルミニウムゲル細粒 440
カンゾウ粗エキス 2016
乾燥組織培養不活化狂犬病ワクチン 1625
乾燥炭酸ナトリウム 1701
乾燥痘そうワクチン 1696
乾燥はぶウマ抗毒素 1090
乾燥BCGワクチン 514
乾燥ボツリヌスウマ抗毒素 563
カンゾウ末 2014
乾燥まむしウマ抗毒素 1296
乾燥硫酸アルミニウムカリウム 441
カンデサルタン シレキセチル 612
カンデサルタン シレキセチル・アムロジピンベシル酸塩錠 615
カンデサルタン シレキセチル錠 613
カンデサルタン シレキセチル・ヒドロクロロチアジド錠 618
カンテン 1940
カンテン末 1941
含糖ペプシン 1662
d-カンフル 611
dl-カンフル 611
肝油 803
カンレノ酸カリウム 1553

キ

希塩酸 1111
キキョウ 2101
キキョウ末 2101
キキョウ流エキス 2102
キクカ 1980
キササゲ 1976
キジツ 2036
キシリトール 1923
キシリトール注射液 1924
キタサマイシン 1226
キタサマイシン酢酸エステル 1227
キタサマイシン酒石酸塩 1228
キナプリル塩酸塩 1617
キナプリル塩酸塩錠 1618
キニジン硫酸塩水和物 1620
キニーネエチル炭酸エステル 1621

2980 *Index in Japanese*

キニーネ塩酸塩水和物　1622
キニーネ硫酸塩水和物　1623
牛脂　1956
吸水クリーム　815
キョウカツ　2077
キョウニン　1946, 2907
キョウニン水　1947
希ヨードチンキ　1171
金チオリンゴ酸ナトリウム　1697

ク

グアイフェネシン　1088
グアナベンズ酢酸塩　1089
グアネチジン硫酸塩　1090
グアヤコールスルホン酸カリウム　1556
クエチアピンフマル酸塩　1613
クエチアピンフマル酸塩細粒　1615
クエチアピンフマル酸塩錠　1615
クエン酸ガリウム(⁶⁷Ga)注射液　1055
クエン酸水和物　769
クエン酸ナトリウム水和物　1704
クコシ　2067
クジン　2155
クジン末　2155
苦味重曹水　2154
苦味チンキ　1961
クラブラン酸カリウム　1554
クラリスロマイシン　770
クラリスロマイシン錠　772
グリクラジド　1068
グリシン　1083
グリセリン　1080
グリセリンカリ液　1082
クリノフィブラート　779
グリベンクラミド　1067
グリメピリド　1069
グリメピリド錠　1070
クリンダマイシン塩酸塩　775
クリンダマイシン塩酸塩カプセル　776
クリンダマイシンリン酸エステル　777
クリンダマイシンリン酸エステル注射液　778
グルカゴン(遺伝子組換え)　1072
グルコン酸カルシウム水和物　598
グルタチオン　1079
L-グルタミン　1078
L-グルタミン酸　1077
クレゾール　816
クレゾール水　816
クレゾール石ケン液　816
クレボプリドリンゴ酸塩　773
クレマスチンフマル酸塩　774
クロカプラミン塩酸塩水和物　780
クロキサシリンナトリウム水和物　800
クロキサゾラム　801
クロコナゾール塩酸塩　817
クロスカルメロースナトリウム　633, 2877

クロスポビドン　818
クロチアゼパム　798
クロチアゼパム錠　798
クロトリマゾール　799
クロナゼパム　787
クロナゼパム細粒　787
クロナゼパム錠　788
クロニジン塩酸塩　789
クロピドグレル硫酸塩　793
クロピドグレル硫酸塩錠　794
クロフィブラート　782
クロフィブラートカプセル　783
クロフェダノール塩酸塩　781
クロベタゾールプロピオン酸エステル　779
クロペラスチン塩酸塩　792
クロペラスチンフェンジゾ酸塩　790
クロペラスチンフェンジゾ酸塩錠　791
クロミフェンクエン酸塩　784
クロミフェンクエン酸塩錠　784
クロミプラミン塩酸塩　785
クロミプラミン塩酸塩錠　786
クロム酸ナトリウム(⁵¹Cr)注射液　1704
クロモグリク酸ナトリウム　1705
クロラゼプ酸二カリウム　796
クロラゼプ酸二カリウムカプセル　797
クロラムフェニコール　728
クロラムフェニコールコハク酸エステルナトリウム　730
クロラムフェニコール・コリスチンメタンスルホン酸ナトリウム点眼液　731
クロラムフェニコールパルミチン酸エステル　729
クロルジアゼポキシド　732
クロルジアゼポキシド散　733
クロルジアゼポキシド錠　734
クロルフェニラミンマレイン酸塩　740
d-クロルフェニラミンマレイン酸塩　743
クロルフェニラミンマレイン酸塩散　741
クロルフェニラミンマレイン酸塩錠　742
クロルフェニラミンマレイン酸塩注射液　741
クロルフェネシンカルバミン酸エステル　738
クロルフェネシンカルバミン酸エステル錠　739
クロルプロパミド　747
クロルプロパミド錠　747
クロルプロマジン塩酸塩　744
クロルプロマジン塩酸塩錠　745
クロルプロマジン塩酸塩注射液　745
クロルヘキシジン塩酸塩　735
クロルヘキシジングルコン酸塩液　735
クロルマジノン酢酸エステル　736

Supplement I, JP XVIII

クロロブタノール　737

ケ

ケイガイ　2133
ケイ酸アルミン酸マグネシウム　1287
ケイ酸マグネシウム　1291
軽質無水ケイ酸　1680
軽質流動パラフィン　1478
桂枝茯苓丸エキス　2058, 2913
ケイヒ　1981
ケイヒ末　1981
ケイヒ油　1982
ケタミン塩酸塩　1221
結晶セルロース　716
ケツメイシ　1976
ケトコナゾール　1221
ケトコナゾール液　1223
ケトコナゾールクリーム　1222
ケトコナゾールローション　1223
ケトチフェンフマル酸塩　1225
ケトプロフェン　1224
ケノデオキシコール酸　727
ゲファルナート　1058
ゲフィチニブ　1059
ケンゴシ　2096
ゲンタマイシン硫酸塩　1064
ゲンタマイシン硫酸塩注射液　1066
ゲンタマイシン硫酸塩点眼液　1067
ゲンタマイシン硫酸塩軟膏　1066
ゲンチアナ　2007
ゲンチアナ・重曹散　2008
ゲンチアナ末　2008
ゲンノショウコ　2009
ゲンノショウコ末　2009

コ

コウイ　2060
コウカ　2121
硬化油　1120
コウジン　2112
合成ケイ酸アルミニウム　443
コウブシ　1994
コウブシ末　1994
コウベイ　1968
コウボク　2067, 2914
コウボク末　2068
ゴオウ　2086
コカイン塩酸塩　802
ゴシツ　1940, 2907
牛車腎気丸エキス　2018, 2911
ゴシュユ　2003
呉茱萸湯エキス　2021, 2912
コデインリン酸塩散1%　804
コデインリン酸塩散10%　805
コデインリン酸塩錠　805
コデインリン酸塩水和物　803
ゴナドレリン酢酸塩　1083
ゴボウシ　1969, 2908
コポビドン　812
ゴマ　2143
ゴマ油　2143

Supplement I, JP XVIII Index in Japanese 2981

ゴミシ 2133
コムギデンプン 1741, 2899
コメデンプン 1740
コリスチンメタンスルホン酸ナトリウム 810
コリスチン硫酸塩 811
コルチゾン酢酸エステル 814
コルヒチン 807
五苓散エキス 2017
コレカルシフェロール 748
コレスチミド 808
コレスチミド顆粒 809
コレスチミド錠 809
コレステロール 749
コロンボ 1972
コロンボ末 1972
コンズランゴ 1987
コンズランゴ流エキス 1988

サ

サイクロセリン 823
サイコ 1968
柴胡桂枝乾姜湯エキス 2916
柴胡桂枝湯エキス 2125
サイシン 1949
柴朴湯エキス 2122
柴苓湯エキス 2128
酢酸 403
酢酸ナトリウム水和物 1696
サッカリン 1663
サッカリンナトリウム水和物 1664
サフラン 2122
サラシ粉 736
サラシミツロウ 1956
サラゾスルファピリジン 1666
サリチル酸 1667
サリチル酸精 1669
サリチル酸ナトリウム 1725
サリチル酸絆創膏 1668
サリチル・ミョウバン散 1670
サリチル酸メチル 1346
ザルトプロフェン 1925
ザルトプロフェン錠 1926
サルブタモール硫酸塩 1667
サルポグレラート塩酸塩 1671
サルポグレラート塩酸塩細粒 1672, 2898
サルポグレラート塩酸塩錠 1674
酸化亜鉛 1928
酸化カルシウム 601
酸化チタン 1835
酸化マグネシウム 1290
サンキライ 2153
サンキライ末 2154
サンザシ 1993
三酸化二ヒ素 484
サンシシ 2006, 2910
サンシシ末 2006
サンシュユ 1990, 2909
サンショウ 2041
サンショウ末 2042
酸素 1462

サンソウニン 2042
サントニン 1671
サンヤク 1999
サンヤク末 1999

シ

ジアスターゼ 842
ジアスターゼ・重曹散 843
ジアゼパム 843
ジアゼパム錠 844
シアナミド 819
シアノコバラミン 820
シアノコバラミン注射液 821
ジエチルカルバマジンクエン酸塩 849
ジエチルカルバマジンクエン酸塩錠 849
ジオウ 2113
歯科用アンチホルミン 475
歯科用トリオジンクパスタ 1877
歯科用パラホルムパスタ 1479
歯科用フェノール・カンフル 1508
歯科用ヨード・グリセリン 1172
シクラシリン 751
ジクロキサシリンナトリウム水和物 848
シクロスポリン 752
ジクロフェナクナトリウム 846
ジクロフェナクナトリウム坐剤 847
シクロペントラート塩酸塩 821
シクロホスファミド錠 822
シクロホスファミド水和物 822
シゴカ 2000
ジゴキシン 853
ジゴキシン錠 855
ジゴキシン注射液 854
ジコッピ 2067
シコン 2064
次硝酸ビスマス 556
ジスチグミン臭化物 875
ジスチグミン臭化物錠 876
L-シスチン 826
L-システイン 825
L-システイン塩酸塩水和物 826
シスプラチン 766
ジスルフィラム 877
ジソピラミド 875
シタグリプチンリン酸塩錠 1692
シタグリプチンリン酸塩水和物 1691
シタラビン 827
シチコリン 767
シツリシ 2165
ジドブジン 1927
ジドロゲステロン 907
ジドロゲステロン錠 908
シノキサシン 762
シノキサシンカプセル 762
ジノプロスト 869
ジヒドロエルゴタミンメシル酸塩 859
ジヒドロエルゴトキシンメシル酸塩 860

ジヒドロコデインリン酸塩 857
ジヒドロコデインリン酸塩散1% 857
ジヒドロコデインリン酸塩散10% 858
ジピリダモール 874
ジフェニドール塩酸塩 850
ジフェンヒドラミン 870
ジフェンヒドラミン塩酸塩 871
ジフェンヒドラミン・バレリル尿素散 871
ジフェンヒドラミン・フェノール・亜鉛華リニメント 872
ジブカイン塩酸塩 846
ジフテリアトキソイド 873
ジフルコルトロン吉草酸エステル 852
シプロフロキサシン 763
シプロフロキサシン塩酸塩水和物 765
シプロヘプタジン塩酸塩水和物 824
ジフロラゾン酢酸エステル 851
ジベカシン硫酸塩 845
ジベカシン硫酸塩点眼液 845
シベレスタットナトリウム水和物 1694
シベンゾリンコハク酸塩 750
シベンゾリンコハク酸塩錠 750
シメチジン 761
ジメモルファンリン酸塩 865
ジメルカプロール 867
ジメルカプロール注射液 868
ジメンヒドリナート 866
ジメンヒドリナート錠 866
次没食子酸ビスマス 555
ジモルホラミン 868
ジモルホラミン注射液 869
シャカンゾウ 2105, 2916
弱アヘンアルカロイド・スコポラミン注射液 1452
シャクヤク 2093
芍薬甘草湯エキス 2143
シャクヤク末 2094
ジャショウシ 1985, 2909
シャゼンシ 2100
シャゼンソウ 2100, 2916
臭化カリウム 1552
臭化ナトリウム 1700
十全大補湯エキス 2043
ジュウヤク 2035
シュクシャ 1945
シュクシャ末 1945
酒石酸 1780
ショウキョウ 2009, 2910
ショウキョウ末 2010, 2911
小柴胡湯エキス 2147
硝酸イソソルビド 1205
硝酸イソソルビド錠 1205
硝酸銀 1686
硝酸銀点眼液 1687
常水 1919
ショウズク 1975, 2908
小青竜湯エキス 2150

焼セッコウ 2023
消毒用エタノール 966
消毒用フェノール 1507
消毒用フェノール水 1508
ショウマ 1980, 2908
ジョサマイシン 1212
ジョサマイシン錠 1213
ジョサマイシンプロピオン酸エステル 1214
シラザプリル錠 755
シラザプリル水和物 755
シラスタチンナトリウム 753
ジラゼプ塩酸塩水和物 862
ジルチアゼム塩酸塩 863
ジルチアゼム塩酸塩徐放カプセル 864
シルニジピン 757
シルニジピン錠 758
シロスタゾール 759
シロスタゾール錠 760
シロップ用アシクロビル 412
シロップ用クラリスロマイシン 771
シロップ用セファトリジンプロピレングリコール 655
シロップ用セファドロキシル 647
シロップ用セファレキシン 651
シロップ用セフポドキシム プロキセチル 696
シロップ用セフロキサジン 700
シロップ用トラニラスト 1856
シロップ用ファロペネムナトリウム 994
シロップ用ペミロラストカリウム 1489
シロップ用ホスホマイシンカルシウム 1042
シロドシン 1681
シロドシン口腔内崩壊錠 1683
シロドシン錠 1684
シンイ 2069
シンギ 2031
親水クリーム 815
親水ワセリン 1502
診断用クエン酸ナトリウム液 1705
シンバスタチン 1688
シンバスタチン錠 1689
真武湯エキス 2145, 2920

ス

水酸化カリウム 1556
水酸化カルシウム 598
水酸化ナトリウム 1712
スキサメトニウム塩化物水和物 1764
スキサメトニウム塩化物注射液 1765
スクラルファート水和物 1746
スコポラミン臭化水素酸塩水和物 1676
ステアリルアルコール 1744
ステアリン酸 1743, 2899
ステアリン酸カルシウム 609
ステアリン酸ポリオキシル40 1550
ステアリン酸マグネシウム 1292,

2886
ストレプトマイシン硫酸塩 1745
スピラマイシン酢酸エステル 1736
スピロノラクトン 1737
スピロノラクトン錠 1737
スペクチノマイシン塩酸塩水和物 1734
スリンダク 1757
スルタミシリントシル酸塩錠 1762
スルタミシリントシル酸塩水和物 1761
スルチアム 1764
スルバクタムナトリウム 1749
スルピリド 1758
スルピリドカプセル 1758
スルピリド錠 1759
スルピリン水和物 1760
スルピリン注射液 1760
スルファジアジン銀 1751
スルファメチゾール 1752
スルファメトキサゾール 1753
スルファモノメトキシン水和物 1713
スルフイソキサゾール 1754
スルベニシリンナトリウム 1750
スルホブロモフタレインナトリウム 1755
スルホブロモフタレインナトリウム注射液 1756

セ

成人用沈降ジフテリアトキソイド 873
精製水 1919
精製水(容器入り) 1919
精製ゼラチン 1062
精製セラック 1679
精製デヒドロコール酸 832
精製白糖 1748
精製ヒアルロン酸ナトリウム 1709
精製ヒアルロン酸ナトリウム注射液 1710
精製ヒアルロン酸ナトリウム点眼液 1711
精製ブドウ糖 1075
精製ラノリン 2061
生理食塩液 1703
石油ベンジン 1503
セタノール 722
セチリジン塩酸塩 723
セチリジン塩酸塩錠 724
セッコウ 2023
セトチアミン塩酸塩水和物 725
セトラキサート塩酸塩 726
セネガ 2140
セネガシロップ 2140
セネガ末 2140
セファクロル 640
セファクロルカプセル 641
セファクロル細粒 644
セファクロル複合顆粒 642
セファゾリンナトリウム 656
セファゾリンナトリウム水和物 658

セファトリジンプロピレングリコール 654
セファドロキシル 645
セファドロキシルカプセル 646
セファレキシン 647
セファレキシンカプセル 649
セファレキシン複合顆粒 650
セファロチンナトリウム 652
セフィキシムカプセル 673
セフィキシム細粒 674
セフィキシム水和物 672
セフェピム塩酸塩水和物 669
セフォジジムナトリウム 679
セフォゾプラン塩酸塩 691
セフォタキシムナトリウム 684
セフォチアム塩酸塩 689
セフォチアム ヘキセチル塩酸塩 687
セフォテタン 685
セフォペラゾンナトリウム 681
セフカペン ピボキシル塩酸塩細粒 662
セフカペン ピボキシル塩酸塩錠 663
セフカペン ピボキシル塩酸塩水和物 660
セフジトレン ピボキシル 667
セフジトレン ピボキシル細粒 668
セフジトレン ピボキシル錠 668
セフジニル 664
セフジニルカプセル 665
セフジニル細粒 666
セフスロジンナトリウム 701
セフタジジム水和物 702
セフチゾキシムナトリウム 709
セフチブテン水和物 707
セフテラム ピボキシル 704
セフテラム ピボキシル細粒 706
セフテラム ピボキシル錠 706
セフトリアキソンナトリウム水和物 710
セフピラミドナトリウム 692
セフピロム硫酸塩 694
セフブペラゾンナトリウム 659
セフポドキシム プロキセチル 695
セフポドキシム プロキセチル錠 697
セフミノクスナトリウム水和物 678
セフメタゾールナトリウム 677
セフメノキシム塩酸塩 675
セフロキサジン水和物 698
セフロキシム アキセチル 712
セボフルラン 1677
セラセフェート 715
ゼラチン 1060
L-セリン 1677
セルモロイキン(遺伝子組換え) 719
セレコキシブ 714
センキュウ 1985
センキュウ末 1986
ゼンコ 2095
センコツ 2077
センソ 2159

Supplement I, JP XVIII

Index in Japanese   2983

センナ 2141, 2920
センナ末 2142, 2920
センブリ 2157
センブリ・重曹散 2158
センブリ末 2158

ソ

ソウジュツ 1951
ソウジュツ末 1951
ソウハクヒ 2076
ゾニサミド 1933
ゾニサミド錠 1934
ゾピクロン 1935
ゾピクロン錠 1936
ソボク 2132
ソヨウ 2095
ソルビタンセスキオレイン酸エステル 1732
ゾルピデム酒石酸塩 1931
ゾルピデム酒石酸塩錠 1932
D-ソルビトール 1733
D-ソルビトール液 1733

タ

ダイオウ 2113
大黄甘草湯エキス 1995
ダイオウ末 2114
大柴胡湯エキス 1996
ダイズ油 2156
タイソウ 2042
ダウノルビシン塩酸塩 829
タウリン 1780
タカルシトール水和物 1766
タカルシトール軟膏 1768
タカルシトールローション 1767
タクシャ 1941
タクシャ末 1942
タクロリムスカプセル 1770
タクロリムス水和物 1769
タゾバクタム 1781
ダナゾール 828
タムスロシン塩酸塩 1778
タムスロシン塩酸塩徐放錠 1779
タモキシフェンクエン酸塩 1777
タランピシリン塩酸塩 1771
タルク 1772
タルチレリン口腔内崩壊錠 1774
タルチレリン錠 1775
タルチレリン水和物 1773
炭酸カリウム 1553
炭酸水素ナトリウム 1698
炭酸水素ナトリウム注射液 1699
炭酸ナトリウム水和物 1701
炭酸マグネシウム 1289
炭酸リチウム 1271
単シロップ 1688
タンジン 2131
ダントロレンナトリウム水和物 828
単軟膏 2153
タンニン酸 1780
タンニン酸アルブミン 424

タンニン酸ジフェンヒドラミン 872
タンニン酸ベルベリン 534

チ

チアプリド塩酸塩 1826
チアプリド塩酸塩錠 1826
チアマゾール 1814
チアマゾール錠 1815
チアミラールナトリウム 1818
チアミン塩化物塩酸塩 1815
チアミン塩化物塩酸塩散 1817
チアミン塩化物塩酸塩注射液 1816
チアミン硝化物 1817
チアラミド塩酸塩 1827
チアラミド塩酸塩錠 1828
チアントール 1820
チオペンタールナトリウム 1821
チオリダジン塩酸塩 1823
チオ硫酸ナトリウム水和物 1727
チオ硫酸ナトリウム注射液 1727
チクセツニンジン 2090
チクセツニンジン末 2091
チクロピジン塩酸塩 1829
チクロピジン塩酸塩錠 1829
チザニジン塩酸塩 1836
窒素 1428
チニダゾール 1832
チペピジンヒベンズ酸塩 1833
チペピジンヒベンズ酸塩錠 1834
チメピジウム臭化物水和物 1830
チモ 1945
チモール 1825
チモロールマレイン酸塩 1831
注射用アシクロビル 410
注射用アズトレオナム 507
注射用アセチルコリン塩化物 406
注射用アミカシン硫酸塩 448
注射用アムホテリシン B 466, 2868
注射用アンピシリンナトリウム 471
注射用アンピシリンナトリウム・スルバクタムナトリウム 471, 2868
注射用イダルビシン塩酸塩 1137
注射用イミペネム・シラスタチンナトリウム 1145, 2884
注射用オザグレルナトリウム 1470
注射用シベレスタットナトリウム 1695
注射用水 1920
注射用水（容器入り） 1920
注射用スキサメトニウム塩化物 1766
注射用ストレプトマイシン硫酸塩 1746
注射用スペクチノマイシン塩酸塩 1735, 2899
注射用セファゾリンナトリウム 657
注射用セファロチンナトリウム 653
注射用セフェピム塩酸塩 671
注射用セフォゾプラン塩酸塩 692
注射用セフォチアム塩酸塩 690
注射用セフォペラゾンナトリウム 682
注射用セフォペラゾンナトリウム・ス

ルバクタムナトリウム 683, 2878
注射用セフタジジム 704
注射用セフメタゾールナトリウム 678
注射用タゾバクタム・ピペラシリン 1782
注射用チアミラールナトリウム 1819
注射用チオペンタールナトリウム 1822
注射用テセロイキン（遺伝子組換え） 1789
注射用テモゾロミド 2902
注射用ドキソルビシン塩酸塩 900
注射用ドセタキセル 880
注射用ドリペネム 889
注射用ナルトグラスチム（遺伝子組換え） 1405, 2891
注射用パニペネム・ベタミプロン 1473
注射用バンコマイシン塩酸塩 1904
注射用ヒト絨毛性性腺刺激ホルモン 1086
注射用ヒドララジン塩酸塩 1109
注射用ピペラシリンナトリウム 1534
注射用ビンブラスチン硫酸塩 1908
注射用ファモチジン 990
注射用フェニトインナトリウム 1514
注射用プレドニゾロンコハク酸エステルナトリウム 1576
注射用フロモキセフナトリウム 1016
注射用ペプロマイシン硫酸塩 1496
注射用ベンジルペニシリンカリウム 528
注射用ホスホマイシンナトリウム 1044
注射用ボリコナゾール 1915
注射用マイトマイシン C 1372
注射用ミノサイクリン塩酸塩 1366
注射用メトトレキサート 1333
注射用メロペネム 1322
注射用ロキサチジン酢酸エステル塩酸塩 1659
チョウジ 1984, 2909
チョウジ末 1984
チョウジ油 1984, 2909
チョウトウコウ 2168, 2921
釣藤散エキス 1977
チョレイ 2104
チョレイ末 2104
L-チロシン 1883
チンク油 1929
沈降ジフテリア破傷風混合トキソイド 873
沈降精製百日せきジフテリア破傷風混合ワクチン 873
沈降精製百日せきワクチン 1500
沈降炭酸カルシウム 594
沈降炭酸カルシウム細粒 594
沈降炭酸カルシウム錠 595
沈降破傷風トキソイド 1812
沈降 B 型肝炎ワクチン 1106
チンピ 1983

2984　*Index in Japanese*　　　　　　　　　　　　　　　　　　　　　　　　　　*Supplement I, JP XVIII*

ツ

ツバキ油　1972
ツロブテロール　1881
ツロブテロール塩酸塩　1883
ツロブテロール経皮吸収型テープ
　　1882

テ

テイコプラニン　1791
低置換度ヒドロキシプロピルセルロー
　　ス　1124
テオフィリン　1813
テガフール　1790
デキサメタゾン　836
デキストラン40　837
デキストラン40注射液　838
デキストラン70　839
デキストラン硫酸エステルナトリウム
　　イオウ5　840
デキストラン硫酸エステルナトリウム
　　イオウ18　840
デキストリン　841
デキストロメトルファン臭化水素酸塩
　　水和物　841
テストステロンエナント酸エステル
　　1809
テストステロンエナント酸エステル注
　　射液　1810
テストステロンプロピオン酸エステル
　　1810
テストステロンプロピオン酸エステル
　　注射液　1811
デスラノシド　835
デスラノシド注射液　836
テセロイキン(遺伝子組換え)　1784
テトラカイン塩酸塩　1812
テトラサイクリン塩酸塩　1812
デヒドロコール酸　832
デヒドロコール酸注射液　833
デフェロキサミンメシル酸塩　831
テプレノン　1802
テプレノンカプセル　1804
デメチルクロルテトラサイクリン塩酸
　　塩　834
テモカプリル塩酸塩　1800
テモカプリル塩酸塩錠　1801
テモゾロミド　2900
テモゾロミドカプセル　2901
テルビナフィン塩酸塩　1805
テルビナフィン塩酸塩液　1806
テルビナフィン塩酸塩クリーム　1806
テルビナフィン塩酸塩錠　1807
テルビナフィン塩酸塩スプレー　1807
テルブタリン硫酸塩　1808
テルミサルタン　1794
テルミサルタン・アムロジピンベシル
　　酸塩錠　1795
テルミサルタン錠　1797
テルミサルタン・ヒドロクロロチアジ
　　ド錠　1798

テレビン油　2168
天然ケイ酸アルミニウム　442
デンプングリコール酸ナトリウム
　　1725
テンマ　2007
テンモンドウ　1950

ト

桃核承気湯エキス　2160, 2921
トウガシ　1959
トウガラシ　1973
トウガラシ・サリチル酸精　1975
トウガラシチンキ　1974
トウガラシ末　1973
トウキ　2039
当帰芍薬散エキス　2162
トウキ末　2039
トウジン　1986
透析用ヘパリンナトリウム液　1105
トウニン　2091, 2915
トウニン末　2092, 2915
トウヒ　1960
トウヒシロップ　2084
トウヒチンキ　2084
トウモロコシデンプン　1738
トウモロコシ油　1990
ドキサゾシンメシル酸塩　896
ドキサゾシンメシル酸塩錠　897
ドキサプラム塩酸塩水和物　895
ドキシサイクリン塩酸塩錠　903
ドキシサイクリン塩酸塩水和物　901
ドキシフルリジン　898
ドキシフルリジンカプセル　898
ドキソルビシン塩酸塩　899
ドクカツ　1947
トコフェロール　1838
トコフェロールコハク酸エステルカル
　　シウム　1840
トコフェロール酢酸エステル　1839
トコフェロールニコチン酸エステル
　　1841
トコン　2036
トコンシロップ　2038
トコン末　2037
トスフロキサシントシル酸塩錠　1848
トスフロキサシントシル酸塩水和物
　　1846
ドセタキセル水和物　878
ドセタキセル注射液　879
トチュウ　2002
トドララジン塩酸塩水和物　1842
ドネペジル塩酸塩　882
ドネペジル塩酸塩細粒　883
ドネペジル塩酸塩錠　884
ドパミン塩酸塩　886
ドパミン塩酸塩注射液　886
トフィソパム　1843
ドブタミン塩酸塩　877
トブラマイシン　1837
トブラマイシン注射液　1838
トラガント　2165
トラガント末　2165

トラニラスト　1853
トラニラストカプセル　1854
トラニラスト細粒　1855
トラニラスト点眼液　1856
トラネキサム酸　1850
トラネキサム酸カプセル　1851
トラネキサム酸錠　1852
トラネキサム酸注射液　1852
トラピジル　1857
トラマドール塩酸塩　1849
トリアゾラム　1862
トリアムシノロン　1860
トリアムシノロンアセトニド　1861
トリアムテレン　1862
トリエンチン塩酸塩　1869
トリエンチン塩酸塩カプセル　1870
トリクロホスナトリウム　1868
トリクロホスナトリウムシロップ
　　1869
トリクロルメチアジド　1864
トリクロルメチアジド錠　1865
トリコマイシン　1867
L-トリプトファン　1880
トリヘキシフェニジル塩酸塩　1870
トリヘキシフェニジル塩酸塩錠　1871
ドリペネム水和物　887
トリメタジオン　1875
トリメタジジン塩酸塩　1873
トリメタジジン塩酸塩錠　1874
トリメトキノール塩酸塩水和物　1876
トリメブチンマレイン酸塩　1872
ドルゾラミド塩酸塩　891
ドルゾラミド塩酸塩・チモロールマレ
　　イン酸塩点眼液　893
ドルゾラミド塩酸塩点眼液　892
トルナフタート　1844
トルナフタート液　1845
トルブタミド　1843
トルブタミド錠　1844
トルペリゾン塩酸塩　1846
L-トレオニン　1823
トレハロース水和物　1858
トレピブトン　1859
ドロキシドパ　905
ドロキシドパカプセル　906
ドロキシドパ細粒　906
トロキシピド　1878
トロキシピド細粒　1878
トロキシピド錠　1879
トロピカミド　1877
ドロペリドール　904
トロンビン　1824
豚脂　2062
ドンペリドン　881

ナ

ナイスタチン　1440
ナタネ油　2111
ナテグリニド　1406
ナテグリニド錠　1407
ナドロール　1394
ナファゾリン塩酸塩　1400

Supplement I, JP XVIII　　　　　　　　　　　　　　　　　　　　*Index in Japanese*　　2985

ナファゾリン・クロルフェニラミン液
　　1401
ナファゾリン硝酸塩　1401
ナファモスタットメシル酸塩　1395
ナフトピジル　1396
ナフトピジル口腔内崩壊錠　1397
ナフトピジル錠　1398
ナブメトン　1392
ナブメトン錠　1393
ナプロキセン　1402
ナリジクス酸　1399
ナルトグラスチム（遺伝子組換え）
　　1403, 2891
ナロキソン塩酸塩　1400

ニ

ニガキ　2099, 2915
ニガキ末　2099, 2916
ニカルジピン塩酸塩　1410
ニカルジピン塩酸塩注射液　1410
ニクジュヨウ　1982
ニクズク　2078, 2915
ニコチン酸　1418
ニコチン酸アミド　1417
ニコチン酸注射液　1419
ニコモール　1415
ニコモール錠　1416
ニコランジル　1417
ニザチジン　1431
ニザチジンカプセル　1432
二酸化炭素　627
ニセリトロール　1414
ニセルゴリン　1411
ニセルゴリン散　1412
ニセルゴリン錠　1413
二相性イソフェンインスリン　ヒト
　　（遺伝子組換え）水性懸濁注射液
　　1159, 2886
ニトラゼパム　1426
ニトレンジピン　1426
ニトレンジピン錠　1427
ニトログリセリン錠　1429
ニフェジピン　1420
ニフェジピン細粒　1422
ニフェジピン徐放カプセル　1422
ニフェジピン腸溶細粒　1420
乳酸　1232
L-乳酸　1232
乳酸カルシウム水和物　599
L-乳酸ナトリウム液　1715
L-乳酸ナトリウムリンゲル液　1716
乳糖水和物　1234
尿素　1890
ニルバジピン　1423
ニルバジピン錠　1424
ニンジン　2011
ニンジン末　2012
ニンドウ　2066

ネ

ネオスチグミンメチル硫酸塩　1408

ネオスチグミンメチル硫酸塩注射液
　　1409

ノ

濃グリセリン　1081
濃ベンザルコニウム塩化物液50　520
ノスカピン　1439
ノスカピン塩酸塩水和物　1439
ノルアドレナリン　1433
ノルアドレナリン注射液　1433
ノルエチステロン　1434
ノルゲストレル　1435
ノルゲストレル・エチニルエストラジ
　　オール錠　1436
ノルトリプチリン塩酸塩　1437
ノルトリプチリン塩酸塩錠　1438
ノルフロキサシン　1434

ハ

バイモ　2005
バカンピシリン塩酸塩　508
バクガ　2069
白色セラック　1679
白色軟膏　1921
白色ワセリン　1501, 2892
白糖　1748
バクモンドウ　2081
麦門冬湯エキス　1953
バクロフェン　510
バクロフェン錠　511
バシトラシン　509
パズフロキサシンメシル酸塩　1485
パズフロキサシンメシル酸塩注射液
　　1486
バソプレシン注射液　1904
八味地黄丸エキス　2024, 2912
ハチミツ　2035
ハッカ　2072
ハッカ水　2073
ハッカ油　2072
パップ用複方オウバク散　2098
パニペネム　1471
パパベリン塩酸塩　1475
パパベリン塩酸塩注射液　1476
ハマボウフウ　2013, 2911
バメタン硫酸塩　512
パラアミノサリチル酸カルシウム顆粒
　　604
パラアミノサリチル酸カルシウム水和
　　物　603
パラオキシ安息香酸エチル　979, 2880
パラオキシ安息香酸ブチル　584, 2875
パラオキシ安息香酸プロピル　1601,
　　2896
パラオキシ安息香酸メチル　1343,
　　2890
バラシクロビル塩酸塩　1894
バラシクロビル塩酸塩錠　1896
パラフィン　1476
パラホルムアルデヒド　1478
L-バリン　1897

バルサルタン　1898
バルサルタン錠　1899
バルサルタン・ヒドロクロロチアジド
　　錠　1900
パルナパリンナトリウム　1480
バルビタール　512
バルプロ酸ナトリウム　1728
バルプロ酸ナトリウム錠　1731
バルプロ酸ナトリウム徐放錠A　1729
バルプロ酸ナトリウム徐放錠B　1730
バルプロ酸ナトリウムシロップ　1731
バレイショデンプン　1739
ハロキサゾラム　1095
パロキセチン塩酸塩錠　1483
パロキセチン塩酸塩水和物　1482
ハロタン　1094
ハロペリドール　1090
ハロペリドール細粒　1091
ハロペリドール錠　1093
ハロペリドール注射液　1092
パンクレアチン　1470
パンクロニウム臭化物　1471
ハンゲ　2100
半夏厚朴湯エキス　2027, 2913
半夏瀉心湯エキス　2028
バンコマイシン塩酸塩　1902
パンテチン　1475
パントテン酸カルシウム　602

ヒ

ピオグリタゾン塩酸塩　1522
ピオグリタゾン塩酸塩・グリメピリド
　　錠　1524
ピオグリタゾン塩酸塩錠　1523
ピオグリタゾン塩酸塩・メトホルミン
　　塩酸塩錠　1527
ビオチン　552
ビカルタミド　549
ビカルタミド錠　2872
ピコスルファートナトリウム水和物
　　1720
ビサコジル　554
ビサコジル坐剤　554
L-ヒスチジン　1106
L-ヒスチジン塩酸塩水和物　1107
ビソプロロールフマル酸塩　556
ビソプロロールフマル酸塩錠　557
ピタバスタチンカルシウム口腔内崩壊
　　錠　1541
ピタバスタチンカルシウム錠　1543
ピタバスタチンカルシウム水和物
　　1540
ビタミンA油　1910
ヒト下垂体性性腺刺激ホルモン　1087
ヒト絨毛性性腺刺激ホルモン　1085
人全血液　1921
人免疫グロブリン　1109
ヒドララジン塩酸塩　1109
ヒドララジン塩酸塩散　1110
ヒドララジン塩酸塩錠　1110
ヒドロキシエチルセルロース　1121
ヒドロキシジン塩酸塩　1125

ヒドロキシジンパモ酸塩 1126
ヒドロキシプロピルセルロース 1123
ヒドロキソコバラミン酢酸塩 1120
ヒドロクロロチアジド 1112
ヒドロコタルニン塩酸塩水和物 1119
ヒドロコルチゾン 1113
ヒドロコルチゾンコハク酸エステル 1118
ヒドロコルチゾンコハク酸エステルナトリウム 1117
ヒドロコルチゾン酢酸エステル 1114
ヒドロコルチゾン・ジフェンヒドラミン軟膏 1115
ヒドロコルチゾン酪酸エステル 1115
ヒドロコルチゾンリン酸エステルナトリウム 1116
ピブメシリナム塩酸塩 1545
ピブメシリナム塩酸塩錠 1546
ヒプロメロース 1127
ヒプロメロースカプセル 622
ヒプロメロース酢酸エステルコハク酸エステル 1129
ヒプロメロースフタル酸エステル 1131, 2883
ピペミド酸水和物 1530
ピペラシリン水和物 1530
ピペラシリンナトリウム 1532
ピペラジンアジピン酸塩 1534
ピペラジンリン酸塩錠 1535
ピペラジンリン酸塩水和物 1535
ビペリデン塩酸塩 553
ビホナゾール 552
ヒマシ油 1976
ピマリシン 1520
ヒメクロモン 1127
ピモジド 1521
ビャクゴウ 2063
ビャクシ 1946
ビャクジュツ 1952
ビャクジュツ末 1952
白虎加人参湯エキス 1969
氷酢酸 404
ピラジナミド 1608
ピラルビシン 1536
ピランテルパモ酸塩 1607
ピリドキサールリン酸エステル水和物 1609
ピリドキシン塩酸塩 1611
ピリドキシン塩酸塩注射液 1611
ピリドスチグミン臭化物 1609
ピルシカイニド塩酸塩カプセル 1519
ピルシカイニド塩酸塩水和物 1518
ピレノキシン 1537
ピレンゼピン塩酸塩水和物 1538
ピロ亜硫酸ナトリウム 1722
ピロカルピン塩酸塩 1516
ピロカルピン塩酸塩錠 1516
ピロキシカム 1539
ピロキシリン 1612
ピロールニトリン 1612
ビワヨウ 2066
ビンクリスチン硫酸塩 1909
ピンドロール 1522

ビンブラスチン硫酸塩 1907
ビンロウジ 1948

フ

ファモチジン 988
ファモチジン散 991
ファモチジン錠 992
ファモチジン注射液 989
ファロペネムナトリウム錠 995
ファロペネムナトリウム水和物 993
フィトナジオン 1515
フィルグラスチム(遺伝子組換え) 1007
フィルグラスチム(遺伝子組換え)注射液 1009
フェキソフェナジン塩酸塩 1004
フェキソフェナジン塩酸塩錠 1005
フェニトイン 1512
フェニトイン散 1513
フェニトイン錠 1513
L-フェニルアラニン 1510
フェニルブタゾン 1511
フェニレフリン塩酸塩 1512
フェネチシリンカリウム 1503
フェノバルビタール 1504
フェノバルビタール散10% 1505
フェノバルビタール錠 1506
フェノフィブラート 1001
フェノフィブラート錠 1002
フェノール 1507
フェノール・亜鉛華リニメント 1509
フェノール水 1508
フェノールスルホンフタレイン 1509
フェノールスルホンフタレイン注射液 1510
フェルビナク 996
フェルビナクテープ 997
フェルビナクパップ 997
フェロジピン 998
フェロジピン錠 999
フェンタニルクエン酸塩 1003
フェンブフェン 1000
複方アクリノール・チンク油 416
複方オキシコドン・アトロピン注射液 1460
複方オキシコドン注射液 1460
複方サリチル酸精 1669
複方サリチル酸メチル精 1347
複方ジアスターゼ・重曹散 843
複方ダイオウ・センナ散 2115
複方チアントール・サリチル酸液 1820
複方ヨード・グリセリン 1171
複方ロートエキス・ジアスターゼ散 2136
ブクモロール塩酸塩 572
ブクリョウ 2105
ブクリョウ末 2105
ブシ 2106
フシジン酸ナトリウム 1707
ブシ末 2108
ブシラミン 570

ブシラミン錠 570
ブスルファン 580
ブチルスコポラミン臭化物 1675
ブデソニド 2873
ブテナフィン塩酸塩 580
ブテナフィン塩酸塩液 582
ブテナフィン塩酸塩クリーム 581
ブテナフィン塩酸塩スプレー 583
ブドウ酒 1921
ブドウ糖 1073
ブドウ糖水和物 1074
ブドウ糖注射液 1076
フドステイン 1047
フドステイン錠 1048
ブトロピウム臭化物 583, 2875
ブナゾシン塩酸塩 577
ブピバカイン塩酸塩水和物 577
ブフェトロール塩酸塩 572
ブプラノロール塩酸塩 578
ブプレノルフィン塩酸塩 579
ブホルミン塩酸塩 573
ブホルミン塩酸塩錠 575
ブホルミン塩酸塩腸溶錠 574
ブメタニド 576
フラジオマイシン硫酸塩 1045
プラステロン硫酸エステルナトリウム水和物 1564
プラゼパム 1570
プラゼパム錠 1570
プラゾシン塩酸塩 1571
プラノプロフェン 1563
プラバスタチンナトリウム 1564
プラバスタチンナトリウム液 1567
プラバスタチンナトリウム細粒 1566
プラバスタチンナトリウム錠 1568
フラビンアデニンジヌクレオチドナトリウム 1010
フラボキサート塩酸塩 1012
プランルカスト水和物 1562
プリミドン 1578
フルオシノニド 1026
フルオシノロンアセトニド 1025
フルオレセインナトリウム 1027
フルオロウラシル 1029
フルオロメトロン 1028
フルコナゾール 1018
フルコナゾールカプセル 1019
フルコナゾール注射液 1020
フルジアゼパム 1022
フルジアゼパム錠 1022
フルシトシン 1021
フルスルチアミン塩酸塩 1051
フルタミド 1032
フルトプラゼパム 1033
フルトプラゼパム錠 1033
フルドロコルチゾン酢酸エステル 1023
フルニトラゼパム 1024
フルフェナジンエナント酸エステル 1030
フルボキサミンマレイン酸塩 1034
フルボキサミンマレイン酸塩錠 1036
フルラゼパム塩酸塩 1030

Supplement I, JP XVIII　　　　　　　　　　　　　　　*Index in Japanese*　2987

プルラン　1607
プルランカプセル　622
フルルビプロフェン　1031
ブレオマイシン塩酸塩　559
ブレオマイシン硫酸塩　561
フレカイニド酢酸塩　1012
フレカイニド酢酸塩錠　1013
プレドニゾロン　1572
プレドニゾロンコハク酸エステル
　　1576
プレドニゾロン酢酸エステル　1574
プレドニゾロン錠　1573
プレドニゾロンリン酸エステルナトリ
　　ウム　1575
プロカインアミド塩酸塩　1582
プロカインアミド塩酸塩錠　1584
プロカインアミド塩酸塩注射液　1543
プロカイン塩酸塩　1585
プロカイン塩酸塩注射液　1585
プロカテロール塩酸塩水和物　1587
プロカルバジン塩酸塩　1586
プログルミド　1591
プロクロルペラジンマレイン酸塩
　　1588
プロクロルペラジンマレイン酸塩錠
　　1588
プロゲステロン　1589
プロゲステロン注射液　1590
フロセミド　1049
フロセミド錠　1050
フロセミド注射液　1050
プロタミン硫酸塩　1603
プロタミン硫酸塩注射液　1604
プロチオナミド　1605
ブロチゾラム　568
ブロチゾラム錠　568
プロチレリン　1605
プロチレリン酒石酸塩水和物　1606
プロテイン銀　1687
プロテイン銀液　1687
プロパフェノン塩酸塩　1593
プロパフェノン塩酸塩錠　1594
プロパンテリン臭化物　1595
プロピベリン塩酸塩　1596
プロピベリン塩酸塩錠　1597
プロピルチオウラシル　1602
プロピルチオウラシル錠　1603
プロピレングリコール　1600
プロブコール　1580
プロブコール細粒　1581
プロブコール錠　1582
プロプラノロール塩酸塩　1598
プロプラノロール塩酸塩錠　1599
フロプロピオン　1017
フロプロピオンカプセル　1017
プロベネシド　1578
プロベネシド錠　1579
ブロマゼパム　563
ブロムフェナクナトリウム水和物
　　563
ブロムフェナクナトリウム点眼液
　　565
ブロムヘキシン塩酸塩　565, 2873

プロメタジン塩酸塩　1593
フロモキセフナトリウム　1014
ブロモクリプチンメシル酸塩　566
ブロモバレリル尿素　567
L-プロリン　1591
粉末セルロース　719, 2878

ヘ

ベカナマイシン硫酸塩　515
ベクロメタゾンプロピオン酸エステル
　　514
ベザフィブラート　548
ベザフィブラート徐放錠　549
ベタキソロール塩酸塩　546
ベタネコール塩化物　547
ベタヒスチンメシル酸塩　535
ベタヒスチンメシル酸塩錠　536
ベタミプロン　545
ベタメタゾン　538
ベタメタゾン吉草酸エステル　542
ベタメタゾン吉草酸エステル・ゲンタ
　　マイシン硫酸塩クリーム　543
ベタメタゾン吉草酸エステル・ゲンタ
　　マイシン硫酸塩軟膏　544
ベタメタゾンジプロピオン酸エステル
　　540
ベタメタゾン錠　539
ベタメタゾンリン酸エステルナトリウ
　　ム　541
ペチジン塩酸塩　1500
ペチジン塩酸塩注射液　1501
ベニジピン塩酸塩　516
ベニジピン塩酸塩錠　516
ヘパリンカルシウム　1096
ヘパリンナトリウム　1100
ヘパリンナトリウム注射液　1104
ペプロマイシン硫酸塩　1494
ベポタスチンベシル酸塩　529
ベポタスチンベシル酸塩錠　530
ペミロラストカリウム　1486
ペミロラストカリウム錠　1489
ペミロラストカリウム点眼液　1487
ベラドンナエキス　1958
ベラドンナコン　1957
ベラドンナ総アルカロイド　1958
ベラパミル塩酸塩　1905
ベラパミル塩酸塩錠　1907
ベラパミル塩酸塩注射液　1906
ベラプロストナトリウム　531
ベラプロストナトリウム錠　532
ペルフェナジン　1497
ペルフェナジン錠　1497
ペルフェナジンマレイン酸塩　1498
ペルフェナジンマレイン酸塩錠　1499
ベルベリン塩化物水和物　533
ベンザルコニウム塩化物　519
ベンザルコニウム塩化物液　520
ベンジルアルコール　523, 2872
ベンジルペニシリンカリウム　527
ベンジルペニシリンベンザチン水和物
　　525
ヘンズ　2000

ベンズブロマロン　521
ベンゼトニウム塩化物　522
ベンゼトニウム塩化物液　522
ベンセラジド塩酸塩　518
ペンタゾシン　1491
ペントキシベリンクエン酸塩　1493
ベントナイト　519
ペントバルビタールカルシウム　1491
ペントバルビタールカルシウム錠
　　1492
ペンブトロール硫酸塩　1490

ホ

ボウイ　2153, 2920
防已黄耆湯エキス　1966
ボウコン　2036
ホウ酸　562
ホウ砂　1700
ボウショウ　2155
抱水クロラール　728
ボウフウ　2132
防風通聖散エキス　1961
ボクソク　2111
ボグリボース　1911
ボグリボース口腔内崩壊錠　2904
ボグリボース錠　1912, 2905
ホスホマイシンカルシウム水和物
　　1040
ホスホマイシンナトリウム　1043
ボタンピ　2073
ボタンピ末　2074
補中益気湯エキス　2032
ポビドン　1559
ポビドンヨード　1561
ホマトロピン臭化水素酸塩　1107
ホミカ　2078
ホミカエキス　2079
ホミカエキス散　2080
ホミカチンキ　2080
ホモクロルシクリジン塩酸塩　1108
ポラプレジンク　1546
ポラプレジンク顆粒　1548
ボリコナゾール　1913
ボリコナゾール錠　1916
ポリスチレンスルホン酸カルシウム
　　607
ポリスチレンスルホン酸ナトリウム
　　1721
ポリソルベート80　1550, 2894
ホリナートカルシウム水和物　597
ポリミキシンB硫酸塩　1549
ホルマリン　1039
ホルマリン水　1039
ホルモテロールフマル酸塩水和物
　　1040, 2881
ボレイ　2090
ボレイ末　2090

マ

マイトマイシンC　1371
マオウ　2001

2988　Index in Japanese

麻黄湯エキス　2070, 2914
マクリ　1998
マクロゴール400　1284
マクロゴール1500　1284
マクロゴール4000　1285
マクロゴール6000　1285
マクロゴール20000　1286
マクロゴール軟膏　1286
マシニン　2031
麻酔用エーテル　968
マニジピン塩酸塩　1296
マニジピン塩酸塩錠　1297
マプロチリン塩酸塩　1300
マルトース水和物　1295
D-マンニトール　1298, 2888
D-マンニトール注射液　1300

ミ

ミグリトール　1361
ミグリトール錠　1362
ミグレニン　1363
ミクロノマイシン硫酸塩　1358
ミコナゾール　1357
ミコナゾール硝酸塩　1358
ミゾリビン　1372
ミゾリビン錠　1373
ミチグリニドカルシウム錠　1369
ミチグリニドカルシウム水和物　1368
ミツロウ　1956
ミデカマイシン　1359
ミデカマイシン酢酸エステル　1360
ミノサイクリン塩酸塩　1364
ミノサイクリン塩酸塩顆粒　1365
ミノサイクリン塩酸塩錠　1367
ミョウバン水　439

ム

無コウイ大建中湯エキス　2075, 2914
無水アンピシリン　467
無水エタノール　965, 2880
無水カフェイン　588
無水クエン酸　768
無水乳糖　1233
無水ボウショウ　2154
無水リン酸水素カルシウム　604
ムピロシンカルシウム水和物　1390
ムピロシンカルシウム軟膏　1392

メ

メキシレチン塩酸塩　1356
メキタジン　1319
メキタジン錠　1319
メグルミン　1310
メクロフェノキサート塩酸塩　1301
メコバラミン　1302
メコバラミン錠　1303
メサラジン　1323
メサラジン徐放錠　1325
メストラノール　1326
メタケイ酸アルミン酸マグネシウム

1288
メダゼパム　1304
メタンフェタミン塩酸塩　1330
L-メチオニン　1331
メチクラン　1349
メチラポン　1355
dl-メチルエフェドリン塩酸塩　1340
dl-メチルエフェドリン塩酸塩散10%
　1341
メチルエルゴメトリンマレイン酸塩
　1342
メチルエルゴメトリンマレイン酸塩錠
　1342
メチルジゴキシン　1350
メチルセルロース　1336
メチルテストステロン　1347
メチルテストステロン錠　1348
メチルドパ錠　1339
メチルドパ水和物　1338
メチルプレドニゾロン　1344
メチルプレドニゾロンコハク酸エステ
　ル　1345
メチルベナクチジウム臭化物　1336
滅菌精製水(容器入り)　1920
メテノロンエナント酸エステル　1328
メテノロンエナント酸エステル注射液
　1328
メテノロン酢酸エステル　1327
メトキサレン　1335
メトクロプラミド　1351
メトクロプラミド錠　1351
メトトレキサート　1331
メトトレキサートカプセル　1332
メトトレキサート錠　1334
メトプロロール酒石酸塩　1352
メトプロロール酒石酸塩錠　1353
メトホルミン塩酸塩　1329
メトホルミン塩酸塩錠　1329
メドロキシプロゲステロン酢酸エステ
　ル　1306
メトロニダゾール　1354
メトロニダゾール錠　1354
メナテトレノン　1314
メピチオスタン　1316
メピバカイン塩酸塩　1317
メピバカイン塩酸塩注射液　1318
メフェナム酸　1307
メフルシド　1309
メフルシド錠　1310
メフロキン塩酸塩　1308
メペンゾラート臭化物　1316
メルカプトプリン水和物　1320
メルファラン　1313
メロペネム水和物　1321
dl-メントール　1315, 2889
l-メントール　1315, 2890

モ

木クレオソート　2171
モクツウ　1941, 2907
モサプリドクエン酸塩散　1388
モサプリドクエン酸塩錠　1389

モサプリドクエン酸塩水和物　1387
モッコウ　2132
モノステアリン酸アルミニウム　440
モノステアリン酸グリセリン　1082,
　2883
モルヒネ・アトロピン注射液　1385
モルヒネ塩酸塩錠　1384
モルヒネ塩酸塩水和物　1382
モルヒネ塩酸塩注射液　1383
モルヒネ硫酸塩水和物　1386
モンテルカストナトリウム　1334
モンテルカストナトリウム顆粒　1379
モンテルカストナトリウム錠　1380
モンテルカストナトリウムチュアブル
　錠　1377

ヤ

ヤクチ　1960, 2908
ヤクモソウ　2063, 2913
薬用石ケン　1306
薬用炭　1305
ヤシ油　1986

ユ

ユウタン　1955
ユーカリ油　2002
輸血用クエン酸ナトリウム注射液
　1704
ユビデカレノン　1886

ヨ

ヨウ化カリウム　1557
ヨウ化ナトリウム　1713
ヨウ化ナトリウム(^{123}I)カプセル
　1714
ヨウ化ナトリウム(^{131}I)液　1714
ヨウ化ナトリウム(^{131}I)カプセル
　1714
ヨウ化人血清アルブミン(^{131}I)注射液
　1169
ヨウ化ヒプル酸ナトリウム(^{131}I)注射
　液　1714
葉酸　1037
葉酸錠　1038
葉酸注射液　1037
ヨウ素　1170
ヨクイニン　1987
ヨクイニン末　1987
抑肝散エキス　2173
抑肝散加陳皮半夏エキス　2922
ヨード・サリチル酸・フェノール精
　1173
ヨードチンキ　1170
ヨードホルム　1174

ラ

ラウリル硫酸ナトリウム　1718
ラウロマクロゴール　1246
ラクツロース　1235

Supplement I, JP XVIII　　　　　　　　　　　　　　　　　　　　　*Index in Japanese*　　2989

ラタモキセフナトリウム　1245
ラッカセイ油　2093
ラニチジン塩酸塩　1625
ラノコナゾール　1238
ラノコナゾールクリーム　1239
ラノコナゾール外用液　1240
ラノコナゾール軟膏　1240
ラフチジン　1236
ラフチジン錠　1237
ラベタロール塩酸塩　1230
ラベタロール塩酸塩錠　1231
ラベプラゾールナトリウム　1624
ランソプラゾール　1241
ランソプラゾール腸溶カプセル　1242
ランソプラゾール腸溶性口腔内崩壊錠
　　1243

リ

リオチロニンナトリウム　1267
リオチロニンナトリウム錠　1268
リシノプリル錠　1270
リシノプリル水和物　1269
L-リシン塩酸塩　1282
L-リシン酢酸塩　1281
リスペリドン　1645
リスペリドン細粒　1645
リスペリドン錠　1648
リスペリドン内服液　1647
リセドロン酸ナトリウム錠　1724
リセドロン酸ナトリウム水和物　1722
リゾチーム塩酸塩　1283
六君子湯エキス　2116
リドカイン　1263
リドカイン注射液　1264
リトドリン塩酸塩　1649
リトドリン塩酸塩錠　1651
リトドリン塩酸塩注射液　1650
リバビリン　1632
リバビリンカプセル　1633
リファンピシン　1639
リファンピシンカプセル　1640
リボスタマイシン硫酸塩　1638
リボフラビン　1635
リボフラビン散　1635
リボフラビン酪酸エステル　1636
リボフラビンリン酸エステルナトリウ
　　ム　1637
リボフラビンリン酸エステルナトリウ

　　ム注射液　1638
リマプロスト　アルファデクス　1264
リュウガンニク　2065
リュウコツ　2065
リュウコツ末　2065
硫酸亜鉛水和物　1930
硫酸亜鉛点眼液　1931
硫酸アルミニウムカリウム水和物
　　442
硫酸カリウム　1558
硫酸鉄水和物　1004
硫酸バリウム　513
硫酸マグネシウム水　1295
硫酸マグネシウム水和物　1294
硫酸マグネシウム注射液　1294
リュウタン　2040
リュウタン末　2040
流動パラフィン　1477
リュープロレリン酢酸塩　1252
リョウキョウ　1944
苓桂朮甘湯エキス　2119
リルマザホン塩酸塩錠　1643
リルマザホン塩酸塩水和物　1642
リンゲル液　1644
リンコマイシン塩酸塩水和物　1266
リンコマイシン塩酸塩注射液　1267
リン酸水素カルシウム水和物　605
リン酸水素ナトリウム水和物　1719
リン酸二水素カルシウム水和物　606

レ

レセルピン　1628
レセルピン散0.1%　1630
レセルピン錠　1630
レセルピン注射液　1629
レチノール酢酸エステル　1631
レチノールパルミチン酸エステル
　　1632
レナンピシリン塩酸塩　1246
レノグラスチム(遺伝子組換え)　1248
レバミピド　1626
レバミピド錠　1627
レバロルファン酒石酸塩　1254
レバロルファン酒石酸塩注射液　1254
レボチロキシンナトリウム錠　1262
レボチロキシンナトリウム水和物
　　1261
レボドパ　1255

レボフロキサシン細粒　1257
レボフロキサシン錠　1259
レボフロキサシン水和物　1256
レボフロキサシン注射液　1258
レボフロキサシン点眼液　1258
レボホリナートカルシウム水和物
　　600
レボメプロマジンマレイン酸塩　1261
レンギョウ　2004
レンニク　2077

ロ

L-ロイシン　1251
ロキサチジン酢酸エステル塩酸塩
　　1656
ロキサチジン酢酸エステル塩酸塩徐放
　　カプセル　1657
ロキサチジン酢酸エステル塩酸塩徐放
　　錠　1658
ロキシスロマイシン　1660
ロキシスロマイシン錠　1661
ロキソプロフェンナトリウム錠　1280
ロキソプロフェンナトリウム水和物
　　1279
ロサルタンカリウム　1274
ロサルタンカリウム錠　1275
ロサルタンカリウム・ヒドロクロロチ
　　アジド錠　1276
ロジン　2118
ロスバスタチンカルシウム　1652
ロスバスタチンカルシウム錠　1654
ロック用ヘパリンナトリウム液　1104
ロートエキス　2135
ロートエキス・アネスタミン散　2137
ロートエキス・カーボン散　2136
ロートエキス散　2135
ロートエキス・タンニン坐剤　2138
ロートコン　2133
ロフラゼプ酸エチル　976
ロフラゼプ酸エチル錠　978
ロベンザリットナトリウム　1273
ローヤルゼリー　2119
ロラゼパム　1273

ワ

ワルファリンカリウム　1917
ワルファリンカリウム錠　1918

Addenda

Addenda   1

Relevant notices and communications

Information related to the revision in the Supplement I to the JP 18th Edition

Briefing on drafts of General Tests and General Information related to Chromatography

September 2021

Pharmaceuticals and Medical Devices Agency

Office of Review Management

With the publication of the following four drafts of General Tests and General Information related to Chromatography for public consultation, the information below is provided for your review.

- Draft of new General Test "*<2.00> Chromatography*"
- Draft of new General Information "*<G1-5-181> Control Strategies and Change Control Concepts at Each Stage of Chromatography Lifecycle*"
- Draft of revised General Test "*<2.01> Liquid Chromatography*"
- Draft of revised General Test "*<2.02> Gas Chromatography*"

Harmonization process of G-20 Chromatography by Pharmacopoeia Discussion Group (PDG) has started since 2009. Reviewing the submitted comments on the Stage 2 draft published for the public consultation from July 2017 to October 2017, the Chromatography Working Group (WG) of Japanese Pharmacopoeia (JP) Expert Committee has continuously discussed the draft toward to the harmonization. Since the process reached Stage 3A of the harmonization working procedure, the draft of General Test in the JP *<2.00> Chromatography* based on the Stage 3A draft is published for public consultation. In order to contribute to the proper implementation of the *<2.00>* in the quality control of pharmaceuticals, draft of General Information *<G1-5-181>*, revised draft of General Test *<2.01>* and revised draft of General Test *<2.02>* have also been discussed, and they are published for public consultation simultaneously. Considering the above, when you review these four drafts, we would like to ask you to refer them mutually.

In addition, revised draft of General Information *<G1-2-152> System Suitability* is also under discussion by the Chromatography WG, with the direction that the 3rd chapter "Point to Consider at the Change of Analytical System" in this revised draft is going to be integrated into the *<G1-5-181>*. In the near future, the revised draft of *<G1-2-152>* will be published for public consultation, which will result in listing it in the JP simultaneously along with the above four drafts.

The key points of these four drafts are as follows.

- **Draft of a New General Test: *<2.00> Chromatography***
  - ➢ *<2.00>* is not intended to be applied retrospectively to the monographs listed in JP, but to be applicable to the new monographs after *<2.00>* being listed in JP.

2   *Addenda*

    ➢   Regarding the 4th chapter "Adjustment of chromatographic conditions" in the *<2.00>*, the following points are going to be provided as JP original contents:

        ·   The 4th chapter should be applied to liquid chromatography and gas chromatography, but it should not be applied to thin layer chromatography.

        ·   In cases of some biotechnological/biological products, the 4th chapter is not necessarily applicable.

        ·   Crude drugs and related drugs are not covered in the 4th chapter.

- **Draft of New General Information: *<G1-5-181> Control Strategies and Change Control Concepts at Each Stage of Chromatography Lifecycle***

    ➢   When applying the 4th chapter "Adjustment of chromatographic conditions" in the *<2.00>* to products, in order to perform the appropriate risk assessment, the points to consider for the change control are provided. The draft *of <G1-5-181>* is arranged to promote the effort of the change control, considering the life cycle of analytical procedures which consists of design to development, qualification and continuous verification. This arrangement is made so that the points to consider for the change control can be clearly provided at each stage of chromatography lifecycle.

    ➢   Since the draft of *<G1-5-181>* is positioned as a document that provides technical information from scientific viewpoints, it does not intend to mention any regulatory requirements.

    ➢   It is also taken into consideration that the draft of *<G1-5-181>* will be used as a guide that summarizes the key points for the change control of analytical conditions at the quality tests of pharmaceuticals in public testing institutions.

- **Revised draft of General Test: *<2.01> Liquid Chromatography***

    ➢   In the 6th chapter "System Suitability" in the *<2.01>*, its relationship with the system suitability specified in the *<2.00>* is clarified.

    ➢   Regarding the 7th chapter "Points to Consider on changing the operating conditions" in the *<2.01>*, in terms of international harmonization, it is revised that the change controls based on the appropriate risk assessment will be performed, as shown in the contents of 4th chapter "Adjustment of chromatographic conditions" in the *<2.00>*. In addition, the contents of this chapter duplicate with those of the *<2.00>* are deleted from the *<2.01>*.

    ➢   The 8th chapter "Terminology" in the *<2.01>* is deleted because the terminology related to chromatography in the JP will be provided in the terminology of the *<2.00>*.

- **Revised draft of General Test: *<2.02> Gas Chromatography***

    ➢   Regarding the 7th chapter "Points to Consider on changing the operating conditions" in the *<2.02>*, in terms of international harmonization, it is revised that the change controls based on the appropriate risk assessment will be performed, as shown in the contents of 4th chapter "Adjustment of chromatographic conditions" in the *<2.00>*. In addition, the contents of this chapter duplicate with those of *the <2.00>* are deleted from the *<2.02>*.

Addenda   3

Briefing on New draft of General Information

"Functionality-related Characteristics of Excipients Relevant to Preparations"

⟨*G9-1-181*⟩

September 2021

Pharmaceuticals and Medical Devices Agency

Office of Review Management

Before publication of a proposed new draft to the Japanese Pharmacopoeia (JP) General Information "Functionality-related Characteristics of Excipients Relevant to Preparations" for public consultation, the following background information is provided for your review.

This new General Information explains the physical and chemical properties of excipients, as Functionality Related Characteristics (FRC), which are closely relevant to the improvement of the usefulness of active pharmaceutical ingredients and preparations in the manufacturing process, storage, and use of the preparations.

In addition to the specifications prescribed in each monograph with the main purpose of identifying substances and ensuring quality, test methods that are applied to evaluation of FRC are available for specific excipients. These test methods evaluate physical and chemical properties that are used as not quality requirements but indicators for addition of functions. For example, the water-retaining amount is one of the FRC of the excipients used for appropriately controlling the disintegration property of a pharmaceutical product.

<Policies for drafting this General Information>

- The test methods applied to the evaluation of FRC are not prescribed in each excipient monograph, and the FRC and the applicable test methods shall be provided as examples for each individual item in this General Information.
- Since the test methods included in this General Information are examples and are not mandatory for FRC evaluation, no acceptance criteria are prescribed for the test methods.
- For the time being, the FRC and the test methods applicable to its evaluation included in the General Information are limited to the subjects to PDG harmonization, except those already included in the monographs.

Furthermore, with the addition of this new General Information to the JP, the specifications and the test methods for consistency of Petrolatum and White Petrolatum which are subject to PDG harmonization and whose revised drafts are published for public consultations from September 30, 2019 to December 30, 2019 will be removed from each monograph. For details, please refer to the newly revised drafts in the Additional Revision of the Revision Drafts for the First Supplement to JP18 published in September, 2021.

4   *Addenda*

March 1, 2022

Disclosure of Information about Columns for Japanese Pharmacopoeia
Draft Monographs for Crude Drugs

Office of Review Management,

Pharmaceuticals and Medical Devices Agency

The products in the Official Monographs for Crude Drugs are composed of multicomponent systems as a characteristic of natural products, and the compositions and the quantitative values of constituents are diversified within a certain range due to differences in secondary metabolites, growth environments, cultivation conditions, genetic factors and processing methods of the original plants. For that reason, it is necessary to select column(s) depending on the test sample for assay of each manufacturer or each manufacturers association even for the test of the same monograph. The expert committees for crude drugs gathers the test results of multiple samples and discusses on the draft monograph with the multiple data. It would be valuable to share with the public by disclosing the information about columns that were evaluated in the development of monograph. Thus, please be notified that Office of Review Management, Pharmaceuticals and Medical Devices Agency (PMDA) starts to take a measure to in principle disclose the information about columns, such as the name (model number) of columns, for Japanese Pharmacopoeia (JP) draft monographs (crude drugs) under the following rules:

1. Concerning tests as a whole using columns in the draft monographs (crude drugs), while further ensuring of transparency of the JP revision process is required, the measure mentioned above is to post the information about the columns that were used for acquisition of the data that were referred in the preparation of the drafts on the PMDA website by PMDA at the start of publication of the relevant drafts for public comments.
2. Addition of information about other alternative columns or update of information associated with technological innovation is in principle not to be done.
3. The columns to be disclosed have not been confirmed as applicable to all the samples that could be the subjects to application to the monographs of the relevant drafts.
4. The information about columns are released only when cooperation is provided by the manufactures or manufacturers association who prepared the drafts.

Disclosure History:

Extracts, the crude drugs and preparations to be included Supplement I to the Japanese Pharmacopoeia 18th edition, March 1, 2022.

Extracts, the crude drugs and preparations to be included the Japanese Pharmacopoeia 18th edition, December 2, 2019.

Extracts, the crude drugs and preparations to be included Supplement II to the Japanese Pharmacopoeia 17th edition, June 1, 2018.

Extracts, the crude drugs and preparations to be included Supplement I to the Japanese Pharmacopoeia 17th edition, January 4, 2017.

Extracts, the crude drugs and preparations included the Japanese Pharmacopoeia 17th edition, January 4, 2017.

Extracts, the crude drugs and preparations to be included Supplement I to the Japanese Pharmacopoeia 18th edition

Saikokeishikankyoto Extract: Saikosaponin b_2
(Column: Particle size 5 μm, 4.6 mmID×15 cm)

Brand Name
COSMOSIL 5C$_{18}$-MS-II
Inertsil ODS-3
L-column2 ODS
Mightysil RP-18 GP
TSKgel ODS-100S
TSKgel ODS-120A
TSKgel ODS-80Ts
YMC-Pack ODS-A

Saikokeishikankyoto Extract: Baicalin
(Column: Particle size 5 μm, 4.6 mmID×15 cm)

Brand Name
COSMOSIL 5C$_{18}$-AR-II
COSMOSIL 5C$_{18}$-MS-II
Mightysil RP-18GP
Mightysil RP-18GP Aqua
TSKgel ODS-80Ts
TSKgel ODS-80TsQA
YMC-Pack ODS-A

Saikokeishikankyoto Extract: Glycyrrhizic acid
(Column: Particle size 5 μm, 4.6 mmID×15 cm)

Brand Name
Mightysil RP-18GP
TSKgel ODS-100S
TSKgel ODS-100V
TSKgel ODS-80Ts
TSKgel ODS-80TsQA
YMC-Pack ODS-A
Mightysil RP-18GP

Yokukansankachimpihange Extract: Saikosaponin b_2
(Column: Particle size 5 μm, 4.6 mmID×15 cm)

Brand Name
COSMOSIL 5C$_{18}$-AR-II
Inertsil ODS-4V
Mightysil RP-18GP
TSKgel ODS-100S
TSKgel ODS-80TsQA
YMC-Pack ODS-A

Yokukansankachimpihange Extract: Glycyrrhizic Acid
(Column: Particle size 5 μm, 4.6 mmID×15 cm)

Brand Name
Atlantis dC18
COSMOSIL 5C$_{18}$-AR-II
Develosil ODS-HG-5
TSKgel ODS-100S
TSKgel ODS-80TsQA
YMC-Pack *Pro*-C18

Yokukansankachimpihange Extract: Hesperidin
(Column: Particle size 5 μm, 4.6 mmID×15 cm)

Brand Name
COSMOSIL 5C$_{18}$-AR-II
Develosil ODS-HG-5
Mightysil RP-18GP
TSKgel ODS-100S
TSKgel ODS-100V
TSKgel ODS-80Ts
TSKgel ODS-80TsQA
YMC-Pack ODS-A
YMC-Pack *Pro*-C18

* Described according to the articles listed in the Supplement I to JP 18th Edition.

6   *Addenda*

Revision of General Information "On the Scientific Names of Crude Drugs listed in the JP"

2022. 9

The JP Committee on Crude Drugs

The background to the revision of General Information "On the Scientific Names of Crude Drugs listed in the JP" is explained below as the starting of collecting public comments on the revision.

The scientific names of the original plants of crude drugs listed in the Japanese Pharmacopoeia should be based on the "International Plant Name Index (IPNI)" in the Guideline for drafting The Japanese Pharmacopoeia. (Partially omitted) Family names are determined to follow the new Engler's classification system. On the other hand, in plant taxonomy it is now common to use the APG system, which is based on DNA information, instead of the systems such as the New Engler and Cronquist systems, which are based on morphological characteristics. This divergence is mainly due to the fact that the JP is not an academic text but an ordinance, and the adoption of the classification system that is currently undergoing revision has been postponed in order to avoid frequent amendments to the description. However, more than 20 years have passed since the first publication of the APG classification system, during that time it has matured into a reliable new classification system, by the accumulation of analysis data and three revisions, and is now used not only in specialized research fields but also in botanical illustrations for the general public. In view of this situation, we have decided to revise the JP general information "On the Scientific Names of Crude Drugs listed in the JP" and add family names in the APG classification. The following arrangement has been made for the revision.

1. In the existing general information, Japanese family names were described, but the Japanese family names have been deleted as only Latin names are given in the monographs.
2. In the Articles 18.5 and 18.6 of the International Code of Nomenclature for Algae, Fungi and Plants (Shenzhen Code) 2018, it is clearly stated that family names that have long been used conventionally, such as Leguminosae, Labiatae, etc., are treated as officially published names and these names are used as the official names. In addition, as the Article 18.5 also contains alternative names for the nine family names concerned, they are given in the style of "full name/alternative name". Example: Leguminosae/Fabaceae.
3. The family names of source species of crude drugs derived from gymnosperms, algae and fungi which are not included in the APG classification system are based on Yonekura, "Updated Syllabus of Vascular Plant Families (Hokuryukan)" and the Global Biodiversity Information Facility (GBIF: https://www.gbif.org). Ephedra Herb, Rosin, Digenea, Polyporus Sclerotium, Poria Sclerotium, Oyster Shell, etc. fall under this category, but none of them differ from the current description of the JP. These items that do not fall under the APG classification are marked with a mark (#) in the table.

In addition to the revised general information, extracted items with different family names in the new Engler and APG classification systems is attached as a reference material for the convenience of confirmation work when opinions are collected.

Addenda 7

Information about Columns for Japanese Pharmacopoeia Draft Monographs (Chemical Drug)

Pharmaceuticals and Medical Devices Agency

Office of Review Management

March 1, 2023

In accordance with the policy for "Disclosure of Information about Columns for Japanese Pharmacopoeia Draft Monographs (by Division of Pharmacopoeia and Standards for Drugs, Office of Standards and Guidelines Development, Pharmaceuticals and Medical Devices Agency, dated March 1, 2016)" (see Annex), the information about the columns that were used for acquisition of the data that were referred in the preparation of the drafts for public comments is as follows:

Posting Date	Monograph	Test	Brand Name
December 24, 2021	Voglibose Tablets	Identification	DOWEX™ 50W × 2 100-200 Mesh (H) Cation Exchange Resin
			DOWEX™ 50W × 4 100-200 Mesh (H) Cation Exchange Resin
December 1, 2021	Enviomycin Sulfate	Content ratio of the active principle	InertSustain AQ-C18 HP
September 1, 2021	Anastrozole Tablets	Uniformity of dosage unit, Dissolution, Assay	Hicrom RPB
September 1, 2021	Bicalutamide Tablets	Assay	Spherisorb ODS2
June 1, 2021	Voglibose Orally Disintegrating Tablets	Uniformity of dosage unit, Dissolution, Assay	YMC-Pack Polyamine II
March 1, 2021	Budesonide	Purity (2) Related substances, Isomer ratio, Assay	Hypersil ODS C18 or Discovery HS C18
September 1, 2020	Temozolomide	Purity (2) Related substances, Assay	Spherisorb ODS2 5 µm 150 mm × 4.6 mm
		Purity (3) Acetonitrile	J&W DB-WAX, 30 m × 0.53 mm fused silica, 1.0 µm film thickness
September 1, 2020	Temozolomide Capsules	Identification, Purity Related substances, Uniformity of dosage units, Assay	Spherisorb ODS2 5 µm 150 mm × 4.6 mm
September 1, 2020	Temozolomide for Injection	Identification, Purity Related substances, Assay	Spherisorb ODS2 5 µm 150 mm × 4.6 mm
June 1, 2020	Anastrozole	Purity (2) Related substances, Assay	Hichrom RPB
June 1, 2020	Formoterol Fumarate Hydrate	Purity (2) Related substances	Zorbax SB-C8
		Purity (2) Diastereomer	Asahipak ODP-50
March 2, 2020	Oxybutynin Hydrochloride	Purity (2) Related substances	Symmetry C8

* Described according to the articles listed in the Supplement I to JP 18th Edition.

* Articles deferred for listing in the Supplement I to JP 18th Edition: Sucrose (published in September 1, 2020).

8   *Addenda*

Annex

March 1, 2016

Disclosure of Information about Columns for Japanese Pharmacopoeia Draft Monographs

Division of Pharmacopoeia and Standards for Drugs,
Office of Standards and Guidelines Development,
Pharmaceuticals and Medical Devices Agency

Please be notified that the division of Pharmacopoeia and Standards for Drugs, Office of Standards and Guidelines Development, Pharmaceuticals and Medical Devices Agency (PMDA) starts to take a measure to in principle disclose the information about columns, such as the name (model number) of columns, for Japanese Pharmacopoeia (JP) draft monographs (hereinafter excluding the draft monographs for crude drugs) under the following rules:

1. Concerning tests as a whole using columns in the draft monographs, while further ensuring of transparency of the JP revision process is required, the measure mentioned above is to post the information about the columns that were used for acquisition of the data that were referred in the preparation of the drafts on the PMDA website by PMDA at the start of publication of the relevant drafts for public comments.

2. This disclosure is principally provided for ensuring of enhancement of public comments by wide sharing of the information 1 above with stakeholders other than the manufacturers who prepared the drafts at the time of publication for public comments. Thus, addition of information about other alternative columns or update of information associated with technological innovation is in principle not to be done.

3. The columns to be disclosed have not been confirmed as applicable to all the samples that could be the subjects to application to the monographs of the relevant drafts.

4. The information about columns are released only when cooperation is provided by the manufactures who prepared the drafts.

Addenda 9

The monographs revised in the Supplement I to JP 18 and their revised sections

Please refer to p.2845 for revision to remove Heavy Metals Test and Individual Metal Impurity Test from Japanese Pharmacopoeia (JP) Official Monographs, accompanying the application of Control of Elemental Impurities.

Title (Japanese title)		Section	Page
Amphotericin B for Injection （注射用アムホテリシンB）	Add.		2868
	Rev.	Uniformity of dosage units	
	Del.		
Amphotericin B Tablets （アムホテリシンB錠）	Add.		2868
	Rev.	Uniformity of dosage units	
	Del.		
Ampicillin Sodium and Sulbactam Sodium for Injection （注射用アンピシリンナトリウム・スルバクタムナトリウム）	Add.		2868
	Rev.	Uniformity of dosage units	
	Del.		
Benzyl Alcohol （ベンジルアルコール）	Add.		2872
	Rev.	Identification	
	Del.		
Bromhexine Hydrochloride （ブロムヘキシン塩酸塩）	Add.		2873
	Rev.	Purity	
	Del.		
Butropium Bromide （ブトロピウム臭化物）	Add.		2875
	Rev.	Assay	
	Del.		
Butyl Parahydroxybenzoate （パラオキシ安息香酸ブチル）	Add.		2875
	Rev.	International Harmonization, Purity, Assay	
	Del.		
Croscarmellose Sodium （クロスカルメロースナトリウム）	Add.		2877
	Rev.	Identification, Purity, Residue on ignition, Containers and storage	
	Del.		
Cefoperazone Sodium and Sulbactam Sodium for Injection （注射用セフォペラゾンナトリウム・スルバクタムナトリウム）	Add.		2878
	Rev.	Uniformity of dosage units	
	Del.		
Powdered Cellulose （粉末セルロース）	Add.		2878
	Rev.	International Harmonization, Identification, Purity	
	Del.		
Enviomycin Sulfate （エンビオマイシン硫酸塩）	Add.		2879
	Rev.	Content ratio of the active principle	
	Del.		
Epoetin Beta (Genetical Recombination) （エポエチン　ベータ（遺伝子組換え））	Add.		2879
	Rev.	Identification	
	Del.		
Ethanol （エタノール）	Add.		2880
	Rev.	International Harmonization, Containers and storage, Shelf life	
	Del.		
Anhydrous Ethanol （無水エタノール）	Add.		2880
	Rev.	International Harmonization, Containers and storage, Shelf life	
	Del.		

Ethyl Parahydroxybenzoate （パラオキシ安息香酸エチル）	Add.		2880
	Rev.	International Harmonization, Purity, Assay	
	Del.		
Formoterol Fumarate Hydrate （ホルモテロールフマル酸塩水和物）	Add.	Purity (Diastereomer), Others (Related substance)	2881
	Rev.	Chemical name, Purity (Related substances),	
	Del.		
Glyceryl Monostearate （モノステアリン酸グリセリン）	Add.		2883
	Rev.		
	Del.	Identification (1)	
Hypromellose Phthalate （ヒプロメロースフタル酸エステル）	Add.		2883
	Rev.	International Harmonization, Description, Viscosity, Purity	
	Del.		
Imipenem and Cilastatin Sodium for Injection （注射用イミペネム・シラスタチンナトリウム）	Add.		2884
	Rev.	Uniformity of dosage units	
	Del.		
Insulin Human (Genetical Recombination) （インスリン　ヒト（遺伝子組換え））	Add.		2884
	Rev.	Identification, Assay	
	Del.		
Insulin Human (Genetical Recombination) Injection （インスリン　ヒト（遺伝子組換え）注射液）	Add.		2885
	Rev.	Assay	
	Del.		
Isophane Insulin Human (Genetical Recombination) Injectable Aqueous Suspension （イソフェンインスリン　ヒト（遺伝子組換え）水性懸濁注射液）	Add.		2885
	Rev.	Purity, Assay	
	Del.		
Biphasic Isophane Insulin Human (Genetical Recombination) Injectable Aqueous Suspension （二相性イソフェンインスリン　ヒト（遺伝子組換え）水性懸濁注射液）	Add.		2886
	Rev.	Assay	
	Del.		
Magnesium Stearate （ステアリン酸マグネシウム）	Add.		2886
	Rev.	International Harmonization, Identification, Purity, Relative content of stearic acid and palmitic acid, Assay	
	Del.		
D-Mannitol （D-マンニトール）	Add.		2888
	Rev.	International Harmonization, Purity, Assay	
	Del.		
dl-Menthol （dl-メントール）	Add.		2889
	Rev.		
	Del.	Storage	
l-Menthol （l-メントール）	Add.		2890
	Rev.		
	Del.	Storage	
Methyl Parahydroxybenzoate （パラオキシ安息香酸メチル）	Add.		2890
	Rev.	International Harmonization, Purity, Assay	
	Del.		
White Petrolatum （白色ワセリン）	Add.	International Harmonization, Identification (IR), Purity (Polycyclic aromatic hydrocarbons)	2892
	Rev.	Origin/limits of content, Description, Melting point, Purity, Containers and storage	
	Del.	Purity (Sulfur compound, Organic acids, Fats and fatty oils or resins	

Addenda 11

Title	Section		Page
Yellow Petrolatum （黄色ワセリン）	Add.	International Harmonization, Identification (IR), Purity (Polycyclic aromatic hydrocarbons)	2893
	Rev.	Origin/limits of content, Description, Melting point, Purity, Containers and storage	
	Del.	Purity (Sulfur compound, Organic acids, Fats and fatty oils or resins	
Polysorbate 80 （ポリソルベート80）	Add.		2894
	Rev.	International Harmonization, Composition of fatty acids, Acid value, Purity, Residue on ignition	
	Del.		
Propyl Parahydroxybenzoate （パラオキシ安息香酸プロピル）	Add.		2896
	Rev.	International Harmonization, Purity, Assay	
	Del.		
Sarpogrelate Hydrochloride Fine Granules （サルポグレラート塩酸塩細粒）	Add.		2898
	Rev.	Uniformity of dosage units, Assay	
	Del.		
Sodium Chloride （塩化ナトリウム）	Add.		2898
	Rev.	Identification	
	Del.		
Spectinomycin Hydrochloride for Injection （注射用スペクチノマイシン塩酸塩）	Add.		2899
	Rev.	Uniformity of dosage units	
	Del.		
Wheat Starch （コムギデンプン）	Add.		2899
	Rev.	Purity	
	Del.		
Stearic Acid （ステアリン酸）	Add.		2899
	Rev	Congealing point	
	Del.		
Voglibose Tablets （ボグリボース錠）	Add.		2905
	Rev	Identification	
	Del.		

Crude Drugs

Title (Japanese title)	Section		Page
Achyranthes Root （ゴシツ）	Add.		2907
	Rev.	Identification	
	Del.		
Akebia Stem （モクツウ）	Add.		2907
	Rev.	Origin/limits of content	
	Del.		
Apricot Kernel （キョウニン）	Add.		2907
	Rev.	Assay	
	Del.		
Artemisia Capillaris Flower （インチンコウ）	Add.		2907
	Rev.	Description	
	Del.		
Artemisia Leaf （ガイヨウ）	Add.		2907
	Rev.	Description	
	Del.		

12 Addenda

Bearberry Leaf	Add.		
	Rev.	Description, Assay	2908
（ウワウルシ）	Del.		
Bitter Cardamon	Add.	Identification	
	Rev.		2908
（ヤクチ）	Del.		
Burdock Fruit	Add.		
	Rev.	Description	2908
（ゴボウシ）	Del.		
Cardamon	Add.		
	Rev.	Japanese commonly used name	2908
（ショウズク）	Del.		
Cimicifuga Rhizome	Add.		
	Rev.	Purity	2908
（ショウマ）	Del.		
Clove	Add.		
	Rev.	Origin/limits of content	2909
（チョウジ）	Del.		
Clove Oil	Add.		
	Rev.	Origin/limits of content	2909
（チョウジ油）	Del.		
Cnidium Monnieri Fruit	Add.		
	Rev.	Latin name	2909
（ジャショウシ）	Del.		
Cornus Fruit	Add.		
	Rev.	Assay	2909
（サンシュユ）	Del.		
Corydalis Tuber	Add.		
	Rev.	Assay	2909
（エンゴサク）	Del.		
Powdered Corydalis Tuber	Add.		
	Rev.	Assay	2910
（エンゴサク末）	Del.		
Gardenia Fruit	Add.		
	Rev.	Origin/limits of content	2910
（サンシシ）	Del.		
Ginger	Add.		
	Rev.	Assay	2910
（ショウキョウ）	Del.		
Powdered Ginger	Add.		
	Rev.	Assay	2911
（ショウキョウ末）	Del.		
Glehnia Root and Rhizome	Add.		
	Rev.	Origin/limits of content	2911
（ハマボウフウ）	Del.		
Goshajinkigan Extract	Add.		
	Rev.	Assay	2911
（牛車腎気丸エキス）	Del.		
Goshuyuto Extract	Add.		
	Rev.	Assay	2912
（呉茱萸湯エキス）	Del.		
Hachimijiogan Extract	Add.		
	Rev.	Assay	2912
（八味地黄丸エキス）	Del.		
Hangekobokuto Extract	Add.		
	Rev.	Assay	2913
（半夏厚朴湯エキス）	Del.		

	Add.		
Keishibukuryogan Extract	Rev.	Assay	2913
（桂枝茯苓丸エキス）	Del.		
	Add.		
Leonurus Herb	Rev.	Description	2913
（ヤクモソウ）	Del.		
	Add.		
Magnolia Bark	Rev.	Origin/limits of content	2914
（コウボク）	Del.		
	Add.		
Maoto Extract	Rev.	Assay	2914
（麻黄湯エキス）	Del.		
	Add.		
Mukoi-Daikenchuto Extract	Rev.	Assay	2914
（無コウイ大建中湯エキス）	Del.		
	Add.		
Nutmeg	Rev.	Japanese commonly used name	2915
（ニクズク）	Del.		
	Add.		
Peach Kernel	Rev.	Assay	2915
（トウニン）	Del.		
	Add.		
Powdered Peach Kernel	Rev.	Assay	2915
（トウニン末）	Del.		
	Add.	Identification	
Picrasma Wood	Rev.		2915
（ニガキ）	Del.		
	Add.	Identification	
Powdered Picrasma Wood	Rev.		2916
（ニガキ末）	Del.		
	Add.		
Plantago Herb	Rev.	Description	2916
（シャゼンソウ）	Del.		
	Add.		
Prepared Glycyrrhiza	Rev.	Description	2916
（シャカンゾウ）	Del.		
	Add.		
Processed Ginger	Rev.	Assay	2916
（カンキョウ）	Del.		
	Add.		
Senna Leaf	Rev.	Description, Identification	2920
（センナ）	Del.		
	Add.		
Powdered Senna Leaf	Rev.	Identification	2920
（センナ末）	Del.		
	Add.		
Shimbuto Extract	Rev.	Assay	2920
（真武湯エキス）	Del.		
	Add.		
Sinomenium Stem and Rhizome	Rev.	Origin/limits of content	2920
（ボウイ）	Del.		
	Add.		
Tokakujokito Extract	Rev.	Assay	2921
（桃核承気湯エキス）	Del.		

14 Addenda

	Add.		
Turmeric	Rev.	Description	2921
（ウコン）	Del.		
Uncaria Hook	Add.		
	Rev.	Assay	2921
（チョウトウコウ）	Del.		

PMRJ Reference Standards Ordering Information for Foreign Users

Pharmaceutical and Medical Device Regulatory Science Society of Japan (PMRJ) has been registered by the Minister of Health, Labour and Welfare as an organization that produces and distributes Japanese Pharmacopoeia (JP) Reference Standards and other compendial reference standards of Japan. Those reference standards serve as national standards in the qualitative and quantitative evaluation of the quality of pharmaceuticals and other products, and thereby play a critical role by providing the basis for guaranteeing the reliability and objectivity of test results. PMRJ engages in its reference standard work with full awareness of its great responsibility to produce and distribute such reference standards with assurance of their quality.

Steps for Ordering PMRJ Reference Standards

1. Visit PMRJ Reference Standards Online Store < https://www.pmrj-ec.jp/aec/user/?lang=en >.
2. Please fill in the required items of the quotation form.
3. Upon receipt of your inquiry, we will send you our proforma invoice.
4. Please send us your purchase order subject to your acceptance of our Terms and Conditions.
5. Upon receipt of your purchase order, we will send you our order confirmation and invoice necessary for your remittance.
6. Please remit us the full invoice amount as soon as you receive our order confirmation and Invoice.
   Notes:
   (1) You need to bear all transaction fees, namely not only bank charges originating from the payment by wire transfer outside Japan but also bank charges incurred in Japan for credit of the full invoice amount to our designated account.
   (2) Please instruct your bank to select "OUR" or "DEBT" in the column with 71A "DETAILS OF CHARGES" of the application for remittance so that the full invoice amount can be credited with our designated account.
7. After our receipt of the full invoice amount, we will ship out your order subject to our securing the necessary cargo space.
   Notes:
   (1) The risk of loss for all reference standards purchased by Customer shall pass to the Customer at the point of delivery to the carrier.

For further information;

Please visit PMRJ Pharmaceutical Reference Standards Center website <https://www.pmrj-rs.jp/en> or contact Customer Service at jprslab-std@pmrj.jp

Pharmaceutical and Medical Device Regulatory Science Society of Japan
Pharmaceutical Reference Standards Center

2-1-2, Hiranomachi, Chuo-ku, Osaka 541-0046, Japan
Email: jprslab-std@pmrj.jp   Tel: +81-6-6221-3444

Pharmaceutical Reference Standards Center   https://www.pmrj-rs.jp/en
PMRJ Reference Standards Online Store   https://www.pmrj-ec.jp/aec/user/?lang=en

Revised April 2021

16   *Addenda*

Pharmaceutical and Medical Device Regulatory Science Society of Japan (PMRJ)   Rev. June 1, 2023

PMRJ Reference Standards Catalog

Please visit PMRJ Pharmaceutical Reference Standards Center website <https://www.pmrj-rs.jp/en> to check the ordering instruction.
In addition, please find a leaflet of each reference standard on the webpage for the reference standard prior to use.

1. Japanese Pharmacopoeia Reference Standards

Product Code	Reference Standard (RS)	Unit Quantity	Storage Temperature	Shipping Conditions	Price
1005000021	Acetaminophen RS	300 mg	≤25°C	A	JPY 18,334
1169000021	Acetanilide for Apparatus Suitability RS	200 mg	≤25°C	A	JPY 10,476
1170000021	Acetophenetidine for Apparatus Suitability RS	200 mg	≤25°C	A	JPY 10,476
1001500021	Aciclovir RS	100 mg	≤25°C	A	JPY 15,715
1006000021	Adrenaline Bitartrate for Purity RS	50 mg	≤8°C	AU	JPY 13,776
1011500021	Alendronate Sodium RS	150 mg	≤25°C	A	JPY 24,096
1011000021	Alprostadil RS	10 mg	≤5°C	R	JPY 66,838
7000040021	Amikacin Sulfate RS	100 mg	−20 – −30°C	F	JPY 40,028
1114000021	p-Aminobenzoyl Glutamic Acid for Purity RS	500 mg	≤25°C	A	JPY 29,582
1008000021	Amitriptyline Hydrochloride RS	100 mg	≤25°C	AU	JPY 21,359
1012000021	Amlexanox RS	300 mg	≤8°C	A	JPY 38,762
1010000021	Amlodipine Besilate RS	150 mg	≤25°C	A	JPY 66,250
7000110021	Ampicillin RS	100 mg	−20 – −30°C	F	JPY 40,129
1007500021	Anastrozole RS	300 mg	≤8°C	AU	JPY 27,230
1106000021	Anhydrous Lactose for Identification RS	50 mg	≤25°C	A	JPY 12,815
1002000021	Ascorbic Acid RS	1 g	≤25°C	A	JPY 21,145
1003000021	Aspirin RS	300 mg	≤25°C	A	JPY 16,019
1005800021	Atorvastatin Calcium RS	150 mg	≤8°C	A	JPY 17,809
1007000021	Atropine Sulfate RS	250 mg	≤25°C	AU	JPY 21,359
1034700021	Auranofin RS	100 mg	≤8°C	AU	JPY 41,905
1001000021	Azathioprine RS	600 mg	≤25°C	A	JPY 34,175
7000020021	Azithromycin RS	100 mg	−20 – −30°C	F	JPY 40,129
1112000021	Baclofen RS	800 mg	≤8°C	AU	JPY 34,175
1111000021	Baicalin RS	30 mg	≤8°C	A	JPY 30,381
1145000021	Beclometasone Dipropionate RS	100 mg	≤25°C	A	JPY 20,638
1151000021	Berberine Chloride RS	30 mg	≤25°C	A	JPY 33,943
1146000021	Betamethasone RS	100 mg	≤25°C	A	JPY 17,915
1148000021	Betamethasone Sodium Phosphate RS	100 mg	≤8°C	A	JPY 18,647
1147000021	Betamethasone Valerate RS	100 mg	≤25°C	AU	JPY 20,428
1114900021	Bicalutamide RS	100 mg	≤8°C	AU	JPY 13,400
1115000021	Bisacodyl RS	100 mg	≤25°C	A	JPY 21,359
1143300021	Bromfenac Sodium RS	150 mg	≤8°C	AU	JPY 29,119
1128200021	Budesonide RS	120 mg	≤8°C	RU	JPY 38,460
1114200021	Butyl Parahydroxybenzoate RS	200 mg	≤8°C	A	JPY 37,715
1036500021	Cabergoline RS	100 mg	−20 – −30°C	F	JPY 155,740
1035000021	Caffeine RS	300 mg	≤25°C	AU	JPY 26,699
1171000021	Caffeine for Apparatus Suitability RS	200 mg	≤25°C	AU	JPY 10,476
1039500021	Calcitonin Salmon RS	See leaflet	≤−20°C	F	JPY 74,381
1154000021	Calcium Folinate RS	250 mg	≤25°C	A	JPY 21,359
1069000021	Calcium Oxalate Monohydrate for Calibration of Apparatus RS	100 mg	≤25°C	A	JPY 23,047
1114600021	Calcium Pantothenate RS	1.1 g	≤8°C	A	JPY 41,905
1037000021	Camostat Mesilate RS	200 mg	≤25°C	A	JPY 26,699
1042000021	d-Camphor RS	300 mg	≤25°C	AU	JPY 18,019
1043000021	dl-Camphor RS	300 mg	≤25°C	AU	JPY 16,762
1040000021	Carbidopa RS	200 mg	≤25°C	A	JPY 34,175
1040500021	Carboplatin RS	100 mg	≤8°C	AU	JPY 28,285
1039800021	L-Carnosine RS	100 mg	≤8°C	A	JPY 28,182

Addenda 17

 Pharmaceutical and Medical Device Regulatory Science Society of Japan (PMRJ)

Rev. June 1, 2023

Product Code	Reference Standard (RS)	Unit Quantity	Storage Temperature	Shipping Conditions	Price
7000370021	Cefaclor RS	100 mg	−20 − −30°C	F	JPY 40,129
7000410021	Cefalexin RS	100 mg	−20 − −30°C	F	JPY 40,129
7000390021	Cefazolin RS	100 mg	−20 − −30°C	F	JPY 40,129
7000440021	Cefepime Dihydrochloride RS	100 mg	−20 − −30°C	F	JPY 40,129
7000630021	Cefmetazole RS	100 mg	−20 − −30°C	F	JPY 40,129
7000460021	Cefotiam Hydrochloride RS	100 mg	−20 − −30°C	F	JPY 40,129
7000590021	Ceftriaxone Sodium RS	100 mg	−20 − −30°C	F	JPY 40,129
1076700021	Celecoxib RS	320 mg	≤8°C	AU	JPY 16,600
1076000021	Cellacefate for Identification RS	50 mg	≤25°C	A	JPY 12,815
1076500021	Microcrystalline Cellulose for Identification RS	50 mg	≤8°C	A	JPY 12,579
1075300021	Cetotiamine Hydrochloride RS	150 mg	≤8°C	A	JPY 41,905
1052000021	Chlordiazepoxide RS	500 mg	≤25°C	N/A	JPY 34,175
1054000021	Chlormadinone Acetate RS	100 mg	≤25°C	A	JPY 16,657
1053000021	Chlorpheniramine Maleate RS	400 mg	≤25°C	AU	JPY 26,699
1059000021	Cholecalciferol RS	100 mg	≤8°C	RU	JPY 21,476
1063000021	Ciclosporin RS	100 mg	≤25°C	A	JPY 26,699
1070600021	Cilnidipine RS	200 mg	≤8°C	A	JPY 40,679
1071000021	Cilostazol RS	450 mg	≤25°C	A	JPY 26,191
1068520021	Ciprofloxacin RS	250 mg	≤8°C	A	JPY 27,062
1066000021	Cisplatin RS	150 mg	≤8°C	AU	JPY 26,191
1066600021	Citicoline RS	150 mg	≤8°C	A	JPY 28,509
7000220021	Clarithromycin RS	100 mg	−20 − −30°C	F	JPY 40,129
7000240021	Clindamycin Phosphate RS	100 mg	−20 − −30°C	F	JPY 40,129
1050000021	Clobetasol Propionate RS	50 mg	≤25°C	A	JPY 18,857
1049000021	Clofibrate RS	800 mg	≤25°C	A	JPY 26,699
1051000021	Clomifene Citrate RS	200 mg	≤25°C	A	JPY 21,359
1048900021	Clopidogrel Sulfate RS	200 mg	≤8°C	AU	JPY 35,466
1058000021	Cortisone Acetate RS	100 mg	≤25°C	A	JPY 15,271
1060000021	Cyanocobalamin RS	200 mg	≤8°C	A	JPY 14,204
1078600021	Danazol RS	100 mg	≤25°C	A	JPY 19,905
1086000021	Deferoxamine Mesilate RS	200 mg	≤25°C	A	JPY 21,359
1085000021	Deslanoside RS	100 mg	≤25°C	AU	JPY 20,638
1083000021	Dexamethasone RS	100 mg	≤25°C	A	JPY 18,124
1061000021	Diethylcarbamazine Citrate RS	200 mg	≤25°C	AU	JPY 26,699
1068530021	Diflorasone Diacetate RS	100 mg	≤8°C	A	JPY 41,026
1068500021	Diflucortolone Valerate RS	100 mg	≤25°C	A	JPY 18,753
1065000021	Digoxin RS	50 mg	≤25°C	AU	JPY 19,800
1068000021	Dihydroergotoxine Mesilate RS	100 mg	≤25°C	A	JPY 36,876
1091000021	Dobutamine Hydrochloride RS	300 mg	≤25°C	A	JPY 26,699
1090300021	Docetaxel RS	370 mg	≤8°C	A	JPY 74,528
1090500021	Donepezil Hydrochloride RS	450 mg	≤8°C	AU	JPY 15,715
7000700021	Doripenem RS	150 mg	−20 − −30°C	F	JPY 146,484
1097800021	Dorzolamide Hydrochloride RS	80 mg	≤8°C	A	JPY 62,857
1086800021	Doxazosin Mesilate RS	200 mg	≤25°C	A	JPY 18,857
7000680021	Doxorubicin Hydrochloride RS	100 mg	−20 − −30°C	F	JPY 35,138
1026000021	Edrophonium Chloride RS	200 mg	≤25°C	A	JPY 26,699
1029000021	Elcatonin RS	See leaflet	≤−20°C	F	JPY 46,515
1027000021	Enalapril Maleate RS	200 mg	≤25°C	A	JPY 22,000
1032000021	Endotoxin RS	See leaflet	≤8°C	A	JPY 23,047
1031800021	Entacapone RS	210 mg	≤8°C	A	JPY 74,301
1031830021	Entacapone Related Substance A for System Suitability RS	10 mg	≤8°C	A	JPY 14,025
1027800021	Epalrestat RS	280 mg	≤8°C	A	JPY 47,143
7000170021	Epirubicin Hydrochloride RS	100 mg	−20 − −30°C	F	JPY 40,129
1028000021	Epitiostanol RS	100 mg	≤8°C	R	JPY 13,724
1028100021	Eplerenone RS	150 mg	≤8°C	A	JPY 66,250
1028200021	Epoetin Alfa RS	0.05 mL	−80°C	F	JPY 56,572

18   *Addenda*

 PMRJ   Pharmaceutical and Medical Device Regulatory Science Society of Japan (PMRJ)   Rev. June 1, 2023

Product Code	Reference Standard (RS)	Unit Quantity	Storage Temperature	Shipping Conditions	Price
1028250021	Epoetin Beta RS	0.25 mL	−80°C	F	JPY 53,428
1030000021	Ergocalciferol RS	100 mg	≤8°C	RU	JPY 21,791
1031000021	Ergometrine Maleate RS	50 mg	≤8°C	N/A	JPY 16,339
1028700021	Eribulin Mesilate RS	50 mg	−80°C	FU	JPY 414,360
1028730021	Eribulin Mesilate Related Substance C for System Suitability RS	5 mg	−80°C	F	JPY 223,150
1021000021	Estradiol Benzoate RS	50 mg	≤25°C	A	JPY 15,593
1022000021	Estriol RS	100 mg	≤25°C	A	JPY 15,296
1024000021	Ethenzamide RS	300 mg	≤25°C	A	JPY 17,496
1023000021	Ethinylestradiol RS	100 mg	≤25°C	AU	JPY 21,359
1009000021	Ethyl Aminobenzoate RS	250 mg	≤25°C	AU	JPY 21,359
1013000021	Ethyl Icosapentate RS	240 mg	−20 − −30°C	F	JPY 68,096
1188800021	Ethyl Loflazepate RS	100 mg	≤8°C	N/A	JPY 86,160
1114100021	Ethyl Parahydroxybenzoate RS	200 mg	≤8°C	A	JPY 37,715
1025000021	Etoposide RS	100 mg	≤8°C	A	JPY 26,191
1127900021	Fenofibrate RS	200 mg	≤8°C	A	JPY 38,880
1127800021	Fexofenadine Hydrochloride RS	100 mg	≤25°C	A	JPY 22,000
1127500021	Filgrastim RS	1 mL	−80°C	F	JPY 110,000
1135400021	Fludrocortisone Acetate RS	100 mg	≤8°C	A	JPY 60,762
1133000021	Fluocinolone Acetonide RS	50 mg	≤25°C	A	JPY 20,009
1132000021	Fluocinonide RS	100 mg	≤25°C	AU	JPY 21,791
1134000021	Fluorometholone RS	100 mg	≤25°C	A	JPY 20,638
1135200021	Flutamide RS	150 mg	≤8°C	AU	JPY 32,476
1135600021	Fluvoxamine Maleate RS	350 mg	≤25°C	AU	JPY 29,334
1176000021	Folic Acid RS	500 mg	≤25°C	A	JPY 18,262
7000830021	Fradiomycin Sulfate RS	200 mg	−20 − −30°C	F	JPY 38,602
1141000021	Furosemide RS	200 mg	≤25°C	A	JPY 26,191
1135000021	Fursultiamine Hydrochloride RS	200 mg	≤25°C	A	JPY 26,699
1036000021	Gabexate Mesilate RS	200 mg	≤25°C	A	JPY 26,699
1034900021	Gatifloxacin RS	500 mg	≤8°C	A	JPY 66,250
1055500021	Gefarnate RS	170 mg	≤8°C	A	JPY 78,572
1055700021	Gefitinib RS	160 mg	≤8°C	AU	JPY 103,200
1045000021	Ginsenoside Rb$_1$ RS	15 mg	−20 − −30°C	F	JPY 55,524
1046000021	Ginsenoside Rg$_1$ RS	15 mg	−20 − −30°C	F	JPY 58,000
1044000021	Gitoxin for Purity RS	10 mg	≤25°C	AU	JPY 20,115
1048200021	Glimepiride RS	200 mg	≤25°C	A	JPY 48,191
1048400021	Glucagon RS	See leaflet	−20 − −30°C	F	JPY 45,350
1128300021	Glucose RS	1 g	≤8°C	A	JPY 12,151
1048500021	D-Glucuronolactone RS	100 mg	≤8°C	A	JPY 10,476
1048000021	Glycyrrhizic Acid RS	30 mg	≤8°C	A	JPY 37,400
1057000021	Gonadorelin Acetate RS	50 mg	−20 − −30°C	F	JPY 68,096
1047000021	Guaifenesin RS	200 mg	≤25°C	A	JPY 26,191
1149000021	Heparin Sodium RS	See leaflet	≤8°C	A	JPY 36,562
1149010021	Heparin Sodium for Identification RS	100 mg	≤8°C	A	JPY 18,857
1056000021	High-molecular Mass Urokinase RS	See leaflet	−20 − −30°C	F	JPY 26,191
1118000021	Human Chorionic Gonadotrophin RS	See leaflet	≤−20°C	F	JPY 42,324
1117000021	Human Menopausal Gonadotrophin RS	See leaflet	≤−20°C	F	JPY 47,457
1119000021	Hydrochlorothiazide RS	100 mg	≤25°C	A	JPY 16,972
1120000021	Hydrocortisone RS	100 mg	≤25°C	A	JPY 17,809
1122000021	Hydrocortisone Acetate RS	100 mg	≤8°C	A	JPY 18,019
1123000021	Hydrocortisone Sodium Phosphate RS	100 mg	≤8°C	A	JPY 18,228
1121000021	Hydrocortisone Succinate RS	100 mg	≤25°C	A	JPY 19,276
1115600021	Hydroxyethylcellulose for Identification RS	50 mg	≤8°C	A	JPY 23,019
1015000021	Idoxuridine RS	100 mg	≤25°C	A	JPY 16,019
1016000021	Imipramine Hydrochloride RS	200 mg	≤25°C	A	JPY 26,699
1017500021	Indapamide RS	200 mg	≤8°C	A	JPY 63,905
1019000021	Indometacin RS	350 mg	≤25°C	AU	JPY 26,699
1017010021	Insulin Aspart RS	See leaflet	−20 − −30°C	F	JPY 52,291

Pharmaceutical and Medical Device Regulatory Science Society of Japan (PMRJ)   Rev. June 1, 2023

Product Code	Reference Standard (RS)	Unit Quantity	Storage Temperature	Shipping Conditions	Price
1017020021	Insulin Glargine RS	See leaflet	≤−20°C	F	JPY 78,500
1116000021	Insulin Human RS	See leaflet	−20 − −30°C	F	JPY 33,943
1018000021	Interleukin-2 RS	See leaflet	−80°C	F	JPY 26,191
1015500021	Ipriflavone RS	100 mg	≤25°C	A	JPY 34,572
1014000021	Isoflurane RS	18 mL	≤8°C	R	JPY 40,857
1014300021	Isomalt RS	1.5 g	≤8°C	A	JPY 54,165
1038000021	Kallidinogenase RS	See leaflet	−20 − −30°C	F	JPY 17,705
1105000021	Lactose for Identification RS	50 mg	≤25°C	A	JPY 10,680
1177000021	Lactulose RS	1.5 g	≤25°C	A	JPY 26,699
1179100021	Lanoconazole RS	190 mg	≤8°C	A	JPY 117,252
1179600021	Lansoprazole RS	200 mg	≤8°C	A	JPY 25,229
1186200021	Lenograstim RS	1 mL	−80°C	F	JPY 74,381
1183100021	Leuprorelin Acetate RS	300 mg	−20 − −30°C	F	JPY 257,250
1183000021	Limaprost RS	10 mg	−20 − −30°C	FU	JPY 68,096
1188500021	Losartan Potassium RS	100 mg	≤25°C	A	JPY 19,905
1082000021	Low-molecular Mass Heparin RS	See leaflet	≤8°C	R	JPY 36,143
1188000021	Loxoprofen RS	200 mg	≤8°C	A	JPY 22,427
1180000021	Lysozyme RS	500 mg	≤8°C	A	JPY 34,572
1156000021	Maltose RS	300 mg	≤25°C	A	JPY 34,175
1155000021	Manidipine Hydrochloride RS	250 mg	≤8°C	AU	JPY 60,762
1156300021	D-Mannitol RS	4.6 g	≤8°C	A	JPY 36,240
1159000021	Mecobalamin RS	450 mg	≤25°C	A	JPY 26,191
1167500021	Medroxyprogesterone Acetate RS	150 mg	≤8°C	A	JPY 58,147
1168000021	Menatetrenone RS	300 mg	≤8°C	R	JPY 26,191
7000960021	Meropenem RS	100 mg	−20 − −30°C	F	JPY 40,129
1160000021	Mestranol RS	100 mg	≤25°C	A	JPY 16,134
1167000021	Methotrexate RS	800 mg	≤8°C	AU	JPY 20,825
1166000021	Methoxsalen RS	200 mg	≤25°C	A	JPY 16,447
1164000021	Methyldopa RS	400 mg	≤25°C	A	JPY 26,699
1161000021	Methylergometrine Maleate RS	50 mg	≤25°C	A	JPY 19,485
1114300021	Methyl Parahydroxybenzoate RS	200 mg	≤8°C	AU	JPY 37,715
1165000021	Methylprednisolone Succinate RS	100 mg	≤25°C	A	JPY 26,191
1163000021	Methyltestosterone RS	100 mg	≤25°C	A	JPY 21,359
1162000021	Metildigoxin RS	50 mg	≤25°C	AU	JPY 16,343
1158000021	Mexiletine Hydrochloride RS	100 mg	≤25°C	AU	JPY 16,019
1156700021	Miglitol RS	200 mg	≤8°C	A	JPY 42,422
7000940021	Minocycline Hydrochloride RS	100 mg	−20 − −30°C	F	JPY 40,129
1157300021	Mitiglinide Calcium RS	360 mg	≤8°C	A	JPY 99,254
1157000021	Mizoribine RS	300 mg	≤8°C	A	JPY 49,238
1168460021	Montelukast for System Suitability RS	5 mg	≤8°C	A	JPY 27,062
1168400021	Montelukast Dicyclohexylamine RS	120 mg	≤8°C	A	JPY 22,428
1168490021	Montelukast Racemate for System Suitability RS	5 mg	≤8°C	A	JPY 32,094
1168430021	Montelukast Sodium for Identification RS	50 mg	≤8°C	A	JPY 18,415
1101000021	Nabumetone RS	200 mg	≤8°C	A	JPY 56,572
1100500021	Nateglinide RS	170 mg	≤25°C	A	JPY 57,619
1108000021	Neostigmine Methylsulfate RS	100 mg	≤25°C	A	JPY 26,191
1103000021	Nicotinamide RS	500 mg	≤25°C	A	JPY 18,262
1102000021	Nicotinic Acid RS	500 mg	≤25°C	A	JPY 16,767
1107000021	Nilvadipine RS	250 mg	≤8°C	A	JPY 31,428
1104000021	Nizatidine RS	150 mg	≤25°C	A	JPY 48,191
1109000021	Noradrenaline Bitartrate RS	50 mg	≤8°C	AU	JPY 15,271
1110000021	Norgestrel RS	350 mg	≤25°C	A	JPY 34,175
1034800021	Olmesartan Medoxomil RS	200 mg	≤8°C	A	JPY 47,029
1039000021	Over-sulfated Chondroitin Sulfate for System Suitability RS	See leaflet	≤8°C	A	JPY 11,524
1033000021	Oxytocin RS	See leaflet	−20 − −30°C	F	JPY 10,476
1034000021	Ozagrel Sodium RS	100 mg	≤25°C	A	JPY 18,857

Addenda 19

20 *Addenda*

 Pharmaceutical and Medical Device Regulatory Science Society of Japan (PMRJ)   Rev. June 1, 2023

Product Code	Reference Standard (RS)	Unit Quantity	Storage Temperature	Shipping Conditions	Price
1144000021	Paeoniflorin RS	20 mg	≤8°C	A	JPY 35,515
1114500021	Paroxetine Hydrochloride RS	200 mg	≤8°C	AU	JPY 31,742
1112800021	Pazufloxacin Mesilate RS	150 mg	≤8°C	A	JPY 111,365
1149200021	Pemirolast Potassium RS	200 mg	≤25°C	A	JPY 41,905
1152000021	Pentobarbital RS	100 mg	≤25°C	N/A	JPY 26,191
1150000021	Perphenazine RS	100 mg	≤25°C	A	JPY 21,359
1127000021	Phytonadione RS	200 mg	≤8°C	A	JPY 66,000
1114800021	Pioglitazone Hydrochloride RS	160 mg	≤8°C	AU	JPY 27,238
7000820021	Piperacillin RS	100 mg	−20 − −30°C	F	JPY 40,129
1115500021	Pitavastatin Methylbenzylamine RS	100 mg	≤8°C	A	JPY 76,338
1070000021	Potassium Sucrose Octasulfate RS	1 g	−20 − −30°C	F	JPY 18,857
1153000021	Povidone for Identification RS	50 mg	≤8°C	A	JPY 14,951
1129400021	Pranlukast RS	100 mg	≤8°C	A	JPY 72,465
1129000021	Pravastatin 1,1,3,3-Tetramethylbutylammonium RS	200 mg	−20 − −30°C	F	JPY 26,191
1128600021	Prazosin Hydrochloride RS	100 mg	≤25°C	A	JPY 28,285
1136000021	Prednisolone RS	100 mg	≤25°C	A	JPY 17,496
1138000021	Prednisolone Acetate RS	100 mg	≤25°C	A	JPY 17,705
1137000021	Prednisolone Succinate RS	150 mg	≤25°C	A	JPY 21,359
1130000021	Primidone RS	300 mg	≤25°C	A	JPY 17,600
1143000021	Probenecid RS	500 mg	≤25°C	A	JPY 34,175
1142600021	Probucol RS	300 mg	≤25°C	A	JPY 35,619
1139000021	Prochlorperazine Maleate RS	500 mg	≤25°C	A	JPY 34,175
1140000021	Progesterone RS	150 mg	≤25°C	A	JPY 26,191
1142400021	Propiverine Hydrochloride RS	200 mg	≤25°C	A	JPY 26,191
1114250021	Propyl Parahydroxybenzoate RS	200 mg	≤8°C	A	JPY 37,715
1128000021	Puerarin RS	20 mg	≤8°C	A	JPY 36,457
1123800021	Pyridoxal Phosphate RS	200 mg	≤8°C	A	JPY 50,651
1124000021	Pyridoxine Hydrochloride RS	200 mg	≤25°C	A	JPY 25,631
1047200021	Quetiapine Fumarate RS	170 mg	≤8°C	AU	JPY 27,238
1179200021	Rabeprazole Sodium RS	1.35 g	≤8°C	A	JPY 48,191
1179000021	Ranitidine Hydrochloride RS	100 mg	≤25°C	A	JPY 26,191
1184000021	Reserpine RS	50 mg	≤25°C	A	JPY 30,650
1059700021	Residual Solvents Class 1 RS	1.2 mL/ampoule (3 ampoules/box)	Room Temperature	A	JPY 54,898
1059800021	Residual Solvents Class 2A RS	1.2 mL/ampoule (3 ampoules/box)	Room Temperature	A	JPY 73,250
1059850021	Residual Solvents Class 2B RS	1.2 mL/ampoule (3 ampoules/box)	Room Temperature	A	JPY 59,462
1059860021	Residual Solvents Class 2C RS	1.2 mL/ampoule (3 ampoules/box)	Room Temperature	A	JPY 50,468
1059900021	Residual Solvents for System Suitability RS	1.2 mL/ampoule (3 ampoules/box)	Room Temperature	A	JPY 48,706
1185000021	Retinol Acetate RS	200 mg/capsule (5 capsules/bottle)	≤8°C	A	JPY 19,381
1186000021	Retinol Palmitate RS	200 mg/capsule (5 capsules/bottle)	≤8°C	A	JPY 18,334
1181700021	Ribavirin RS	150 mg	≤8°C	A	JPY 54,746
1182000021	Riboflavin RS	200 mg	≤25°C	A	JPY 20,612
1183500021	Rilmazafone Hydrochloride RS	200 mg	≤8°C	A	JPY 115,040
1179900021	Risedronic Acid RS	200 mg	≤25°C	A	JPY 45,047
1181000021	Ritodrine Hydrochloride RS	250 mg	≤25°C	A	JPY 66,250
1188600021	Rosuvastatin Calcium RS	400 mg	−20 − −30°C	FU	JPY 43,320
1187000021	Roxatidine Acetate Hydrochloride RS	300 mg	≤25°C	A	JPY 54,476
7000990021	Roxithromycin RS	100 mg	−20 − −30°C	FU	JPY 40,129
1041000021	Saccharated Pepsin RS	5 g	≤8°C	A	JPY 26,505
1059100021	Saccharin RS	100 mg	≤8°C	A	JPY 31,900
1059150021	Saccharin Sodium RS	100 mg	≤8°C	A	JPY 29,310
1059500021	Sarpogrelate Hydrochloride RS	350 mg	≤8°C	A	JPY 24,096
1073000021	Scopolamine Hydrobromide RS	200 mg	≤25°C	AU	JPY 26,699
1077000021	Sennoside A RS	20 mg	≤8°C	A	JPY 34,362

Pharmaceutical and Medical Device Regulatory Science Society of Japan (PMRJ) Rev. June 1, 2023

Product Code	Reference Standard (RS)	Unit Quantity	Storage Temperature	Shipping Conditions	Price
1078000021	Sennoside B RS	20 mg	≤8°C	A	JPY 33,105
1075500021	Sevoflurane RS	18 mL	≤8°C	RU	JPY 53,428
1071100021	Silodosin RS	250 mg	≤8°C	A	JPY 90,465
1071500021	Simvastatin RS	100 mg	−20 − −30°C	FU	JPY 26,191
1066500021	Sitagliptin Phosphate RS	130 mg	≤8°C	A	JPY 20,869
1066510021	Sitagliptin Phosphate for System Suitability RS	15 mg	≤8°C	A	JPY 29,191
1068600021	Sivelestat RS	120 mg	−20 − −30°C	F	JPY 95,092
1074000021	Spironolactone RS	200 mg	≤25°C	A	JPY 26,191
7000350021	Sulbactam RS	100 mg	−20 − −30°C	F	JPY 40,129
1075000021	Sulfadiazine Silver RS	300 mg	≤25°C	A	JPY 21,359
1172000021	Sulfanilamide for Apparatus Suitability RS	200 mg	≤25°C	A	JPY 10,476
1173000021	Sulfapyridine for Apparatus Suitability RS	200 mg	≤25°C	A	JPY 10,476
1072000021	Swertiamarin RS	20 mg	≤8°C	A	JPY 35,724
1078300021	Tacalcitol RS	4 mg	−20 − −30°C	FU	JPY 138,285
1078400021	Tacrolimus RS	100 mg	≤8°C	AU	JPY 30,381
7000650021	Tazobactam RS	100 mg	−20 − −30°C	F	JPY 40,129
1086400021	Temozolomide RS	100 mg	≤8°C	A	JPY 68,040
1086200021	Teprenone RS	170 mg	−20 − −30°C	F	JPY 29,334
1084000021	Testosterone Propionate RS	50 mg	≤25°C	A	JPY 19,591
1080000021	Thiamine Chloride Hydrochloride RS	1 g	≤25°C	A	JPY 20,292
1079000021	Thiamylal RS	100 mg	≤25°C	A	JPY 26,191
1100000021	Thrombin RS	30 mg	−20 − −30°C	F	JPY 45,991
1080500021	Timolol Maleate RS	120 mg	≤8°C	A	JPY 33,690
1087000021	Tocopherol RS	150 mg	≤8°C	A	JPY 22,628
1089000021	Tocopherol Acetate RS	150 mg	≤8°C	A	JPY 22,524
1090000021	Tocopherol Nicotinate RS	150 mg	≤8°C	R	JPY 24,724
1088000021	Tocopherol Succinate RS	150 mg	≤8°C	R	JPY 22,524
1099000021	Tolbutamide RS	200 mg	≤25°C	A	JPY 26,699
1098000021	Tolnaftate RS	200 mg	≤25°C	A	JPY 17,391
1090200021	Tosufloxacin Tosilate RS	350 mg	≤8°C	A	JPY 38,762
1093000021	Tranexamic Acid RS	200 mg	≤25°C	A	JPY 26,191
1099500021	Trehalose RS	600 mg	≤25°C	A	JPY 72,285
1094000021	Triamcinolone RS	100 mg	≤25°C	A	JPY 20,219
1095000021	Triamcinolone Acetonide RS	100 mg	≤25°C	A	JPY 20,219
1093500021	Triazolam RS	200 mg	≤8°C	N/A	JPY 33,890
1096000021	Trichlormethiazide RS	250 mg	≤25°C	A	JPY 47,143
1097000021	Trihexyphenidyl Hydrochloride RS	300 mg	≤25°C	A	JPY 34,175
1099600021	Troxipide RS	250 mg	≤25°C	A	JPY 28,285
1081000021	Tyrosine for Digestion Test RS	500 mg	≤25°C	A	JPY 13,563
1175000021	Ubidecarenone RS	150 mg	≤8°C	A	JPY 26,699
1020000021	Ulinastatin RS	See leaflet	−20 − −30°C	F	JPY 38,553
1114340021	Valaciclovir Hydrochloride RS	150 mg	≤8°C	A	JPY 41,179
1114400021	Valsartan RS	350 mg	≤8°C	A	JPY 22,000
7000800021	Vancomycin Hydrochloride RS	500 mg	−20 − −30°C	F	JPY 38,602
1174000021	Vanillin for Apparatus Suitability RS	200 mg	≤25°C	A	JPY 10,476
1113000021	Vasopressin RS	See leaflet	−20 − −30°C	F	JPY 57,619
1126000021	Vinblastine Sulfate RS	50 mg	−20 − −30°C	F	JPY 26,699
1125000021	Vincristine Sulfate RS	80 mg	−20 − −30°C	FU	JPY 67,047
1153700021	Voriconazole RS	200 mg	≤8°C	AU	JPY 66,250
1189000021	Warfarin Potassium RS	350 mg	≤25°C	AU	JPY 26,191
1067000021	Zidovudine RS	200 mg	≤25°C	A	JPY 40,857
1078200021	Zonisamide RS	200 mg	≤8°C	A	JPY 163,238

22   *Addenda*

PMRJ   Pharmaceutical and Medical Device Regulatory Science Society of Japan (PMRJ)   Rev. June 1, 2023

2. Official Non-pharmacopoeial Reference Standards*

* Former National Institute of Health Sciences Reference Standards

2-1. Reference Standards for Assays and Tests of Japanese Pharmaceutical Codex

Product Code	Reference Standard (RS)	Unit Quantity	Storage Temperature	Shipping Conditions	Price
2002000021	Estradiol RS	50 mg	≤25°C	AU	JPY 20,009
2003000021	Estrone RS	50 mg	≤25°C	A	JPY 20,009
2005000021	Fludroxycortide RS	100 mg	≤25°C	A	JPY 24,200
2001000021	Indocianine Green RS	300 mg	≤8°C	A	JPY 18,962

2-2. Other Reference Standards

Product Code	Reference Standard (RS)	Unit Quantity	Storage Temperature	Shipping Conditions	Price
3001000021	Human Growth Hormone RS	See leaflet	−20 – −30°C	F	JPY 44,734

3. Ministerial Ordinance coal-tar color for TLC Reference Standards

Product Code	Reference Standard (RS)	Unit Quantity	Storage Temperature	Shipping Conditions	Price
4001000021	Blue No. 1 for TLC RS	100 mg	≤25°C	A	JPY 13,619
4002000021	Blue No. 2 for TLC RS	100 mg	≤25°C	A	JPY 13,619
4035000021	Green No. 3 for TLC RS	100 mg	≤25°C	A	JPY 13,619
4036000021	Green No. 402 for TLC RS	100 mg	≤25°C	A	JPY 13,619
4031000021	Orange No. 203 for TLC RS	100 mg	≤25°C	A	JPY 13,619
4032000021	Orange No. 205 for TLC RS	100 mg	≤25°C	A	JPY 13,619
4033000021	Orange No. 402 for TLC RS	100 mg	≤25°C	A	JPY 13,619
4034000021	Orange No. 403 for TLC RS	100 mg	≤25°C	A	JPY 13,619
4003000021	Red No. 2 for TLC RS	100 mg	≤25°C	A	JPY 13,619
4004000021	Red No. 3 for TLC RS	100 mg	≤25°C	A	JPY 13,619
4005000021	Red No. 102 for TLC RS	100 mg	≤25°C	A	JPY 13,619
4006000021	Red No. 104 (1) for TLC RS	100 mg	≤25°C	A	JPY 13,619
4007000021	Red No. 105 (1) for TLC RS	100 mg	≤25°C	A	JPY 13,619
4008000021	Red No. 106 for TLC RS	100 mg	≤25°C	A	JPY 13,619
4009000021	Red No. 202 for TLC RS	100 mg	≤25°C	A	JPY 13,619
4010000021	Red No. 203 for TLC RS	100 mg	≤25°C	A	JPY 13,619
4011000021	Red No. 204 for TLC RS	100 mg	≤25°C	AU	JPY 13,619
4012000021	Red No. 218 for TLC RS	100 mg	≤25°C	A	JPY 13,619
4013000021	Red No. 221 for TLC RS	100 mg	≤25°C	AU	JPY 13,619
4014000021	Red No. 223 for TLC RS	100 mg	≤25°C	A	JPY 13,619
4015000021	Red No. 230 (1) for TLC RS	100 mg	≤25°C	A	JPY 13,619
4016000021	Red No. 230 (2) for TLC RS	100 mg	≤25°C	A	JPY 13,619
4017000021	Red No. 231 for TLC RS	100 mg	≤25°C	A	JPY 13,619
4018000021	Red No. 232 for TLC RS	100 mg	≤25°C	A	JPY 13,619
4019000021	Red No. 502 for TLC RS	100 mg	≤25°C	A	JPY 13,619
4020000021	Red No. 503 for TLC RS	100 mg	≤25°C	A	JPY 13,619
4021000021	Red No. 504 for TLC RS	100 mg	≤25°C	A	JPY 13,619
4022000021	Red No. 505 for TLC RS	100 mg	≤25°C	A	JPY 13,619
4023000021	Red No. 506 for TLC RS	100 mg	≤25°C	A	JPY 13,619
4024000021	Yellow No. 4 for TLC RS	100 mg	≤25°C	A	JPY 13,619
4025000021	Yellow No. 5 for TLC RS	100 mg	≤25°C	A	JPY 13,619
4026000021	Yellow No. 201 for TLC RS	100 mg	≤25°C	A	JPY 13,619
4027000021	Yellow No. 401 for TLC RS	100 mg	≤25°C	A	JPY 13,619
4028000021	Yellow No. 403 (1) for TLC RS	100 mg	≤25°C	A	JPY 13,619
4029000021	Yellow No. 404 for TLC RS	100 mg	≤25°C	A	JPY 13,619
4030000021	Yellow No. 405 for TLC RS	100 mg	≤25°C	A	JPY 13,619

Addenda **23**

PMRJ Pharmaceutical and Medical Device Regulatory Science Society of Japan (PMRJ) Rev. June 1, 2023

4. Japan's Specifications and Standards for Food Additives Reference Standards

Product Code	Reference Standard (RS)	Unit Quantity	Storage Temperature	Shipping Conditions	Price
5002000021	Food Blue No. 1 RS	100 mg	≤25°C	A	JPY 13,619
5003000021	Food Blue No. 2 RS	100 mg	≤25°C	A	JPY 13,619
5013000021	Food Green No. 3 RS	100 mg	≤25°C	A	JPY 13,619
5004000021	Food Red No. 2 RS	100 mg	≤25°C	A	JPY 13,619
5005000021	Food Red No. 3 RS	100 mg	≤25°C	A	JPY 13,619
5006000021	Food Red No. 40 RS	100 mg	≤25°C	A	JPY 13,619
5007000021	Food Red No. 102 RS	100 mg	≤25°C	A	JPY 13,619
5008000021	Food Red No. 104 RS	100 mg	≤25°C	A	JPY 13,619
5009000021	Food Red No. 105 RS	100 mg	≤25°C	A	JPY 13,619
5010000021	Food Red No. 106 RS	100 mg	≤25°C	A	JPY 13,619
5011000021	Food Yellow No. 4 RS	100 mg	≤25°C	A	JPY 13,619
5012000021	Food Yellow No. 5 RS	100 mg	≤25°C	A	JPY 13,619
5015000021	Natamycin RS	150 mg	≤8°C	R	JPY 68,409
5014000021	Nisin RS	500 mg	−20 – −30°C	F	JPY 60,343
5001000021	Xylitol RS	3.7 g	≤25°C	A	JPY 31,428

5. Other Reference Standards

Product Code	Reference Standard (RS)	Unit Quantity	Storage Temperature	Shipping Conditions	Price
8005000021	IMWP RS on Favipiravir	100 mg	≤8°C	A	JPY 18,380

* This reference standard (IMWP RS on Favipiravir) is used for quantification of favipiravir and confirmation of system suitability for the International Meeting of World Pharmacopoeias (IMWP) monographs on Favipiravir and on Favipiravir tablets.

The storage temperatures are defined as follows:

Room Temperature	: 1 – 30°C
≤25°C	: 1 – 25°C
≤5°C	: Refrigerate (1 – 5°C)
≤8°C	: Refrigerate (1 – 8°C)
≤−20°C	: Freeze (≤−20°C)
−20 – −30°C	: ≤−20°C. Avoid storage below −30°C because the container may not withstand such low temperatures.
−80°C	: Freeze (−80°C ± 10°C)

Shipping Conditions

A	: at ambient temperature
R	: kept refrigerated
F	: kept frozen (with Dry-Ice)
AU	: at ambient temperature, dangerous goods
RU	: kept refrigerated, dangerous goods
FU	: kept frozen (with Dry-Ice), dangerous goods
N/A	: Not available for overseas shipping

Terms and Conditions

Acceptance

All sales are subject to, and expressly conditioned on, these Terms and Conditions and Customer's assent to these Terms and Conditions. These Terms and Conditions are controlling and any additional or inconsistent terms and conditions in any acknowledgement, purchase order, or acceptance documents requested from, or provided by the Customer are expressly rejected.

Purchase Orders

All Reference Standards are subject to availability. Please note that some items may not be available depending on the destination country or region.

Purchase orders may be placed by Customer in electronic submission through PMRJ Reference Standards Online Store. PMRJ will not accept any order by telephone or facsimile. All purchase orders are subject to acceptance by PMRJ. Prices of all Reference Standards are either on-CPT (Incoterms 2020) basis or on EXW (Incoterms 2020) basis. The risk of loss for all Reference Standards purchased by Customer shall pass to the Customer at the point of delivery to the carrier. The Customer is responsible for paying all customs duties, taxes, and tariffs levied for importation of the Reference Standards.

Prices and Package Sizes

Prices and package sizes of Reference Standards are subject to change without notice. The latest price for each Reference Standard can be checked on our website. PMRJ shall not provide any discount.

Payment

Payment shall be made in advance by Customer in Japanese yen by wire transfer. No credit card payment option is available.

If payment is not confirmed within 45 days from the date of invoice, the order will be cancelled automatically. Customer needs to bear all transaction fees, namely not only bank charges originating from the payment by wire transfer outside Japan but also bank charges incurred in Japan for credit of the full invoice amount to PMRJ's designated account, as well as any customs duties, taxes, and tariffs levied for the importation of the Reference Standards.

Returns and Cancellations

All sales of PMRJ products are final. PMRJ products may not be returned for exchange or refund. The Customer that refuses delivery or refuses to pay customs and duties charges for exports from Japan are financially responsible for the total cost of the PMRJ products shipped.

Shipping

PMRJ reserves the right to change the shipping method of any order to meet the importing requirements of the ship-to country. PMRJ will not ship any Reference Standards to post office boxes.

Pharmaceutical and Medical Device Regulatory Science Society of Japan
Pharmaceutical Reference Standards Center

Terms and Conditions

Compliance with Law

By purchasing PMRJ products, Customer agrees to comply with all applicable provisions of any national or local law, and all orders, rules, and regulations, including but not limited to Japanese economic sanctions and controlled substances laws and regulations.

PMRJ products are subject to Japanese export control laws and regulations and may require an export license or applicable license exception prior to exportation from Japan.

Indemnification

Customers shall bear all risk of theft, loss, or damage not caused by PMRJ for all PMRJ products acquired pursuant to these Terms and Conditions. Customers agree to indemnify, defend, and hold PMRJ, its officers, trustees, and employees, harmless from all loss, liability, claims, or expenses (including reasonable attorney's fees) arising out of the Customer's use of the Reference Standards, including but not limited to liabilities arising from bodily injury, including death, or property damage to any person, unless caused by the negligent or intentional act or omission of PMRJ.

Suitability for Use

Customers purchasing Reference Standards must use them for the tests and assays prescribed in the monograph of the Japanese Pharmacopoeia and other official compendia for pharmaceuticals, excipients and food additives. The Reference Standards are analytical reagents and are not to be used for diagnostic or drug purposes or for administration to humans or animals. Customers must use and store the Reference Standards in accordance with the directions in the accompanying leaflet.

Applicable Law

These Terms and Conditions shall be governed by and interpreted in accordance with the laws of Japan. In the event of litigation or other proceedings by PMRJ to enforce or defend any term and condition, Customer agrees to pay all costs and expenses sustained by PMRJ, including, but not limited to, reasonable attorney's fees.

Force Majeure

PMRJ shall not be responsible for delays or failure in delivery, if the supply of the Reference Standards is hindered by occurrence beyond PMRJ's reasonable control including, but not limited to any act of God, civil commotion, unavailability, or shortages of materials.

Severability

If any provision of these terms and conditions is deemed unlawful, void, or unenforceable for any reason whatsoever, then that provision is severed and shall not in any way affect the validity and enforceability of the remaining provisions.

Pharmaceutical and Medical Device Regulatory Science Society of Japan
Pharmaceutical Reference Standards Center

Terms and Conditions

Entire Agreement

Nothing contained in any purchase order or Customer issued document will in any way serve to modify or add any terms and conditions to the sales of product by PMRJ to the Customer pursuant to these Terms and Conditions. The parties agree that the terms and conditions of any order for product placed by any Customer shall be governed only by these Terms and Conditions. These Terms and Conditions are a full and complete statement of the obligations of the parties relating to the subject matter hereof, and supersede all previous agreements, understandings, negotiations, and proposals. No provisions of these Terms and Conditions shall be deemed waived, amended, or modified by any party unless such waiver, amendment, or modification shall be in writing and signed by an officer or other authorized representative of all parties.

Revised. April 2022

Addenda 27

PMRJ Reference Standards Information for Users

Pharmaceutical and Medical Device Regulatory Science Society of Japan (PMRJ) has been registered by the Minister of Health, Labour and Welfare as an organization that produces and distributes Japanese Pharmacopoeia (JP) Reference Standards and other compendial reference standards of Japan.

How to Order PMRJ Reference Standards

Please visit PMRJ Reference Standards Online Store < https://www.pmrj-ec.jp/aec/user/?lang=en> and request for a quotation.

Usage

1. All the reference standards distributed by PMRJ are analytical reagents. They are not drugs or clinical diagnostic drugs, so they must not be used in humans or animals.

2. The reference standards distributed by PMRJ are guaranteed to be suitable for uses specified in the official compendia. The specified uses are given in the Intended Uses section of the leaflet for each reference standard. Please be aware that the quality of the reference standards is not guaranteed if they are used in tests other than those in which their use is specified.

3. If the official compendium directs that a reference standard be dried, dry a suitable amount of it according to the compendium at the time of use. Some reference standards that have been dried are hygroscopic, so perform weighing operations quickly.

4. If the Unit Quantity section of the leaflet directs that all of the reference standard contents be dissolved before use, do not weigh the reference standard before use.

5. Correction Information

   5.1 Loss on Drying, and Water Content

   If an official compendial test method specifies that an amount of reference standard calculated on the dried or anhydrous basis be weighed, separately determine the loss on drying or water content of the reference standard and calculate the amount of reference standard on the dried or anhydrous basis. However, if the Correction Information section of the leaflet contains a loss on drying or water content value, the weighed amount may be converted to the amount calculated on the dried or anhydrous basis by using the value given in the leaflet. For additional information, please see the FAQ on the PMRJ website.

   5.2 Correction Factors

   For some reference standards, the purity has been calculated by the mass balance method, etc., and is shown as a correction factor to apply when the reference standard is used in quantitative tests. If a correction factor is provided in the Correction Information section of the leaflet for a reference standard, be sure to correct the weighed amount of reference standard by multiplying it by the correction factor when the reference standard is used in the official compendial quantitative tests following the correction factor. When quantitative tests using the reference standard contain directions to convert the reference standard value by calculating on the dried basis, calculating on the anhydrous basis, or calculating on the anhydrous and residual solvent–free basis, perform the correction after performing the applicable conversion.

If a correction factor is not provided in the leaflet, regard the reference standard as 100.0% and do not correct the weighed amount of reference standard. For additional information, please see the FAQ on the PMRJ website.

6. The Safety Data Sheet (SDS) for each reference standard can be accessed from the reference standard's webpage.
7. Test data that are not necessary to use the reference standards are not disclosed, and certificates of analysis for the reference standards are not issued.

Storage

Store each reference standard according to its exterior label and the Storage Conditions section of its leaflet. The reference standards distributed by PMRJ do not have expiration dates. Therefore, order only quantities that can be used immediately, and after receipt of a reference standard, immediately store it at the specified temperature and use it as soon as possible. The quality of a reference standard cannot be guaranteed if (1) significant time has passed since it was shipped, even if it has not been opened, or (2) it has been stored after opening.

The storage temperatures are defined as follows:
- Room Temperature: 1 – 30°C
- ≤25°C: 1 – 25°C
- Refrigerate (≤8°C): 1 – 8°C
- Freeze (≤−20°C): ≤−20°C
- Freeze (−20 – −30°C): ≤−20°C. Avoid storage below −30°C because the container may not withstand such low temperatures.
- Freeze (−80°C): −80°C ± 10°C

For further information

Please visit PMRJ Pharmaceutical Reference Standards Center website <https://www.pmrj-rs.jp/en> or contact Customer Service at jprslab-std@pmrj.jp.

Pharmaceutical and Medical Device Regulatory Science Society of Japan
Pharmaceutical Reference Standards Center

2-1-2, Hiranomachi, Chuo-ku, Osaka 541-0046, Japan
Email: jprslab-std@pmrj.jp   Tel: +81-6-6221-3444

Pharmaceutical Reference Standards Center   https://www.pmrj-rs.jp/en
PMRJ Reference Standards Online Store   https://www.pmrj-ec.jp/aec/user/?lang=en

Revised April 2021